Clinical Uncertainty in Primary Care

Lucia Siegel Sommers • John Launer
Editors

Clinical Uncertainty in Primary Care

The Challenge of Collaborative Engagement

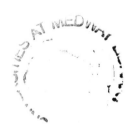

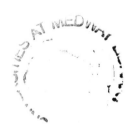

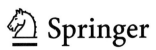 Springer

Editors
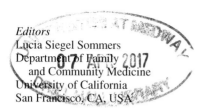
Lucia Siegel Sommers
Department of Family
and Community Medicine
University of California
San Francisco, CA, USA

John Launer
Tavistock Clinic
London, UK

Additional material to this book can be downloaded from
http://extras.springer.com/978-1-4614-6811-0

ISBN 978-1-4614-6811-0 (Hardcover)   ISBN 978-1-4614-6812-7 (eBook)
ISBN 978-1-4939-1275-9 (Softcover)
DOI 10.1007/978-1-4614-6812-7
Springer New York Heidelberg Dordrecht London

Library of Congress Control Number: 2013937177

Printed on acid-free paper

Springer is part of Springer Science+Business Media (www.springer.com)

Foreword

In this book, Lucia Sommers and John Launer, with the accompanying input of their contributing authors, have done a deeply insightful and close-to-exhaustive job of defining clinical uncertainty. They identify its origins, components, and sub-types; demonstrate the ways in which, and the extent to which, it is intrinsic to medicine – to medical science, medical technology, and medical practice; and present a cogent case for its special relationship to primary care practice. More important, they powerfully and convincingly advocate for the intellectual, psychological, interpersonal, and existential value that forming and participating in small groups of primary care physicians, oriented around issues of medical uncertainty, can have for them and, as a consequence, for the way that they relate to their patients and the quality of care that they deliver to them. In "thickly descriptive," ethnographic-like, narrative ways, the authors depict the micro-dynamics of the interactions between physicians that take place in such groups.

Their at-once descriptive and analytic materials vividly suggest how such group dynamics – the support and stimulation that they provide – break through the otherwise solitude of these clinicians, their uncertainty about their uncertainty, and their educationally, psychologically, and culturally influenced propensity to suppose that if they were fully competent, they should be able to function and deal with the quandaries that their practice entail, with self-reliant individualism. In addition, the book identifies extant clinical peer groups of this sort, comments in passing on the interesting sociological fact that they are largely located in northern Europe, and shows the patterned similarities and differences in how they function.

Clinical Uncertainty in Primary Care: The Challenge of Collaborative Engagement not only presents a model of collegial collaboration and support, it also implicitly legitimates it.

Renée C. Fox
Annenberg Professor Emerita of the Social Sciences
University of Pennsylvania

About the Editors and Authors

Lucia Siegel Sommers is an educator and health services researcher with a 40-year history of working with clinician small groups. She holds an undergraduate degree from the University of Pennsylvania; a master's in social work from Bryn Mawr University; a doctorate in public health from the University of California, Berkeley; and completed a 2-year fellowship in health services research at Stanford University. From 1994 through 2001, Lucia was a full-time faculty member in the Internal Medicine Residency Program at St. Mary's Medical Center in San Francisco and Associate Program Director from 1997 to 2001. She is currently an assistant adjunct professor in the Department of Family and Community Medicine at the University of California, San Francisco, where she has taught medical students since 1996 and began the Practice Inquiry Continuing Medical Education Program in 2005. Her published research includes studies focused on the effectiveness of medical audit, nurse–physician collaboration to improve care and reduce costs in hospitals, and interdisciplinary care for the frail elderly in the primary care office setting.

John Launer is a family physician, family therapist, educator, and writer. He graduated in English at Cambridge before studying medicine at London University. After obtaining Membership of the Royal College of General Practitioners with distinction in 1983, he worked for 22 years as a GP in Edmonton, North London, and continues to work as a part-time GP. In 1994, he completed training at the Tavistock Clinic as a family therapist and joined the senior staff there as honorary consultant in general practice and primary care. Since then, his teaching and clinical work have drawn together ideas from family medicine and family therapy, with a focus on narrative and clinical supervision. John is an Associate Dean for Postgraduate Medical Education at London University and has published five previous books as author or editor, including *Narrative-Based Primary Care: A Practical Guide*. He has lectured and run workshops internationally, including in the US, Canada, Scandinavia, Israel, and Japan.

Trisha Greenhalgh is Co-Director of the Global Health, Policy and Innovation Unit at Barts and the London School of Medicine and Dentistry, London, UK. She is dual qualified, having gained a BA in Social and Political Sciences from the University of Cambridge in 1980 and a medical degree from the University of Oxford in 1983. She leads a program of research at the interface between social sciences and medicine which seeks to celebrate and retain the traditional and the humanistic aspects of medicine and health care while also embracing the unparalleled opportunities of contemporary science and technology to improve health outcomes and relieve suffering. Her work covers such diverse themes as reclaiming narrative and literature as legitimate components of the medical curriculum; exploring how "rationing" decisions are made when demand for health care exceeds the resources available; studying the social, political, and ethical implications of new technologies such as networked electronic patient records; and searching for better metaphors than "knowledge translation" to illuminate the complex links between research and clinical practice. She is the author of 140 peer-reviewed publications and 8 textbooks.

Professor Colin Coles is an educationist who has been working in medical education for nearly forty years in Europe and more recently, Africa. He has extensive experience in curriculum design, evaluation and development in undergraduate and postgraduate medical education, as well as in continuing professional development. His current research focuses on the cutting edge of curriculum development, which in health care focuses increasingly on the workplace and the conditions necessary for effective learning there. He holds the position of professor in the Faculty of Education, Health and Social Care at the University of Winchester in the UK, where in 1997 he helped to found a masters degree in education for medical practitioners which now has over 150 registered students. He is an international conference contributor, and advises several professional organizations on educational matters. He publishes widely, and with Della Fish has co-authored books on the development of professional judgement (1998) and curriculum development in medical education (2005).

Henry Jablonski, M.D. (Karolinska Institute), M.Sc. (Stockholm School of Economics (SSE)), is a psychoanalyst and psychiatrist in private practice in Stockholm. His thesis (1971) at the SSE was a critique against cost-benefit analysis and its reductionistic use of quantitative measures in the public health system and a plea for the parallel use of qualitative goal descriptions and a dialogue between doctors, administrators, and politicians. He has led Balint groups for GPs since the mid-1980s and in the past decade also for hospital doctors. He is the President of the International Balint Federation and the Swedish Society of Medical Psychology. His major research project was on voluntary sterilization from a psychoanalytical and family system's perspective. He has written papers on Balint work, film and psychoanalysis, and the role of nature in depression and mourning.

Dorte Kjeldmand has been working as a GP at Eksjö Primary Health Care Center, County of Jönköping, in the southern part of Sweden since 1989 and is a national examiner of specialists in General Practice. She has been a certified Balint group leader since 2000 and leads a number of Balint groups. She is also a researcher in the Department of Public Health and Caring Services, Section of Health Services Research, University of Uppsala, where she did her 2006 dissertation titled "The Doctor, the Task and the Group, Balint Groups as a Means of Developing New Understanding in the Physician-Patient Relationship." In addition to clinical work, she is also a physician teacher and directs training at the internship and residency levels.

John Salinsky is a general practitioner in North West London and a program director of Whittington GP Specialty Education and Training in North London. He is a past general secretary of the International Balint Federation and was editor of the *Journal of the Balint Society* (UK), 1997–2011. He is the author, with Paul Sackin, of *What are you feeling, Doctor? Identifying and avoiding defensive patterns in the consultation* (Radcliffe Medical Press 2000). He has contributed chapters on Balint groups to a number of books and has also written two books on *Medicine and Literature* (Radcliffe Medical Press 2002, 2004).

Heather Armson, M.D., MCE, CCFP, FCFP, is an associate professor and the assistant dean of Continuing Professional Development for family medicine at the University of Calgary. She was previously the director of Practice-Based Small-Group Learning program and is currently the director of research for The Foundation for Medical Practice Education. Her research interests include the processes involved in enhancing practice implementation of new knowledge, including the roles of small-group learning, community of learners, self-assessment, and commitment-to-change.

Ronald MacVicar is a General Practitioner in Inverness in the north of Scotland and the Director of Postgraduate General Practice Education for the North of Scotland Deanery of NHS Education for Scotland (NES). He spent a year on sabbatical in Southern Ontario in 2001–2002 in part to investigate the Practice-Based Small-Group Learning (PBSGL) program which had developed in McMaster University over the previous decade. He has since led the implementation and growth of PBSGL as a core workstream within NES and as an established method of continuing professional development for a substantial proportion of Scottish General Practitioners.

Tina Kenyon, ACSW, is a faculty member at the NH Dartmouth Family Medicine Residency at Concord Hospital and an instructor in the Department of Community and Family Medicine at the Geisel School of Medicine in Dartmouth. Her current areas of interest include curriculum and faculty development, population-based education, and organizational process improvement.

Claudia W. Allen, Ph.D., a licensed clinical psychologist specializing in family therapy, directs the Behavioral Medicine curriculum in the Family Medicine Residency at the University of Virginia. She focuses on supporting trainees and faculty in advancing their personal/professional development and integrating behavioral medicine into their daily practices.

Alan Siegel, M.D., is a core faculty member at Contra Costa Family Medicine Residency in Martinez, California, whose research interests include pediatric obesity group care. He oversees outpatient training for the residents, faculty development and continuing medical education for the faculty, and helps direct a county-wide Healing Through the Arts program.

Charlotte Tulinius, M.D., Ph.D., M.H.P.E., M.R.C.G.P., is Associate Professor of Postgraduate Education at The Research Unit for General Practice, Copenhagen University, Denmark; she also works as the Medical Director of Curriculum at the Royal College of General Practitioners, London, UK. Her professional work has been divided between clinical work, teaching, and research. She did her Ph.D. using ethnographic fieldwork methods to describe the cultural and social meanings of smoking in children's families. Her master's degree in medical education from Maastricht University in the Netherlands led to the research and implementation projects in health professions education she is currently directing with partners in Scandinavia, UK, and East Africa. Her research interests focus on participatory action research in the areas of general practice, faculty development, curriculum development, and the development of methods using reflexivity and the arts for data collection, research communication, and teaching.

Gösta Eliasson, Med. lic., is general practitioner and chair of the Council for Professional Development of the Swedish Association of General Practice. He is a former director of the governmentally-financed Institute of Family Medicine, Stockholm, Sweden, and former academic teacher at the Department of General Practice, University of Gothenburg. His primary interests include undergraduate education, vocational training, postgraduate education, practice visiting/peer review, and cooperation between hospital and primary care. He is the author of over 30 articles and reports including scientific papers on facilitating quality improvement in primary health care by practice visiting (1998) and experiences of CME small group work in general practice in Sweden (1999).

Acknowledgments

As we consider the efforts that have gone into this edited volume from both sides of the Atlantic, we want to express our gratitude toward those colleagues, friends, and family who have helped make it possible. First and foremost, we want to acknowledge the intelligence and alacrity of our chapter authors who joined forces with us for this pioneering collection of essays and reports on the collaborative engagement of clinical uncertainty in primary care. We expect our relationships with all our authors to deepen as we plan future work together.

In the US, a very special thanks goes to Renée Fox who has helped us recognize the unique nature of this "collaborative effort" about collaboration. In England, we especially recognize the responsive support of Trisha Greenhalgh and John Salinsky. Their judgment and editorial skills were indispensable.

Peter Sommers was indefatigable in the careful editing of innumerable drafts of every type of document – chapters, abstracts, on-line documents (in addition to running the Sommers' house over the last few months). In London, Rabbi Lee Wax-Launer and Ruth and David Launer showed the same dedication.

Finally, we wish to recognize the commitment of those clinicians who participate in the small groups described in this book. If we succeed in furthering an international dialogue on the collaborative engagement of clinical uncertainty in the primary care setting, we will have begun to honor their work and dedication.

Contents

Part I
Clinical Uncertainty in Primary Care

Chapter 1
Introduction

Lucia Siegel Sommers

This is a book about primary care clinicians and the clinical uncertainty that is endemic to their work. As long as patients visit their primary care clinicians for front-line help with undifferentiated symptoms, disabling chronic conditions, and for end-of-life decision-making, uncertainty will remain an insistent companion. Advances such as genomic medicine and web-connected populations bring both outsized hopes and unsettling fears. The latest breakthroughs in medical diagnosis and treatment foster increased expectations for certainty. At the same time, a sobering reality clouds the horizon. As Gerrity and her colleagues write, "uncertainty borders the edges of knowledge so that the larger the territory known, the more extensive are the settings in which uncertainty is experienced" (1992).

One definition of uncertainty is "the subjective perception of ignorance" (Han et al. 2011). A more comprehensive definition might be "a subjective perception of not knowing what to think or what to do." For a primary care clinician, this perception can arise out of a simple and commonly encountered experience such as a patient presenting with an unusual set of symptoms that, although worrisome, become the substrate for an ordered investigation with seemingly clear boundaries. Just as likely, this subjective perception of ignorance can arise from a multilayered, existential uncertainty, such as a patient presenting with similar set of symptoms, but this time, evoking memories of failed decision-making, patient suffering, and clinician regret, all of which lead to a loss of confidence in how to proceed. Throughout this book, numerous rich and varied case vignettes provide instructive examples of the breadth of uncertainty as it presents in primary care.

L. Siegel Sommers (✉)
Department of Family and Community Medicine, University of California,
2393 Filbert Street, San Francisco 94123, CA, USA (Residence)
e-mail: Lucia.Sommers@ucsf.edu

L.S. Sommers and J. Launer (eds.), *Clinical Uncertainty in Primary Care: The Challenge of Collaborative Engagement*, DOI 10.1007/978-1-4614-6812-7_1,
© Springer Science+Business Media New York 2013

This book is also about addressing uncertainty in primary care practice, *engaging* it, and what engagement could come to mean for today's primary care clinicians. As recognized by countless clinical theorists and educators, clinical judgment is at the heart of engaging uncertainty. Cassell attests to this when he states, "The key to understanding medical judgment is knowing that it is fundamentally the management of uncertainty" (1991). Employing clinical judgment to engage uncertainty requires clinicians to place the full weight of their knowledge, explicit and tacit, well-honed and still evolving in the service of a single patient's problem and, ideally, to interact with that patient intending to expand knowledge and reason together.

Very importantly, this book is also about a very special form of uncertainty engagement, one that the book's editors and chapter authors have each been privileged to explore over the years – *collaborative engagement with case-based uncertainty in the setting of small groups of clinicians.* We describe this structured small group engagement while at the same time cognizant of a longstanding but generally unspoken tradition in the medical profession: clinicians are expected to work independently in using clinical judgment to address each patient conundrum, seeking help only as they see fit.

Seeking help for case-based uncertainty, particularly for new clinicians, can be a trial and error process of false starts and blind alleys. With repeated effort, over time, clinicians eventually build a contact and information bank they learn to drawn upon. Urgency of patient need and how tired the clinician is at the end of the day (in addition to the volume of chart completions, patient call-backs and other chores) will determine time allotted to 'uncertainty work'. Perhaps one patient daily will demand this special form of mental and emotional gymnastics that entails revisiting the patient narrative, considering what missing data is essential to know, figuring out how to find it, returning to selected details to revise earlier assumptions, and deciding who in the contact bank to call for reviewing one's logic and one's feelings and where to go next. For the other patients seen that day – even those who might benefit from having their cases revisited – there will be no such retrospective review and no reflection with a colleague, let alone a peer group meeting held expressly for that purpose. It is therefore unsurprising that the medical literature on how clinicians make decisions suggests that clinicians develop idiosyncratic practice styles that are often difficult to modify (Wennberg et al. 1982; Eddy 1984).

We believe that small group discussion of challenging patients allows for assessing and continually improving one's practice style alongside those of colleagues, examining its effectiveness and modifying it as necessary to address the patients being discussed. These patients, themselves, become virtual additions to each colleague's clinical experience and part of the group's case repertoire. In the past, because fewer primary care clinicians were available to communities and solo practitioners were situated far from each other, individual clinicians had no choice but to do uncertainty work alone, referring patients as necessary when personalized approaches failed. Today, with more clinicians working in groups in urban areas and clinicians in rural areas connected virtually through electronic media, clinicians have a wider array of options for doing uncertainty work.

It is our purpose in this book, therefore, to offer an option that augments the solo, ad hoc mode of doing uncertainty work with an explicitly shared, collegial one, making it at once accessible for exploration and further development. Collaborative small group work directed to clinical conundrums of all kinds – diagnostic, management, relationship, prognostic, ethical dilemmas, or a mix of all – can provide clinicians with necessary practice for the continuous improvement of judgment, the very judgment they rely upon every day as independent practitioners and that patients count on for high-quality care.

Collaborative Engagement: Describing the Current State of the Art

This book originated when Springer Publishing invited me to edit a volume on the subject of clinical uncertainty in primary care. They made this request based upon their interest in our work on "Practice Inquiry" (PI) in the San Francisco Bay Area since 2002 (Sommers et al. 2007). PI is an ongoing, small group learning and practice change activity within a primary care setting, expressly designed for enhancing clinical judgment through collegial collaboration (See Chapters 9 and 10). I approached John Launer, a primary care physician, family therapist, and educator in London, UK, to join me in the project of editing this book. John had worked with a team of colleagues at the Tavistock Clinic since the mid-1990s to develop Narrative-Based Supervision (NBS), an approach to case-based discussion in groups, based on the ideas of narrative medicine (see Chapters 7 and 8). Together with Jonathan Burton, he had also organized a series of conferences in the late 1990s and early 2000s on "Working Models of Supervision and Support in Primary Care" that in some ways prefigured this volume (Burton and Launer 2003). John and I agreed to collaborate in exploring the ways primary care clinicians around the world engage uncertainty in primary care, with a specific focus on the kinds of peer group discussions we were trying to promote in different ways on opposite sides of the Atlantic.

We were both aware of Balint Groups that were started in England in the 1950s as the progenitor of clinician small group work for addressing challenging patient cases. We also were acquainted with the Problem-Based Small Group Learning Program (PBSGL), begun in the early 1990s at McMaster University in Canada that used evidence-based medicine precepts to discuss cases in clinician small group settings. We were gaining familiarity with nationwide programs both in Denmark and Sweden that relied upon clinician small groups as the educational setting for physician continuing professional development. Where else in Europe and North America, we wondered, could similar work be going on? Who, like us, was seeing merit in a peer group approach to addressing challenging cases in primary care? Who, like us, believed that knowledge and wisdom might best be acquired not only through learning general principles and abstract facts but also through reflection in dialogue with others who faced similar problems?

Who thought that such collaborative engagement – with its emotional commitment and depth of thought – might produce improvement in clinical judgment and professional practice that was more profound and more sustained than other forms of learning? What challenges were they facing and how were they assessing the impact of their group learning methods?

Simultaneous with developing more formal contacts with Balint, PBSGL, and the Danish and Swedish groups, we mounted a purposive email outreach to identify collaborative engagement efforts in Europe and North America. (We use the term "collaborative engagement" to refer to any clinician small group work focused on addressing case-based clinical uncertainty). We sent our inquiry to educators and primary care leaders around the world with whom we were acquainted personally or through their published work and who were likely to be familiar with programs similar to ours; they, in turn, were requested to pass it on to their colleagues. In our query, we described our work (NBS and PI) as examples of collaborative engagement and asked about similar efforts for practicing primary care clinicians that met the following criteria: using small groups of clinicians all of whom have their own patients; coming together on a regular basis; employing a defined discussion format; and discussing actual patient cases that represented clinical uncertainty or related content. We stated that we had a particular interest in forms of collaborative engagement that used a trained facilitator and took place in the clinicians' work setting, but certainly did not wish to exclude models that did not meet these criteria.

We defined case-based clinical uncertainty as "the confusion, conflict, stuckness, unease, and/or discomfort an individual primary care clinician experiences when confronting a predicament in an individual patient who presents a diagnostic, therapeutic, general management, clinician-patient relationship, prognostic, ethical dilemma, or some combination of these dimensions." A focus on uncertainty cases, we added, did not need to make up the clinician group's exclusive focus but should at least represent a significant portion of its work. We emphasized that our interest was primarily in learning about efforts undertaken by established primary care clinicians. Although we valued many approaches to case-based education that we knew were taking place with medical students and residents, our focus was on collaborative engagement being practiced beyond the early years of clinicians' careers.

As the initial set of responses came back, we noted that a number of interesting topics were raised such as how to define "a case," the value of reflective writing about cases, and the overall utility of theoretical models for dealing with uncertainty. Although models for coping with uncertainty and teaching how to manage it were also proposed, unfortunately none of the responses provided accounts of clinicians actually applying these models in groups or even working alone. Hoping to clarify our intentions, we emailed subsequent inquiries with the following sentence added, "What we're really looking for is any material – published or not – that describes how anyone has managed to get practicing clinicians together, systematically, in a group, and applied a method for helping them talk about their 'stuck' cases, that is, those patients for whom they're all out of ideas and don't know where to go next."

Our inquiry was sent to over 75 individuals in North America and Northern Europe in late 2011; 50 responded over a 4-month period. Our outreach identified only one program that met our criteria: the Irish CME network of clinician small groups. Unfortunately, contacts with this program were established too late for its inclusion in the book (O'Riordan 2000). It is important to note that we did not solicit information from southern Europe, South America, Australia, or Asia since we lacked contacts in these locales. Additionally, our publication contract necessitated a short time window for gathering information. Nevertheless, with the information we garnered from our contacts and the colleagues to whom they forwarded our inquiry, we formed a very strong impression: while everyone expressed a belief that collaborative engagement should be a vital form of continuing professional development in primary care, models for doing it are very few indeed, and, outside a very few countries, such collegial work happens rarely and unsystematically.

This finding, although dispiriting, strengthened our resolve to raise the profile of collaborative engagement. Appreciating the contributions of Balint and PBSGL groups as well as the Danish and the Swedish country-wide programs, we saw the need for a book that would bring Narrative-Based Supervision and Practice Inquiry together with these other approaches as embodying the current "state of the art" of collaborative engagement with uncertainty. In publishing this description, we anticipate that programs we did not reach will find us, establish contact, and, in time, a second edition of the book could result.

It is worth noting that primary care clinicians in the UK have a tradition of holding "practice meetings" in their workplace where individual cases are discussed on an occasional or even regular basis. Over the years occasional reports of longstanding groups in the UK have appeared in the literature (Reiss et al. 1981). "Significant event analysis" has often been a method of choice for this work (De Wet et al. 2011). In the mid-2000s the British journal *Work Based Learning in Primary Care* documented several voluntary, self-directed learning groups (Burton 2003).

In addition, the responses to our inquiry told us that the 'long case' discussion, even where it was formerly a UK practice tradition, has given way almost universally to conversations about clinical guidelines, practice systems, money, or other impersonal and administrative matters. Cases, if discussed at all, are more likely to be addressed briefly and in terms of exchanging information. Case discussion, where it does take place, is far more likely to do so in the coffee room or even the corridor, may last a minute or two at most, and be confined to simple questions such as which drug features in the latest guidelines.

In contrast to the UK, primary care clinicians in the US have no tradition of clinical case discussion in the primary care setting despite their working closely together in large and small group practices as health care businesses. If individual patients were discussed at all, it was in the hospital lunch room where physicians would meet after rounding on their patients in the morning and before returning to their offices after lunch. The changes ushered in during the "managed care revolution" of the 1990s ended these discussions as "hospitalists" began to change the relationship primary care physicians had with their patients and their colleagues (McAlearney 2004; Beckman 2009).

Assumptions and Questions

The findings from our inquiry stimulated us to articulate an explicit rationale for clinician small group engagement with case-based clinical uncertainty. First, we saw the value of acknowledging that clinical uncertainty is not something occasional or incidental to primary care. It is intrinsic to practically every moment of every encounter with patients and arguably between professionals as well. Uncertainty is, fundamentally, in the nature of knowledge and the complexity of human interactions. Consequently, how clinicians use judgment to deal with uncertainty is critical. It affects their ability to have meaningful relationships with patients, colleagues, and staff; determines how they self-assess to identify knowledge and skill needs; influences patient outcomes and costs of care; and impacts satisfaction with clinical work.

Secondly, we saw that addressing uncertainty cannot be solely an internal, individual process in the mind of the clinician. It requires interaction, dialogue, and an understanding of knowledge as emergent rather than fixed and as contingent and contextualized rather than general and abstract. This view arises from a particular philosophical view of the world based on a wide range of twentieth-century European thinkers (Bakhtin 1982; Buber 2000; Habermas 1985; Levinas 2006) and American social theorists (Mead 1913; Berger and Luckmann 1967). It is echoed in fields of study as diverse as narrative studies (Ricoeur 1984), complexity (Waldrop 1993; Stacey 2001), and knowledge production (Nonaka and Takeuchi 1995).

All these perspectives are consistent with a range of contemporary approaches to clinical practice including biopsychosocial medicine (Engel 1977), patient-centered medicine (Levenstein et al. 1986), narrative-based medicine (Greenhalgh and Hurwitz 1998; Charon 2006), relationship-centered care (Beach and Inui 2006), interpretive medicine (Reeve 2010), practice-based evidence (Gabbay and Le May 2010), and values-based practice (Fulford et al. 2012). Clinical approaches such as these all involve an understanding that knowledge and meaning emerge through social interaction between clinician and patient and between clinician and clinician. According to all of them, the kinds of inputs to judgment that a clinician requires to address clinical uncertainty are rich and multi-faceted. These judgment inputs include "evidence" derived from randomized clinical trials as well as that grounded in clinical experience. Inputs also include a clinician's knowledge about a patient emerging from a long-term relationship as well as the clinician's self-knowledge derived from reflections on past uncertainties.

Next, through our own small group work with clinicians, we had observed the careful, multi-layered assessment of judgment inputs that results when clinicians discuss their case-based quandaries with colleagues, each of whom brings a unique experiential base to the table. In this collaborative context, managing uncertainty becomes understood as a subtle, tentative, dialogical, and evolutionary process rather than solely a matter of finding and applying the "right" practice guidelines. Collegial deliberations around an individual uncertainty case allow for the careful crafting of decision and management strategies that could well represent departures from evidence-based practice but result, nonetheless, in ones that "makes sense" in *this case* for *this patient*. The deviation from guideline-specified care (e.g., a 'practice variation') could represent "desirable variation" (Miller et al. 2001) and call for "practice-situated judgment" that would ultimately prevent error down the line (Jerak-Zuiderent 2012). The clinician who brought the case, the colleagues who contributed to the conversation, as well as their patients could all benefit from the collaborative, case-based learning. (Edmondson et al. 2009) Another way of framing such activity, very much in tune with current themes in medical education, would be as a form of shared reflective practice, or a collective exercise in mindfulness (Weick et al. 1999).

Lastly, we concluded that achieving this level of competency in uncertainty engagement requires opportunities for regular, case-based, small group discussion among professionals, preferably (but not necessarily) with a skilled and trained facilitator, in the workplace on set-aside time. For such opportunities to occur and be supported within a health care system, they must be envisioned as adding value to the practice lives of participating clinicians and, most importantly, to the patients they care for.

The medical literature offers a mixed picture on the impact of small group, interactive approaches for affecting changes in clinician attitudes and behavior (Marinopoulos et al. 2007; Forsetlund et al. 2009). We, thus, found ourselves speculating about how ongoing, structured collaborative engagement with uncertainty could affect clinician attitudes, clinician behavior, organizational policies, and patient outcomes. Specifically we asked ourselves:

- How could collaborative engagement help clinicians feel better supported in their daily work? Could it lead to improved work satisfaction overall?
- How could collaborative engagement invigorate the primary care specialties, now under significant threat from de-skilling and managerialism? Could it even help reverse the waning interest in primary care as a specialty?
- In what arenas could collaborative engagement be linked to specific clinician practice changes that in turn connect to patient outcomes?
- Do patients whose clinicians become involved in collaborative engagement report higher satisfaction with their care?
- What kinds of organizational policy changes result from collaborative engagement?
- How are non-clinician staff impacted?

For looking ahead to the further development of collaborative engagement, the questions above are important. A focus on value and impact can help steer clear of distractions leading to premature reliance on untested methods or doctrinaire distinctions and encourage sharing and learning across approaches. We are confident that the linkages we have made with Balint, PBSGL, and the Danish and Swedish groups while working on this book will only deepen. Furthermore, as readers come to understand the factors motivating the book's contributors to first develop their collaborative engagement approaches and the benefits accrued, they will consider trying out selected methods in their own settings. Our readers, like us, will then come to appreciate how questions about the impact and value of collaborative engagement must above all be considered in the context that all of us who contributed to this volume originally shared: the need for clinicians to talk together about their patients.

The Need to Talk About Patients and Getting Good at It

The respondents to our email survey did not perceive primary care clinicians as aware of the value, let alone the possibility of sharing case-based uncertainty with peers. In subsequent correspondence with selected respondents, we asked them to speculate on reasons for this. Some believed that the all-consuming, near obsession with efficiency and use of time, particularly in the US, could well discourage whatever natural interest there might be in having scheduled, collegial talk about patients. Two other explanations offered were clinician discomfort in disclosing uncertainty in a formal setting and availability of "curbside" consultation, although the latter was judged to have become less available in recent years. Several respondents pointed out how talking in a structured way about individual uncertainty patients did not fit into any of their current quality assurance/quality improvement forums. This prompted us to ask ourselves, how is it that formal quality improvement activities seem to exclude a focus on challenging patients? (Bishop 2013).

One respondent to our email inquiry, Dr. Jeffrey Borkan, a family physician, anthropologist, and Chair of Family Medicine at Alpert School of Medicine, Brown University, had a more nuanced explanation as to why clinicians seemed to talk about everything else (e.g., practice guidelines and performance targets), but real patients when they come together: "We may not be very good at discussing in an explicit manner what is actually important." In reflecting upon his response, we wondered, what is involved in appreciating the need to talk about one's individual patients as important? Furthermore, what is involved in getting good at talking about them?

Appreciating the need to talk about patients with one's colleagues, we speculated, could come about after experiencing a particular challenging patient. Perplexed after a visit, the clinician might muse wistfully: "How helpful it would be if there were some place where I could take this case to get input from my colleagues." This realization would need to occur for a critical core of clinicians willing to try something new despite initial discomfort. Indeed, this is exactly the realization that seems to have given rise to the six approaches described in this book. In each of them, clinicians appeared to have the need to share their clinical experiences with colleagues coupled with a conviction that such discussion was worth spending precious time during the working day or even outside it. A confluence of events, thus, across these various locales has made talking about real patients a legitimate activity.

"Getting good" at talking with one's colleagues about real patients who present uncertainty is challenging. The experiences described in many of the chapters of this book provide suggestions as well as detailed recipes for taking first steps. In addition to a plentiful number of uncertainty case vignettes, authors describe small group discussion techniques. What these approaches share is a commitment to using a consistent and disciplined method for addressing case discussion. More importantly, they recognize implicitly or explicitly the importance of mutual respect, confidentiality, openness, and trust.

Above all, getting good at talking about uncertainty patients with one's colleagues requires practice. Common to all approaches for collaborative engagement described in this book is the requirement to create a special, regularly scheduled time for clinicians to practice uncertainty engagement *together*. In promoting a rich and varied menu of small group models from which to choose, the book's editors and chapter authors envision this requirement leading to a salutary outcome – primary care clinicians moving from a passive "toleration" of uncertainty to an active, committed engagement.

Uncertainty in the Zeitgeist

Although engaging uncertainty in the ways described in this book may still be uncommon, the formal study of uncertainty in non-medical fields is far more developed. Acknowledgement of "uncertainty" in our culture, especially since the millennium, has gained increasing traction in the news and social media as a way to characterize everything from life on Wall Street to "friending" on Facebook. US military leaders now place "uncertainty," along with "volatility," "complexity," and "ambiguity," into the acronym "VUCA." They envision VUCA as defining the zeitgeist, and they reframe old problems as "VUCA situations" requiring management with tactics that evolve and are flexible (Jacobs 2002).

Has the term "uncertainty" gained similar cachet in the medical literature? To find out, we carried out a specially designed PubMed literature search looking at the frequency of the term "uncertainty" found in either the title or the abstract of a journal article or, starting in 2003, as a Medical Subject Heading (MESH). Using PubMed, we looked at Medline citations in two different sets of journals: the "Core Clinical Journals," a subset of 119 English language clinical journals of interest to practicing clinicians, and a selected group of noncore journals that populated the reference lists of contributors to this book.[1] From 1970 through 2010, the number of 'uncertainty' citations in core and non-core journals doubled on average within each ten year increment. There were 78 core and 12 non-core citations during the 1970–1979 period; these grew to 919 and 482 citations respectively for the 2000–2009 period.

---

[1]These noncore journals publish work in health services research, health care policy, health care professional issues, behavioral medicine, and medical education. We removed references having the terms "uncertainty principle" or "equipoise" in the title or abstract from both searches since these terms identify clinical trial or philosophy of science citations not pertinent to this search.

Although covering a wide array of topics, the increasing number of these citations over the past 40 years gives credence to the need for the focused study of uncertainty as a phenomenon in all domains of clinical practice, not only primary care. What are the uncertainty topics that other medical specialties grapple with? How do non-primary care physicians talk about collaborative engagement? In what other arenas in medicine do clinicians of all specialties have common ground for exploring collaborative engagement of uncertainty? (e.g., the role of uncertainty in medical errors; van den Berge and Mamede 2013) Recognizing the increased interest in clinical uncertainty, we are encouraged that clinicians and researchers may now have better access to resources for funding studies looking specifically at the contexts, strategies, and outcomes of collaborative engagement of uncertainty.

Three Perspectives on Clinical Uncertainty in the Medical Literature

In our analysis of the medical literature, we have identified three theoretical perspectives that address the phenomenon of clinical uncertainty and its companion subject, clinical judgment. These perspectives are briefly described below. Each perspective alone proves insufficient for elucidating the intricacies of patient-clinician encounters marked by clinical uncertainty, but when combined, they offer a comprehensive picture of the challenges.

This short section and attached table are meant to encourage readers to explore this growing body of literature for its contribution to collaborative engagement. In Table. 1.1, we list authors and titles of work that contain characteristics suggestive of one perspective more than another, although often a single categorization is inadequate to characterize an author's position in the referenced piece.

The three main theoretical perspectives are as follows:

1. Uncertainty is a problem resulting from an individual clinician's limitations in medical knowledge and/or in cognitive and affective functioning.

Here, the problem is understood to result from the clinician's not knowing either certain pieces of medical knowledge or medical policies/guidelines of import. It can also result from the clinician's inability to reason properly, use appropriate decision strategies, apply or transfer knowledge, or monitor affective reactions to uncertainty.

Enhancing clinical judgment in the face of uncertainty of this nature involves increasing one's medical knowledge but, just as importantly, knowing how to find and manage knowledge, as well as manage one's cognitions and emotions in the face of uncertainty. In addition, limitations in human reasoning necessitate the use of decision-making strategies such as decision analysis or other probabilistic methods for individual patient decision-making. Monitoring cognitions and affective states are best done with reflective techniques to minimize both cognitive and affective biases.

Table 1.1 Clinical uncertainty in the medical literature: selected readings (see references for full citations)

Uncertainty resulting from individuals' limitations in knowledge, reasoning, and emotional functioning	Uncertainty resulting from how persons interact and form relationships	Uncertainty resulting from living within complex adaptive systems (CAS)
Feinstein AR. Clinical Judgment. 1967	Fox RC. Training for uncertainty. In: The student-physician: Introductory studies in the sociology of medical education. 1957	Marinker M. On the boundary. 1973 (precursor)
	Davis F. Uncertainty in Medical Prognosis Clinical and Functional. 1960	Bursztajn et al. Medical choices, medical chances: How patients, families, and physicians can cope with uncertainty. 1981 (precursor)
Elstein AS. Clinical judgment: psychological research and medical practice. 1976	Light D Jr. Uncertainty and control in professional training. 1979	Griffiths F, Byrne D. General practice and the new science emerging from the theories of 'chaos' and complexity. 1998
Weinstein MC, Fineberg HV. Clinical decision analysis. 1980	Fox RC. The evolution of medical uncertainty. 1980	Wilson T et al. Complexity science: complexity and clinical care. 2001
Wennberg et al. Professional uncertainty and the problem of supplier-induced demand. 1982	Atkinson P. Training for certainty. 1984	Plsek PE, Greenhalgh T. Complexity science: The challenge of complexity in health care. 2001
Eddy DM. Variations in physician practice: the role of uncertainty. 1984	Gutheil TG et al. Malpractice prevention through the sharing of uncertainty. Informed consent and the therapeutic alliance. 1984	Frankford DM et al. Transforming practice organizations to foster lifelong learning and commitment to medical professionalism. 2000
Moskowitz AJ et al. Dealing with uncertainty, risks, and tradeoffs in clinical decisions. A cognitive science approach. 1988	Katz J. Why doctors don't disclose uncertainty. 1984	Miller WL et al. Practice jazz: understanding variation in family practices using complexity science. 2001
Kassirer JP. Our stubborn quest for diagnostic certainty. 1989	Morreim EH. Cost containment: issues of moral conflict and justice for physicians. 1985	McDaniel RR et al. Surprise, Surprise, Surprise! A complexity science view of the unexpected. 2003
Beresford EB. Uncertainty and the shaping of medical decisions. 1991	Gerrity MS et al. Uncertainty and professional work: Perceptions of physicians in clinical practice. 1992.	Innes AD et al. Complex consultations and the 'edge of chaos'. 2005

(continued)

Table 1.1 (continued)

Uncertainty resulting from individuals' limitations in knowledge, reasoning, and emotional functioning	Uncertainty resulting from how persons interact and form relationships	Uncertainty resulting from living within complex adaptive systems (CAS)
McNeil BJ. Shattuck Lecture–Hidden barriers to improvement in the quality of care. 2001	Cassell EJ. The sorcerer's broom. Medicine's rampant technology. 1993	Sturmberg JP. Variability, continuity and trust -towards an understanding of uncertainty in health and health care. 2010
Hall KH. Reviewing intuitive decision-making and uncertainty: the implications for medical education. 2002	Quill TE, Suchman AL. Uncertainty and control: learning to live with medicine's limitations. 1993	Bleakley A. Blunting Occam's razor: aligning medical education with studies of complexity. 2010.
Ghosh AK. On the challenges of using evidence-based information: the role of clinical uncertainty. 2004	Rizzo JA. Physician uncertainty and the art of persuasion. 1993	Srivastava R. Dealing with uncertainty in a time of plenty. 2011
Mamede S et al. Diagnostic errors and reflective practice in medicine. 2007.	Hunter K. "Don't think zebras": uncertainty, interpretation, and the place of paradox in clinical education. 1996	Jerak-Zuiderent S. Certain uncertainties: modes of patient safety in healthcare. 2012.
Djulbegovic B et al. Uncertainty in clinical medicine. In: Philosophy of medicine. 2011	Fox RC. Medical uncertainty revisited. In Handbook of Social Studies in Health and Medicine. 2000	
Chalmers I. Systematic reviews and uncertainties about the effects of treatments. 2010	Epstein RM, Hundert EM. Defining and assessing professional competence. 2002.	
Kent DM. Shah ND. Risk models and patient-centered evidence: should physicians expect one right answer? 2012	Parascandola M et al. Patient autonomy and the challenge of clinical uncertainty. 2002.	
	Balsa AI et al. Clinical uncertainty and healthcare disparities. 2003	
	Han PK et al. Varieties of uncertainty in health care: a conceptual taxonomy. 2011.	
	Han PK. Conceptual, methodological, and ethical problems in communicating uncertainty in clinical evidence. 2013.	
	Politi MC et al. Supporting shared decisions when clinical evidence is low. 2013	

2. Uncertainty is a problem arising from how persons interact and form relationships (e.g., clinician with patient, clinician with clinician, clinician with non-clinician staff).

This problem results when structural and contextual factors pertaining to clinicians, patients, and/or organizations interfere with individuals' capacities to interact. Whether acquiring clinical knowledge, providing direct care, communicating with patients, or working with colleagues and staff, clinicians inhabit worlds where they depend upon human relationships to create meaning in their own lives while working with others who have this same goal.

Enhancing clinical judgment in the face of uncertainty of this nature involves creating different kinds of clinician-patient, clinician-clinician, and clinician-organization/community relationships where there are opportunities for articulation of shared goals, negotiation, collaborative learning, and knowledge creation.

3. Uncertainty is a problem resulting from living within complex adaptive systems (CAS) where varying mixes of natural systems and man-made systems interact and resist control.

This problem results from failing to appreciate how individuals function in their environment in nonlinear, dynamic ways. The resulting relationships and interconnections cause unpredictable shifts from which information and power flow to new system nodes, making control elusive.

Enhancing clinical judgment in the face of uncertainty of this nature involves openness to surprise, moving forward with good enough information, and appreciating variations and instability for surfacing opportunity.

A Note on Terms

Some of the chapters in this book are written by authors familiar with American usage and others by those accustomed to British terms. To assist readers in better understanding key terms used, we offer the following definitions:

Primary Care Physician/General Practitioner

In the US, the term "primary care physician" refers to a physician who completed residency training in either family medicine, general internal medicine, or general pediatrics. In the UK and the European countries described in this book, doctors working in primary care have almost all completed specialty training as family physicians. They are commonly known as general practitioners or GPs and offer first contact care across all of medicine including general pediatrics and general internal medicine, as well as in gynecology and psychiatry.

Primary Care Clinician/Primary Care Team Member

In the US, the term "primary care clinician" includes primary care physicians and also nurse practitioners and physician assistants. In the UK and Europe, people often use the term "primary care team" to describe GPs and those who work alongside them: depending on the location, this might include nurse practitioners, community nurses, midwives, counselors, and other professionals.

Primary Care Office or Clinic/GP Surgery

A primary care office or clinic in the UK and Europe is frequently referred to as a "surgery."

Resident/Registrar

In the UK and Europe, a doctor in specialty training in family medicine is called a "registrar." In the US, a doctor in training is called a "resident."

The Contents of This Book

This book is presented in two parts. Part I includes an introduction by Lucia Sommers (Chapter 1) which describes the purpose of the book in light of clinical uncertainty's pivotal role in primary care.

Trisha Greenhalgh in Chapter 2 titled "Uncertainty and Clinical Method" provides an uncertainty taxonomy that she illustrates with patients from her own primary care practice. She elucidates uncertainty from four distinct perspectives – evidence-based medicine, narrative medicine, case-based reasoning, and technology-infused, multiple actor health care – with an emphasis on the unique contributions of these approaches to engaging uncertainty.

Chapter 3, "Learning about Uncertainty in Professional Practice," by Colin Coles, focuses on how professionals learn to practice, the notion of professional judgment as central to uncertainty engagement, and the role of the educator in supporting clinicians in uncertainty engagement.

Part II of the book first includes descriptions of four different approaches to the challenge of collaborative engagement with uncertainty. Balint Groups, the oldest small group approach, are presented first, followed by the others according to when they were developed. The section concludes with two accounts of national systems of collaborative engagement for primary care clinicians in Denmark and Sweden.

In Chapter 4, "Balint Groups and Peer Supervision," Henry Jablonski, Dorte Kjemand, and John Salinsky describe Balint Group principles and process providing several examples of Balint Groups at work. Chapter 5, "Research on Balint Groups," by the same authors discusses the challenges of Balint Group research, reviews key research findings, and identifies gaps in research to inform future work.

Chapter 6, "The Thistle and the Maple Leaf: PBSGL in Canada and Scotland," by Heather Armson and Ronald MacVicar, reviews the Practice-Based Small-Group Learning (PBSGL) Program, an international program focused on facilitating discussions among clinician peers that highlight real problems in practice and the challenge of integrating evidence-based care with the uncertain problems patients present. The chapter explores the development of the program, the theoretical underpinnings, and lessons learned.

Chapter 7, "Narrative-Based Supervision," written by John Launer, delineates the principles of narrative-based primary care, their application to clinical encounters, the skills involved, how these are used in peer supervision, and the evolution of these principles from an approach to the patient encounter to a method of clinical supervision. In Chapter 8, "Training in Narrative-Based Supervision: Conversations Inviting Change," he describes the training system for Narrative-Based Supervision (NBS) and its context, the approach to teaching supervision skills, and what is known about NBS outcomes.

In Chapter 9, "Practice Inquiry: Uncertainty Learning in Primary Care Practice," Lucia Sommers describes Practice Inquiry (PI) as a set of small group methods designed for engaging clinical uncertainty in the workplace. She explains the need for clinician colleagues to collaborate in addressing individual patient dilemmas, outlines a scenario on how clinician colleagues use PI methods in a group setting, and reviews PI's five essential components: "the colleague group," case-based uncertainty, inputs to judgment, follow-up, and group facilitation. Also described is a hypothetical primary care setting – the "Inquiry Practice" – within which PI and two other inquiry learning methods, "Practice Epidemiology" and "Practice Mining" provide guidance for primary care practice.

Chapter 10, "Using Practice Inquiry to Engage Uncertainty in Residency Education," written by Tina Kenyon, Claudia Allen, and Alan Siegel, describes the use of Practice Inquiry methods for working with postgraduate trainees in three Family Medicine Residency programs: the New Hampshire Dartmouth program, the University of Virginia program, and the Contra Costa County Regional Medical Center program in California. Each program's unique use of Practice Inquiry methods is described. Observations across programs highlight the opportunities and challenges of using Practice Inquiry methods in post graduate medical education. (Although the focus of this book is on collaborative engagement among established primary care clinicians, we include these examples to show how a model developed for that context can be transferred to postgraduate training settings where trainees can acquire collaborative engagement skills early in their careers).

In Chapter 11, "'We're all in the same boat…': Potentials and Tensions When Learning Through Sharing Uncertainty in GP Peer Supervision Groups," Charlotte Tulinius provides examples of Danish GP supervision sessions and discusses common aspects of methods used in these sessions in conjunction with the cultural conditions and perceptions of professionalism supporting these groups. She reviews research results from a study following three Danish GP peer supervision groups over a period of 2 years.

Chapter 12, "Case-Based Learning in Primary Health Care: Strengths and Challenges," contains a review of the Swedish experience with continuing professional and quality development groups called "FQ-groups" written by Gösta Eliasson. He describes how uncertainty is dealt with using case-based methods by providing a group facilitator's description of his group, an overview of FQ-group methods and management concerns, and discussion of these groups' strengths as well as challenges in remaining a viable option for clinical professional development.

An afterword by John Launer completes the book.

References

Atkinson, P. (1984). Training for certainty. *Social Science and Medicine, 19*(9), 949–956.

Bakhtin, M. (1982). *The dialogic imagination: Four essays*. Austin: University of Texas Press.

Balsa, A. I., Seiler, N., McGuire, T. G., et al. (2003). Clinical uncertainty and healthcare disparities. *American Journal of Law and Medicine, 29*(2–3), 203–219.

Beach, M. C., & Inui, M. (2006). Relationship centered care: A constructive reframing. *Journal of General Internal Medicine, 21*, S3–S8.

Beckman, H. (2009). Three degrees of separation. *Annals of Internal Medicine, 151*(12), 890–891.

Beresford, E. B. (1991). Uncertainty and the shaping of medical decisions. *The Hastings Center Report, 21*(4), 6–11.

Berger, P., & Luckmann, T. (1967). *The social construction of reality: A treatise in the sociology of knowledge*. New York: Anchor.

Bishop, T. (2013). Pushing the Outpatient quality envelop. *Journal of the American Medical Association 309*(13), 1353–1354. doi:10.1001/jama.2013.1220.

Bleakley, A. (2010). Blunting Occam's razor: Aligning medical education with studies of complexity. *Journal of Evaluation in Clinical Practice, 16*, 849–855.

Buber, M. (2000). *I and Thou*. New York: Scribner.

Bursztajn, H. J., Feinbloom, R. I., Hamm, R. M., et al. (1981). *Medical choices, medical chances: How patients, families, and physicians can cope with uncertainty*. New York: Routledge.

Burton, J. (2003). Learning groups for health professionals: Models, benefits and problems. *Work Based Learning in Primary Care, 2*, 93–98.

Burton, J., & Launer, J. (2003). *Supervision and support in primary care*. Abingdon: Radcliffe.

Cassell, E. J. (1991). *Doctoring: The nature of primary care medicine*. Oxford/New York: Oxford University Press.

Cassell, E. J. (1993). The sorcerer's broom. Medicine's rampant technology. *Hastings Center Report, 23*(6), 32–39.

Chalmers, I. (2010). Systematic reviews and uncertainties about the effects of treatments. *Cochrane Database System Review, 8*, ED000004.

Charon, R. (2006). *Narrative medicine: Honoring the stories of illness*. Oxford: Oxford University Press.

Davis, F. (1960). Uncertainty in medical prognosis clinical and functional. *American Journal of Sociology, 66*(1), 41–47.

De Wet, C., Bradley, N., & Bowie, P. (2011). Significant event analysis: a comparative study of knowledge, process and attitudes in primary care. *Journal of Evaluation in Clinical Practice, 17*(6), 1207–1215.

Djulbegovic, B., Hozo, I., & Greenland, S. (2011). Uncertainty in clinical medicine. In F. Gifford (Ed.), *Philosophy of medicine (Handbook of the philosophy of science)*. London: Elsevier.

Eddy, D. M. (1984). Variations in physician practice: The role of uncertainty. *Health Affairs (MillBank), 3*(2), 74–89.

Edmondson, R., Pearce, J., & Woerner, M. (2009). Wisdom in clinical reasoning and medical practice. *Theoretical Medicine and Bioethics, 30*, 231–247.

Elstein, A. S. (1976). Clinical judgment: Psychological research and medical practice. *Science, 194*(4266), 696–700.

Engel, G. (1977). The need for a new medical model: A challenge for biomedicine. *Science, 196*, 129–136.

Epstein, R. M., & Hundert, E. M. (2002). Defining and assessing professional competence. *Journal of the American Medical Association, 287*(2), 226–234.

Feinstein, A. R. (1967). *Clinical judgment*. Baltimore: Williams and Wilkins.

Forsetlund, L., Bjørndal, A., Rashidian, A., et al. (2009). Continuing education meetings and workshops: Effects on professional practice and health care outcomes. *Cochrane Database System Review, 15*(2), CD003030.

Fox, R. C. (1957). Training for uncertainty. In R. K. Merton, G. G. Reader, & P. Kendall (Eds.), *The student-physician: Introductory studies in the sociology of medical education*. Cambridge: Harvard University.

Fox, R. C. (1980). The evolution of medical uncertainty. *The Milbank Memorial Fund Quarterly. Health and Society, 58*(1), 1–49.

Fox, R. C. (2000). Medical uncertainty revisited. In G. Albrecht, R. Fitzpatrick, & S. Scrimshaw (Eds.), *Handbook of social studies in health and medicine* (pp. 409–425). London: Sage.

Frankford, D. M., Patterson, M. A., & Konrad, T. R. (2000). Transforming practice organizations to foster lifelong learning and commitment to medical professionalism. *Academic Medicine, 75*(7), 708–717.

Fulford, K. W. M., Peile, E., & Carroll, H. (2012). *Essential values-based practice: Linking science with people*. Cambridge: Cambridge University Press.

Gabbay, J., & LeMay, A. (2010). *Practice-based evidence for healthcare: Clinical mindlines*. London: Routledge.

Gerrity, M. S., Earp, J. A. L., DeVellis, R. F., et al. (1992). Uncertainty and professional work: Perceptions of physicians in clinical practice. *American Journal of Sociology, 97*(4), 1022–1051. (Quote is paraphrase of Blaise Pascal, Thoughts, ed. Brunschvicg, fragment 72, 1670.)

Ghosh, A. K. (2004). On the challenges of using evidence-based information: The role of clinical uncertainty. *The Journal of Laboratory and Clinical Medicine, 144*(2), 60–64.

Greenhalgh, T., & Hurwitz, B. (1998). *Narrative-based medicine: Dialogue and discourse in clinical practice*. London: BMJ Books.

Griffiths, F., & Byrne, D. (1998). General practice and the new science emerging from the theories of 'chaos' and complexity. *British Journal of General Practice, 48*(435), 1697–1699.

Gutheil, T. G., Bursztajn, H., & Brodsky, A. (1984). Malpractice prevention through the sharing of uncertainty. Informed consent and the therapeutic alliance. *The New England Journal of Medicine, 311*(1), 49–51.

Habermas, J. (1985). *The theory of communicative action. Volume 1: Reason and the rationalization of society*. Boston: Beacon.

Hall, K. H. (2002). Reviewing intuitive decision-making and uncertainty: The implications for medical education. *Medical Education, 36*(3), 216–224.

Han, P. K. (2013). Conceptual, methodological, and ethical problems in communicating uncertainty in clinical evidence. *Med Care Res Rev, 70*(1 Suppl), 14S–36S.

Han, P. K., Klein, W. M., & Arora, N. K. (2011). Varieties of uncertainty in health care: A conceptual taxonomy. *Medical Decision Making, 31*(6), 828–838.

Hunter, K. (1996). "Don't think zebras": Uncertainty, interpretation, and the place of paradox in clinical education. *Theoretical Medicine, 17*(3), 225–241.

Innes, A. D., Campion, P. D., & Griffiths, F. E. (2005). Complex consultations and the 'edge of chaos'. *British Journal of General Practice, 55*, 47–52.

Jacobs, T. O. (2002). *Strategic leadership: The competitive edge*. Washington, DC: National Defense University Press.

Jerak-Zuiderent, S. (2012). Certain uncertainties: Modes of patient safety in healthcare. *Social Studies of Science, 42*(5), 732–752.

Kassirer, J. P. (1989). Our stubborn quest for diagnostic certainty. A cause of excessive testing. *The New England Journal of Medicine, 320*(22), 1489–1491.

Katz, J. (1984). Why doctors don't disclose uncertainty. *Hastings Center Report, 14*(1), 35–44.

Kent, D. M., & Shah, N. D. (2012). Risk models and patient-centered evidence: Should physicians expect one right answer? *Journal of the American Medical Association, 307*(15), 1585–1586.

Levenstein, J. H., MacCracken, E. C., McWhinney, I. R., et al. (1986). The patient-centered clinical method. 1. A model for the doctor-patient interaction in family medicine. *Family Practice, 3*, 24–30.

Levinas, E. (2006). *Humanism of the other*. Illinois: University of Illinois Press.

Light, D., Jr. (1979). Uncertainty and control in professional training. *Journal of Health and Social Behavior, 20*(4), 310–322.

Mamede, S., Schmidt, H. G., & Rikers, R. (2007). Diagnostic errors and reflective practice in medicine. *Journal of Evaluation in Clinical Practice, 13*(1), 138–145.

Marinker, M. (1973). On the boundary. *The Journal of the Royal College of General Practitioners, 23*(127), 83–94.

Marinopoulos, S. S., Dorman, T., Ratanawongsa, N., et al. (2007). Effectiveness of continuing medical education. *Evidence Report/Technology Assessment, 149*, 1–69.

McAlearney, A. S. (2004). Hospitalists and family physicians: understanding opportunities and risks. *Journal of Family Practice, 53*(6), 473–81.

McDaniel, R. R., Jr., Jordan, M. E., & Fleeman, B. F. (2003). Surprise, surprise, surprise! A complexity science view of the unexpected. *Health Care Management Review, 28*(3), 266–278.

McNeil, B. J. (2001). Shattuck lecture—hidden barriers to improvement in the quality of care. *The New England Journal of Medicine, 345*(22), 1612–1620.

Mead, G. H. (1913). The social self. *Journal of Philosophy, Psychology and Scientific Methods, 10*, 374–380.

Miller, W. L., McDaniel, R. R., Crabtree, B. F., et al. (2001). Practice jazz: Understanding variation in family practices using complexity science. *Journal of Family Practice, 50*(10), 872–878.

Morreim, E. H. (1985). Cost containment: Issues of moral conflict and justice for physicians. *Theoretical Medicine, 6*, 257–279.

Moskowitz, A. J., Kuipers, B. J., & Kassirer, J. P. (1988). Dealing with uncertainty, risks, and tradeoffs in clinical decisions: A cognitive science approach. *Annals of Internal Medicine, 108*(3), 435–449.

Nonaka, I., & Takeuchi, H. (1995). *The knowledge-creating company*. New York: Oxford University Press.

O'Riordan, M. (2000). Continuing medical education in Irish general practice. *Scandinavian Journal of Primary Health Care, 18*(3), 137–138.

Parascandola, M., Hawkins, J., & Danis, M. (2002). Patient autonomy and the challenge of clinical uncertainty. *Kennedy Institute of Ethics Journal, 12*(3), 245–264.

Plsek, P. E., & Greenhalgh, T. (2001). Complexity science: The challenge of complexity in health care. *British Medical Journal, 323*(7313), 625–628.

Politi, M. C., Lewis, C. L., Frosch, D. L., et al. (2013). Supporting shared decisions when clinical evidence is low. *Medical Care Research and Review, 70*(1 Suppl), 113S–128S.

Quill, T. E., & Suchman, A. L. (1993). Uncertainty and control: Learning to live with medicine's limitations. *Humane Medicine, 9*(2), 109–120.

Reeve, J. (2010). Interpretive medicine: Supporting generalism in a changing primary care world. *Occasional Paper Royal College of General Practitioners, 88*, 1–20.

Reiss, B. B., Berrington, R. M., Stuart, D. R., et al. (1981). Practice educational meetings: a new influence in general practice. *British Medical Journal (Clin Res Ed), 283*(6298),1025–1027.

Ricoeur, P. (1984). *Time and narrative* (Vol. 1). Chicago: University of Chicago Press.

Rizzo, J. A. (1993). Physician uncertainty and the art of persuasion. *Social Science and Medicine, 37*(12), 1451–1459.

Sommers, L. S., Morgan, L., Johnson, L., et al. (2007). Practice inquiry: Clinical uncertainty as a focus for small-group learning and practice improvement. *Journal of General Internal Medicine, 22*(2), 246–252.

Srivastava, R. (2011). Dealing with uncertainty in a time of plenty. *The New England Journal of Medicine, 365*(24), 2252–2253.

Stacey, R. (2001). *Complex responsive processes in organizations: Learning and knowledge creation.* London: Routledge.

Sturmberg, J. P. (2010). Variability, continuity and trust—towards an understanding of uncertainty in health and health care. *Journal of Evaluation in Clinical Practice, 16*(3), 401–402.

van den Berge, K., & Mamede, S. (2013). Cognitive diagnostic error in internal medicine. *European Journal of Internal Medicine*, S0953–6205(13)00090-3. Doi 10.1016/j.ejim.2013.03.006.

Waldrop, M. M. (1993). *Complexity: The emerging science at the edge of order and chaos.* New York: Simon and Shuster.

Weick, E., Sutcliffe, K. M., & Obstfeld, D. (1999). Organizing for high reliability: processes of collective mindfulness. In R. S. Sutton, & B. M. Staw (Eds.), *Research in Organizational Behavior, Volume 1* (pp. 81–125). Stanford: Jai Press.

Weinstein, M. C., & Fineberg, H. V. (1980). *Clinical decision analysis.* Philadelphia: Saunders.

Wennberg, J. E., Barnes, B. A., & Zubkoff, M. (1982). Professional uncertainty and the problem of supplier-induced demand. *Social Science and Medicine, 16*(7), 811–824.

Wilson, T., Holt, T., & Greenhalgh, T. (2001). Complexity science: Complexity and clinical care. *British Medical Journal, 323*(7314), 685–688. Erratum in: *British Medical Journal, 323*(7319), 993.

Chapter 2
Uncertainty and Clinical Method

Trisha Greenhalgh

Prologue

A Friday evening general practice surgery. Four cases, part-fictionalised to protect confidentiality.

Case 1. Lindsay, a 36-year-old woman with a breast lump. She is 7 weeks pregnant with her second child. She had a benign lump removed from this part of the same breast 4 years ago and was told to get any further lumps checked out promptly. She stopped breast feeding 2 months ago. I examine her. She has tender breasts and an ill-defined lump in the upper outer quadrant of the left one, but no 'red flag' signs (such as skin tethering or enlarged lymph nodes).

Case 2. Chris, a 54-year-old man with an itchy rash. For 3 days he has had about ten reddish, blistering and encrusted spots on the left side of his chest and back. He also has three or four on his left thigh and some on both sides of his forehead. If the rash were confined to his trunk, it might be shingles, since it curves down in a crescent shape, but given the wider distribution, it's more likely to be insect bites. He apologises for being here at all. His wife thought it might be an illness, so she made an appointment for him. I am surprised to smell alcohol on Chris's breath, even though it is only 4.30 p.m. A pop-up prompt from my computer reminds me that Chris is a current smoker and that his Framingham risk score for developing cardiovascular disease in the next 10 years is 15%.

T. Greenhalgh (✉)
Centre for Primary Care and Public Health, Blizard Institute,
Barts and The London School of Medicine and Dentistry, Yvonne Carter Building,
58 Turner Street, London E1 2AB, United Kingdom
e-mail: p.greenhalgh@qmul.ac.uk

L.S. Sommers and J. Launer (eds.), *Clinical Uncertainty in Primary Care: The Challenge of Collaborative Engagement*, DOI 10.1007/978-1-4614-6812-7_2,
© Springer Science+Business Media New York 2013

Case 3. Aisha, a 63-year-old British Afghan woman with a painful hip. She has come
to tell me about her experiences in the orthopaedic department. She has had X-rays,
blood tests and scans. A firm diagnosis of advanced osteoarthritis has apparently
been made. Aisha has been advised to have a total hip replacement as soon as possible. She asks me what I think. She is an educated woman and fluent in English, but
she politely rejects my offer of a leaflet and video giving the facts about total hip
replacement. It's not the details of the operation she is interested in but its relevance
to her own situation. I ask what issues are uppermost in her mind. She explains how
much she hates hospitals, how her case was dealt with solely by a doctor in training
rather than the renowned consultant hip surgeon to whom I had referred her and
how her children (who work in medically related professions) feel that she should
have the operation. She has been on the Internet and found out that the small dose
of diclofenac which she takes at night is 'bad for you', but the other painkillers we
have tried are less effective.

Case 4. Faisal, a 24-year-old Iranian man who has booked a double appointment and
attends with a professional interpreter. He thinks he has wax in his ears. I check
them, confirm the wax and explain through the interpreter that he must put in drops
and then see the nurse for syringing. As the interpreter gets up to leave, he hesitates
and mumbles something. The interpreter explains that Faisal says he is depressed.
On questioning, he has been depressed for 5 years. He doesn't want to talk about the
reasons. A letter from the Medical Foundation for Care of Victims of Torture was
scanned onto his electronic record 3 years ago, but I cannot open it because of a
technical fault. Faisal looks at the floor and makes no attempt to elaborate on his
story despite sharp words from the interpreter ('I've told him to answer you, doctor'). I reflect on whether Faisal would be more forthcoming with a different interpreter or a different doctor. The interpreter appears uncomfortable with my apparent
indecision and suggests I put him on Prozac.

I had gone to surgery last Friday intending to collect some cases to illustrate
uncertainty in clinical practice, having planned to start writing this chapter over the
weekend. When I returned, I told my husband I was disappointed: not much uncertainty had been evident today. I would have to try again next week. Yet when I wrote
out each of my 15 encounters as a brief case history, uncertainty was a central feature
of every single one. I wondered why I had been blind to this at the time, even though
I had approached the day's clinic specifically *looking* for examples of uncertainty.

Introduction: Different Perspectives on Uncertainty in Clinical Practice

General practice sits between what Mishler, following Habermas, called the voice
of medicine (i.e. the assumptions, values and logic of a clinico-pathological world
view) and the voice of the lifeworld (i.e. the assumptions, values and logic of a
person-living-in-society world view) (Habermas 1981; Mishler 1984). The general

practitioner, and any other clinician who manages illness in a community context, must be highly trained – up to date with the relevant literature and technically competent – and use this knowledge and skill set in clinical decision-making and care delivery. He or she must also possess the personal qualities that support strong therapeutic relationships – especially the ability to connect at a personal level with the patient and engage with their story.

Uncertainty in clinical method is inherent both to the voice of medicine (the science of clinical decision-making in relation to *diseases*) and to the voice of the lifeworld (the elements of clinical practice to do with the management of *illness*). Both diseases (those textbook entities which we seek to diagnose, treat, prevent and monitor) and illnesses (the lived experiences and symbolic meanings of sickness, healing, coping and dying) unfold in ways we can neither fully predict nor fully control.

Thirty years after Habermas described his 'system' and 'lifeworld' distinction, it is time to add a third voice: the voice of technology – the opportunities, constraints and organisational logic engendered by the ubiquitous use of computers and other information and communication technologies.[1] Paperless consulting, touch-screen self-registration, electronic templates for chronic disease monitoring, Internet-based guidelines and protocols, computer-generated risk scores, online appointment booking, automated data transfer (records, laboratory tests and discharge summaries), telephone consultations, text message reminders, downloadable patient leaflets and digital financial flows are all part of the business as usual of general practice – as is the periodic failure of all these technologies and the idiosyncratic ways in which humans use them. Both staff and patients in the contemporary health care organisation need to be digitally astute and skilled in working around these limitations.

Ironically, given the promise of technology to provide accurate, reliable data at the touch of a button, uncertainty is a particular feature of multi-professional care that is supported by distributed information systems (e.g. a shared computer network which allows different staff members to call up and work on a patient record from their terminal, with automated links to pathology, radiography and outpatient booking services). *Someone* on a multi-professional care team may know an item of information, and/or a data item might be filed *somewhere* on the system, but because of the sheer size and complexity of the socio-technical system, that item may not be accessible or locally meaningful to the member of the team who is currently seeing the patient. As we shall see, the voice of technology does not correspond unproblematically to the harmonised voice of the multi-professional team.

In this chapter, I will review the literature on clinical uncertainty, touching on philosophical, theoretical and empirical perspectives, but I will focus *mainly* on my own clinical perspective – that is, the perspective of a doctor who sees patients, reflects on my practice and strives to make my contribution to a wider team effort. In this chapter, I will summarise four approaches to uncertainty that I find

---

[1] I am indebted to my general practitioner Ph.D. student, Deborah Swinglehurst, for many discussions on 'voice' in the electronic patient record.

particularly relevant to front-line clinical work and especially to clinical judgement. These perspectives overlap considerably but, at a philosophical level, are not fully commensurable with one another.

They are (a) evidence-based medicine, which considers uncertainty in probabilistic (Bayesian) terms; (b) narrative medicine, which considers uncertainty in terms of the open-endedness of the story form and the creative space in which storytelling is performed; (c) medicine as case-based reasoning, which considers uncertainty in terms of situated ethical judgements and tacit knowledge (and which, I feel, overcomes many of the limitations of evidence-based and narrative-based medicine); and (d) multi-professional care, which considers uncertainty in terms of how knowledge, reasoning and action are spread across a network of people and technologies.

I acknowledge that these perspectives do not represent a definitive or complete taxonomy (the psychodynamic approach advocated by Michael Balint might be considered a separate category, though some would classify it as an application of narrative medicine; and a 'critical theory' approach might consider uncertainty from a political power perspective). The four I have chosen might serve as ideal types against which other approaches might be compared and contrasted.

In this chapter, I have used the term 'clinical method' synonymously with 'clinical judgement'. I did this unconsciously, perhaps reflecting the approach that prevailed in the mid-1980s when I first studied general practice and began to be inspired by writers like George Engel, Marshall Marinker, Iain McWhinney and Eliot Mishler (1984; 1978; 1983; 1986). Nowadays, clinical method has taken on a somewhat different meaning, referring not to the situated judgements made by a clinician about a real patient in a real predicament but to a set of transferable clinical skills and task-based procedures (such as how to examine an abdomen), especially when taught to students. When 'clinical method' is given this more contemporary meaning, it is possible to assess it in objective structured clinical examinations (OSCEs) and even do randomised trials in which it is the dependent variable (Murray et al. 1997; Al-Dabbagh and Al-Taee 2005).

When this different meaning of the term was pointed out to me by the editors, I contemplated changing 'clinical method' to 'clinical judgement' throughout this chapter, but after some reflection, I chose to keep the terminology as I had originally used it. To conflate clinical method with context-free performance in an OSCE is an act of reductionism from which academic general practice urgently needs to be redeemed. I want to reclaim the original meaning of the term, and I hope this chapter will illustrate why.

Clinical Method as Evidence-Based Decision-Making

Evidence-based medicine (EBM) is 'the use of mathematical estimates of the risk of benefit and harm, derived from high-quality research on population samples, to inform clinical decision-making in the diagnosis, investigation or management of individual patients.' (Greenhalgh 2010). The expression 'evidence-based medicine' is a relatively new packaging of epidemiological concepts that have been around for decades. EBM was introduced by Sackett and colleagues as a reaction to what they called 'decision-making by anecdote' and which might be more neutrally depicted as replicating the iterative hypothesis-testing of expert diagnosticians (Kassirer et al. 1982).

Proponents of EBM have pointed out the folly of assuming (as we did for centuries) that generations of doctors would become competent merely by watching other doctors make decisions and argued that a more systematic approach to incorporating best research evidence into clinical judgement would reduce inappropriate, wasteful and sometimes overtly harmful variations in practice (Eddy 2005).

Epidemiologists, who generate the science on which EBM is based, look at diseases in populations. They begin with a *sample* – a systematically collected group of people who either have a disease or who might develop it – and they follow this sample to see what happens to them. Sometimes, the sample is allocated at random to receiving treatment A or treatment B, and the outcomes (benefits and harms) compared between the two groups: the much-feted randomised controlled trial. Clinical epidemiology thus generates numbers that inform decisions in prevention, diagnosis, prognosis, treatment and surveillance – such as the sensitivity and specificity of a diagnostic test or the 'number needed to treat' (NNT), an estimate of the efficacy of a drug. This approach rests firmly on objectivist philosophical principles (a) that there is a physical reality independent of the observer; (b) that there are things to be measured and facts to collect; and (c) that the purpose of research is to find valid, reliable, transferable truths ('empirical facts') that can be used to inform decisions by other people in other settings.

From a philosophical perspective, EBM is sometimes considered to be the last bastion of crude empiricism, though Mike Kelly and Tessa Moore have recently argued, based on the philosophy of Hume and Kant, that EBM rests on sophisticated (albeit largely unexamined) reasoning which precedes empirical observation (Kelly and Moore 2012). In their words:

> The principles of the elimination of the possibility of bias in the hierarchy of evidence, of the rule-driven principles of guideline development and appraisal are based on an ideal version of the scientific method, which owe more to the logical precepts of the a priori relations of ideas than they do to messy empirical observation. (p. 10)

When I confirmed the lump that Lindsay had found in her breast, my chain of reasoning included asking myself 'if I took a sample of a thousand women in their 30s, each of whom had a breast lump, in what proportion of them would the lump turn out to be cancerous?' (an estimate of prevalence). Importantly, the answer to this question depends on where the sample of women came from. If the sample were drawn from a specialist breast clinic (say, 1,000 consecutive referrals of breast lumps from general practice), around a quarter of those women would have cancer. But if I took a thousand women in their 30s attending general practice with a breast lump, only around one in 40 would have cancer (Greenhalgh 2010).

Epidemiological research has greatly improved our ability to predict whether a particular patient is likely to develop a particular disease. By following thousands of women prospectively for many years, and carefully recording key data items over time, they have produced sophisticated risk scores in which different factors (a history of a benign breast lump, having a first child late in life, past use of hormonal contraceptives and so on) contribute different amounts to a probability estimate for the development of cancer. This kind of research helps us explain, for example, why Japanese women are less likely to develop breast cancer than British women. It has also informed an emerging science of clinical prediction rules and scoring systems which offer the best combination of symptoms, signs and laboratory tests to 'rule in' or 'rule out' a particular diagnosis or risk state and which, once validated, can be used to help resolve a host of clinical conundrums from diagnosing the cause of a red eye to estimating the risk of falls in an older person (Reilly and Evans 2006).

A clinical prediction score will not tell me whether Lindsay has cancer, but it will reduce the uncertainty around this question. By combining everything I know about her risk factors and the results of my clinical examination, I can estimate that her chance of having breast cancer is rather more than 2.5% (the average level for someone her age seen in general practice). She needs to be referred to a breast clinic, where she is likely to be offered a combination of three tests – examination by a specialist (whose skill in distinguishing benign from suspicious breast lumps on clinical grounds is likely to be greater than mine), an ultrasound examination and a fine needle biopsy (a fourth test, a mammogram X-ray, will probably be omitted because of her pregnancy). Each of these tests alone is incapable of ruling breast cancer in or out with 100% accuracy, but the combination of all three ensures that once all the results are available, Lindsay's doctors will be able to say with confidence *either* that the chance of her having cancer is vanishingly small *or* that she almost certainly does have cancer *or* that there is sufficient residual doubt to justify a prompt operation to remove the lump so that a firm histological diagnosis can be made.

Many readers, especially those who have been trained as doctors since the 1990s, will already be familiar with the principles of EBM and how probabilities derived from epidemiological research are used to produce guidelines and protocols (and, sometimes, programmed into computerised decision support tools) so as to support a scientific, objective and rational approach to clinical decision-making (Eddy 2005). In the language of EBM, a diagnostic test should be sensitive (i.e. it picks up all or very nearly all people who have the disease) and specific (i.e. it excludes all or nearly all people who do not have the disease). A treatment (e.g. drug, operation or lifestyle change) should produce a high level of benefit (e.g. cure or extend life) but a low level of harm (i.e. no serious side effects).

Some diagnostic tests perform extremely well at reducing uncertainty. Take the CAGE questionnaire for example. Faced with a patient who has a possible alcohol-related problem, ask four questions: (a) have you ever felt you needed to Cut down on your drinking? (b) have people Annoyed you by criticising your drinking? (c) have you ever felt Guilty about drinking? and (d) have you ever felt you needed a drink first thing in the morning (Eye-opener) to steady your nerves or to get rid of a hangover? In one study, a CAGE score above or equal to 2 had a sensitivity of 93% and a specificity of 76% for diagnosing a 'problem drinker' (Berandt et al. 1982).

I thought of using this simple score with Chris, but decided against it. I will explain this decision from a narrative medicine perspective in the next section, but to justify it from an EBM perspective, reassuring evidence is emerging that strictly applying *population-based* evidence to *individual* cases produces fewer overall benefits (and more overall harms) than a more nuanced and flexible approach, even if the latter appears less 'evidence-based' (Kent and Shah 2012). Similarly, some treatments are extremely effective and have few downsides. An example is triple therapy (two antibiotics and a proton pump inhibitor) for peptic ulcer disease. For every 1.1 patients given triple therapy, the causative bacterium (helicobacter) will be eradicated in one, and for every 1.8 patients treated, one will remain cured of peptic ulcer 1 year later. Whilst minor side effects with triple therapy are common, serious ones are extremely rare. Thus, whereas 20 years ago there was much uncertainty about how best to treat peptic ulcer, there is now strong consensus (Moore 2009).

However, many diagnostic tests are neither sensitive nor specific, and very few treatments are both highly beneficial and lacking in serious side effects. Herein lies a major – and arguably ineradicable – source of clinical uncertainty. In relation to Faisal, for example, even putting aside whether a diagnosis of depression is either justified or helpful (see section "Clinical Method as Narrative"), epidemiological research has shown that whilst selective serotonin reuptake inhibitors (SSRIs, the class of drug to which Prozac [fluoxetine] belongs) may lead to significant reduction in the symptoms of depression, they also often lead to serious side effects, including an increase in suicidal tendencies and long-term dependence (Cipriani et al. 2010). Far from informing a clear course of action, the epidemiological evidence base on SSRIs merely serves to confirm that the advantages of putting Faisal on this drug *may or may not* be outweighed by the disadvantages.

The EBM community has recognised that in many if not most clinical decisions, there are pros and cons of different options and that different patients may place different values on each option. Much work has been done to develop ways of representing epidemiological research findings diagrammatically so as to support informed, shared decision-making by patients (Han et al. 2011a; Edwards and Elwyn 2010). Aisha, for example, may prefer to tolerate moderate pain and disability than succumb to the surgeon's knife; others with the same symptoms would be keener for an operation.

Would Aisha's uncertainty be helped by formal ways of mapping benefits and risks and asking her to rate her preferences on a scale of nought to five? Perhaps, though I may have to work on her to increase her receptivity to such a task. Working with patients to share uncertainty and address it systematically is not something many clinicians do routinely, though the abstract books of academic conferences are replete with reports of 'tools' intended for use in the clinical consultation for applying essentially Bayesian (probabilistic) reasoning to some clinical scenario or other. The difference between the enthusiasm with which such tools are produced and the reluctance of clinicians to use them in practice would surely be a worthy topic for further research. Indeed, a Ph.D. student of mine had a go at this with diabetes risk scores (Noble et al. 2011).

Let us return to Faisal's unhappiness. A rapidly expanding branch of epidemiology known as 'personalised medicine' seeks to square the circle between population-derived evidence (which can tell us, at best, whether fluoxetine reduces depression symptoms *on average* in people *like* Faisal) and the personal benefit-risk equation in a particular patient (will fluoxetine reduce depression symptoms in *Faisal*, and also, of the many antidepressant drugs available, which is best suited to his particular metabolism?). The epidemiology of personalised medicine (not to be confused with 'evidence-informed individualised care' – that is, the judicious combination of scientific reasoning with deep and intimate knowledge of one's patient (Miles and Loughlin 2011)) works by collecting genetic information and tissue samples as well as conventional risk factors over time, thereby (it is hoped) narrowing the confidence intervals around a prediction of risk or benefit for an individual. The UK Biobank project, for example, has already recruited half a million people and aims to follow them for 20 or more years, leading eventually to several thousand data items for each person (Hewitt 2011).

With the help of such large databases and powerful computer programmes, it is theoretically possible (so the protagonists of personalised medicine believe) that we will reach a point where instead of 'on average' estimates of the likelihood of developing certain conditions or of the benefit or harm of different treatment options, we will be able to say to patients like Lindsay 'your breast cancer is of xx genetic type; given your personal genetic and metabolic profile, the chance of achieving cure with the best treatments currently available is 89%, but the chance that your cancer will subsequently recur is 63%'. Such apparently accurate predictions (a future possibility, some say) have the potential to reduce uncertainty – but they are unnerving and raise important ethical and legal questions about privacy, ownership of data and the regulation of testing (Bourret et al. 2011).

It is beyond the scope of this chapter to pursue the finer points of clinical epidemiology, evidence-based medicine, shared decision-making or the promise of personalised medicine. But it should be clear from this brief account that this approach to clinical method rests on a number of assumptions (Henry 2010; Braude 2009; Djubegovic et al. 2009; Mol 2008). First, it assumes that diseases and risk categories exist and are useful entities – that is, that it is both possible and helpful to sort patients into those who do or do not fulfil the diagnostic criteria for a disease or pre-disease state (breast cancer, peptic ulcer, high cardiovascular risk, 'problem drinking' and so on).

Second, it assumes that clinical method is wholly or mostly to do with the epidemiology-informed tasks of preventing, diagnosing, treating and monitoring disease, and hence with making clinical decisions (should I do this test, that test or no test? Should I prescribe this drug, that drug or no drug? Should I advise my patient to make this or that change to their lifestyle? and so on). Third, it assumes that evidence collected in some other population sample at some other time is more or less transferable to the patient in front of you. Fourth, it assumes that this information (typically derived from a randomised controlled trial or longitudinal cohort study) is at least as valuable as, and should sometimes override, the tacit, intuitive knowledge of the experienced clinician (see section "Clinical Method as Narrative").

Fifth, it assumes that facts and values are separable and that patients' values and preferences are quantifiable, stable over time and readily linked to the diagnostic or treatment options in the clinical decision tree. Finally, the expansion of the evidence base to include genetic material and an increasingly detailed environmental risk profile on hundreds of thousands of research participants rests on the (arguably highly questionable) assumption that this complex system will exhibit linear dynamics, making accurate prediction of individual risk and benefit possible.

These assumptions hold true – or at least, they approximate so closely to the truth that for all practical purposes we can ignore the difference – in some but not all situations. The uncertainty in Lindsay's case (Does she have breast cancer? Should her lump be removed urgently?) and perhaps Aisha's case (What are the benefits and risks of medical and surgical management of moderate osteoarthritis of the hip?) may be substantially reduced by examining the problem through an EBM lens. But the uncertainty in relation to Chris's skin rash will not, since the evidence base for mild, non-specific skin rashes is all but non-existent (Perhaps because virtually all such rashes are self-limiting and this problem would be a low research priority).

And in Faisal's case, where the uncertainty is particularly pressing (What happened to him? Does he have depression? Is depression a helpful or unhelpful category to describe his illness? What are the available non-drug options? Who else is around in his life? Why is his relationship with this professional interpreter so awkward? and so on), only a fraction of this uncertainty will be reduced by recourse to the epidemiological research literature. Furthermore, even assuming a future state in which we will know a lot more than we currently do about the genetics of SSRI response, only the most confident pharmaco-epidemiologist would argue that a full genetic profile will provide the key to eradicating the uncertainty in Faisal's case.

A recent review article in the journal Medical Decision-Making offered a 'new conceptual taxonomy', in which the authors recognised three sources of uncertainty in health care: (a) probability (indeterminacy of future outcome), (b) ambiguity (lack of evidence, contested evidence or imprecision in estimates), and (c) complexity (multiplicity of causal factors and interpretive cues) (Han et al. 2011b). This seems a reasonable way to parse the types of uncertainty which fall *within* the evidence-based medicine paradigm, but it does not engage to any significant degree with the three other perspectives on uncertainty covered in this chapter.

Clinical Method as Narrative

If evidence-based decision-making is the objectivist, disease-oriented perspective on clinical method, narrative medicine is usually thought of as the subjectivist, illness-oriented perspective. Whether a disease or pre-disease state 'really' exists as an objective entity or not, when we are ill or at risk (or believe ourselves to be so), we must make sense of our experience and learn to cope with it via what Mike Bury has called 'rebuilding spoiled identity' (Bury 1991). The illness journey and efforts to manage it unfold against a rich tapestry of symbols, actions and events in the wider world; efforts to manage illness (by patient and professional) have social, cultural and moral dimensions that vary in different contexts and at different times. Narrative medicine, whose cross-disciplinary roots include literary studies, sociology, phenomenology and psychoanalysis, is the art of engagement with the patient as narrator of their personal story and the use of this 'storywork' as a therapeutic force (Charon and Montello 2002; Launer 2002).

Chris has attended my clinic smelling of alcohol. Is he a 'problem drinker'? Whilst one approach to reducing the uncertainty in Chris's case might be to invite him to complete the CAGE questionnaire described briefly in the previous section, another might be to be open to Chris's story in his own words. He tells me that he has had to take a half-day's annual leave to keep this appointment (which had been made by his wife on his behalf) and that rather than 'waste' this enforced leave, he has been watching the football on TV. Intuitively, I compare this story fragment with my stock of past experience of patients who have attended smelling of alcohol (for innocent or pathological reasons) and with my stock of experiences of family and friends who watch the football when on annual leave. Rightly or wrongly, I decide that I have a plausible enough narrative to make CAGE redundant. Perhaps the issue here is not whether prescribed 'good practice' (in this case, the use of an evidence-based assessment instrument) is used but my judgement as an experienced practitioner about whether this instrument is a 'good fit' with the emerging dialogue between patient and clinician. That judgement – the essence of what is often referred to as 'narrative [based] medicine' – is aesthetic, ethical and (above all) intuitive.

The narrative approach originated within, and remains most widely used and researched, in relation to mental health is the so-called talking therapies. Especially in relation to patients whose unhappiness or confusion is linked to the contexts and complexities of their lives, many authors have questioned whether it is useful to manage illness by assigning a disease category ('depression', 'anxiety', 'post-traumatic stress disorder') and linking treatment to those categories (Launer 2002; Heath 1998). Rather, these authors propose, the clinician's central role may be to serve as the audience for the story – that is, as the active listener whose concern and questioning shape the narrative and work towards it acquiring coherence and purpose.

The skilled narrative clinician notes the genre of the story (perhaps using Art Frank's widely cited taxonomy of illness narrative – restitution, tragedy, quest, chaos (Frank 1995)), its characterisation (does the patient depict him or herself as hero, victim, bystander etc.; is the surgeon a hero or villain; do family members play supportive or destructive roles?), its setting (is the story primarily set in the home, the workplace, the community etc.?), the key actions and events (what happens – and by whose agency?) and how a plot is woven through the use of literary devices (metaphor, imagery, tropes). Thus, the clinician learns *how and in what way the person is ill* and, by active listening, helps co-construct a healing or coping narrative (Greenhalgh and Hurwitz 1999).

Physical illness (including chronic illness and cancer), while often readily classifiable as disease, can also be thought of as primarily a challenge of sense-making and identity [re]construction (Bury 1991; Frank 1995; Mattingly 1998). Frank has written powerfully about his own cancer journey and the crucial role of the clinician as witness to the suffering of the individual with 'deep illness' (Frank 1998). My own team recently showed that the narratives of people with diabetes can be analysed in two ways, revealing both a biomedical perspective (the various tasks of self-management including disease monitoring, planning and monitoring the diabetes diet, managing medication, taking exercise, accessing health care, looking after feet and so on) and also a narrative perspective in which these 'biomedical' tasks acquire social meaning and moral worth in the patient's 'lifeworld' (Greenhalgh et al. 2011). 'Self-management' is as much about socio-emotional work as it is about monitoring biomarkers (Hinder and Greenhalgh 2012).

Engagement of the health professional with the patient's narrative is thus not an *alternative* to considering the biomedical aspects of care, but a means by which the science of caring for the person who is ill comes to make sense to both patient and clinician. This engagement also has an ethical dimension, representing as it does the professional and human commitment to acting in the patient's interests. As Charon and Montello have put it, 'the singular case emerges only in the act of narrating it and duties are incurred in the act of hearing it' (Charon and Montello 2002).

Aisha's case shows not only how a narrative approach is relevant to the entirety of the illness journey (the unfolding of the over-arching story of worsening arthritis – a story which will be built and understood through continuity of care), but also how it may help reduce uncertainty at particular steps in that journey. In this particular consultation, Aisha faces a decision: to undergo the hip replacement operation or not. But she is clear that she does not want to know any more facts and figures about the operation, which is why I am not convinced that a 'shared decision-making' framework will work in her case. Perhaps, we should explore how the pain and disability of an arthritic hip are affecting her role in her family and community. Perhaps, I should invite the story of how Aisha came to hate hospitals or of how her grown-up children have responded to the unfolding of her illness journey. Thus, through dialogue, Aisha and I might co-construct a narrative of *today's* plight in relation to her chronic illness.

Faisal's case highlights how a purely 'subjectivist' narrative medicine approach isn't going to get us very far with complex cases. For sure, Faisal (newly registered with my practice) has a story to tell, but he doesn't want to tell it. Faisal's asylum seeker status, the letter from a charity specialising in victims of torture, his averted eyes and burdened body language all suggest the need for intimacy, trust, continuity of care, a common vocabulary and an ethical commitment on the part of the listener as preconditions for beginning his storywork. Yet the interpersonal dynamics of this awkward tripartite consultation provide none of these contextual conditions. My role as clinician is *not* to attempt to extract his painful story with the assistance of this interpreter (who, for all her professional qualifications and shared cultural background, appears oddly disengaged from Faisal's predicament) but somehow to bear witness to his suffering *despite* her presence. I must also work within the constraints of the here and now to create some possibilities for a more productive consultation sometime in the future.

It is not Faisal's untold story (narrative as noun) that is the issue here but the dynamics of the telling – and the not telling (narrative as verb). The Russian philosopher and literary critic Michael Bakhtin emphasised that whenever a story is told, it is shaped by the listener or (imagined) reader, since every utterance is made in response to, or in anticipation of, the utterance of another human being (Bakhtin 1981). Contemporary narrative scholars have moved beyond a narrow focus on the text (i.e. on studying the structural elements of the story) to consider the teller-listener relationship and the act of storytelling (Riessman 2008). In this *performative* framing, narrative medicine is not a purely subjectivist phenomenon. Rather, the story is a practical accomplishment, a product of the dynamic, teller-listener interaction. And it is in this performative space rather than in the narrative itself that the scope for resolving uncertainty lies (Charon and Montello 2002; Mattingly 1998; Malterud 2006).

A number of related streams of academic work are worth mentioning here. First, there is work on the therapeutic relationship, including Frankel's notion of 'relationship-centred care' (Frankel 2004) and earlier seminal work on the same theme by Michael Balint (1957) and Carl Rogers (1951). In contrast to approaches which emphasise tasks and processes, these authors have argued that relationship conditions offered by the clinician (empathy, congruence and unconditional positive regard) are in and of themselves therapeutic and that this relationship creates the preconditions for effective communication (perhaps, co-construction of a narrative). Balint encouraged general practitioners to reflect in groups on clinical cases, sharing stories of the stories they had co-constructed with their patients and using their fellow practitioners as a critical audience to suggest potential therapeutic options.

Clinical Method as Case-Based Reasoning

It is worth reflecting here on why, as my Friday evening clinic unfolded in real time, I experienced little in the way of conscious feelings of uncertainty. This is at least partly because as an experienced clinician working in a familiar setting and most of my patients were known to me, my reasoning was predominantly intuitive (Greenhalgh 2002). That is not to say I was especially knowledgeable about the clinical topics I was encountering, but that I was processing multiple sources of information rapidly and largely unconsciously – and doing what normally works (Dreyfus and Dreyfus 1986; Benner 1984).

As Kathryn Montgomery has shrewdly observed, 'Clinicians' lack of curiosity about clinical thinking (with its concomitant appeal to science) turns out to be characteristic of all practice, an apparently unavoidable consequence of the requirement that practitioners act despite uncertainty' (p. 193) (Montgomery 2009). As clinical practice becomes ever more rationalised and protocol-driven, and as professional development shifts further from reflecting on the curious features of individual cases in favour of achievement of specific learning targets, the question arises: are we in danger of retreating even further from the intuitive side of our expertise?

In relation to Lindsay's case, for example, it was only afterwards that I became conscious of a memory of a lecture on breast cancer in pregnancy some 30 years ago at medical school. In it, we had been reminded that whilst breast cancer in pregnancy is rare, when it occurs it is rapidly progressive, and we should therefore refer any suspected cases urgently (Amant et al. 2012). This snippet of wisdom from an experienced (and probably now long dead) professor of surgery was overlaid by more recent and more conscious memories of evidence-based guidelines for referral of breast lumps in non-pregnant women – and by the rhetorical power of the story within a story of how Lindsay had previously been advised to present without delay should a lump recur in this part of her breast.

The notion of tacit knowledge is relevant here. As Polanyi observed, tacit knowledge is embodied, tied to individuals, impossible to codify or measure objectively and hard to transmit to others (Polanyi 1962). It functions at the periphery of attention and – in Henry's words – 'forms a largely taken-for-granted foundation that makes the information on which the clinician focuses directly, such as the patient's story and the significance of her [clinical examination], possible' (Henry 2010). This is the knowledge that comes from years of walking the wards, consulting in clinic and visiting patients in their homes – and above all, the knowledge which is built by accumulating *cases* (Cox 2001). It is this, rather than an encyclopaedic knowledge of all the relevant guidelines, which defines the difference between the expert and the novice clinician. And it is this tacit dimension, necessarily accessed intuitively, which informs that elusive judgement on what is the *right* thing to do for Lindsay, Chris, Aisha and Faisal.

That the knowledge needed to enact the clinical encounter is often tacit, context-bound and ephemeral rather than codifiable, transferable and enduring often goes under-recognised and under-explored by academic commentators on clinical method. In Faisal's case, for example, I made a judgement not to pursue his symptoms of depression exhaustively in this particular encounter. Rather, I chose to try to convey to him that I was open to developing a therapeutic relationship and working on his narrative at some other time in the future (perhaps with a different interpreter). Designers of electronic records may miss the crucial importance of such situated communication and produce artefacts (such as pop-up prompts or inflexible templates in electronic records) that fit poorly with the subtle micro-detail of clinical work.

The ubiquitous pop-up prompt, whilst driven by 'evidence-based' guidelines, complicates and potentially disrupts the delicate interpersonal interaction on which the clinician-patient consultation has traditionally depended (Balint and Norrell 1983). It is difficult enough to build a therapeutic relationship with Faisal across a language barrier, especially given the limitations of his illness, my own limited understanding of his circumstances and the nature of the cultural support on offer, but this would surely be made even more difficult if Faisal knew I was being prompted (and financially incentivised) to 'offer Chlamydia testing'. Moreover, I deliberately did not enter Faisal's 'depression' as a new coded item on his electronic record. Had I done so, a template would have been triggered which would have included a structured questionnaire on mental health symptoms. Failure to get Faisal to complete that questionnaire and enter his score in the appropriate box would have led to my practice incurring a financial penalty in the pay-for-performance Quality and Outcomes Framework used in the UK (Roland 2004).

Whilst inscribing evidence-based guidelines in technology is not in and of itself a 'bad thing', the voice of technology can be a two-edged sword when subtle emotional work is being done in the consultation. The technological voice must be actively and reflexively managed (and where appropriate, subverted or worked around) as part of case-based reasoning rather than allowed to direct the encounter whatever else is going on in it (Swinglehurst et al. 2011).

Evidence-based and narrative-based approaches to clinical method may on one level be analytically separated (and based on very different philosophical assumptions), but they are not mutually exclusive nor should they be considered in a simplistic zero-sum relationship in which more of one presumes less of the other. There is no evidence that clinicians who try to practise in an evidence-based way necessarily undergo attrition of their humanitarian values nor that the use of evidence-based guidelines and protocols produces a 'science-based meritocracy on the patient ward' (Timmermans and Angell 2001). In Aisha's case, a skilled application of clinical method would combine the narrative approach to reducing uncertainty (e.g. drawing out her story of why she is so opposed to hip surgery) with an evidence-based approach to optimising medical management of her pain and disability.

Those who seek a philosophically commensurate alignment of evidence-based and narrative-based clinical methods should read Montgomery's excellent book 'How Doctors Think' (Montgomery 2006). Drawing on Aristotle, she argues that despite its own emphatic claims to the contrary, medicine is not a science at all – and nor, incidentally, is it an art. Medicine is a *practice* – specifically, an uncertain, paradox-laden, judgement-dependent, science-using, technology-supported practice. As such, and despite the extensive pathophysiological and epidemiological evidence base that informs it, medicine is comparable to the practice of law or making of ethical judgements. In every case, the practitioner must reason not from the general to the particular but from the particular to the general – abduction rather than deduction. The question facing every practitioner, every time they encounter a case, is 'What is it best to do, for this individual, at this time, given these circumstances?'

The good clinician must draw, as the founding fathers of evidence-based medicine famously pointed out, conscientiously and judiciously on the best research evidence on offer and make optimal use of available technologies (Sackett et al. 1996). But because the case is a singular one, because the predicament affects a real individual in the inescapable reality of the here and now and because this person has life projects and commitments and things at stake, a clinical judgement is fundamentally a practical and moral one, informed but not determined by scientific evidence. The skilled practice of medicine is not merely about knowing the rules but about deciding *which* rule is most relevant to the particular situation at hand. Illness may be a narrative, but just as in law, just as in literature, there is no text that is self-interpreting (Montgomery 2006).

As Montgomery points out, Aristotle distinguished three kinds of knowledge: *episteme* (factual knowledge), *techne* (technical knowledge or skill) and *phronesis* (practical wisdom). Clinical method involves not merely the skilled use of the senses to inform diagnosis but also the application of practical wisdom to draw judiciously on science (the evidence base) and technology (e.g. point-of-care prompts or inbuilt templates) when making here-and-now practical, ethical judgements in a particular case. Precisely how these different knowledges are woven together to manage and support the patient depends on the particularities of the case – and it occurred in different ways as I consulted with Lindsay, Chris, Aisha and Faisal.

Clinical Method as Multi-professional Collaborative Work

The input of a doctor to a twenty-first-century consultation usually both presupposes and contributes to a wider package of inter-professional care. When I saw Lindsay, she had already had a telephone consultation with a nurse practitioner and been advised to attend for an 'on the day' emergency appointment. When Chris registered with my practice a year ago, he had had an interview with a health care assistant, who had collected and entered a standard dataset of items such as weight, height, blood pressure and smoking status. More recently, the practice manager had contacted Chris to check missing data items so as to complete his Framingham risk score (a task which attracts an incentive payment for practices). These data items had been combined in an automated algorithm to produce a 'high risk' alert, which triggered the pop-up prompt in Chris's electronic record at the point of care. Aisha's record included an electronically transferred letter from the doctor in the orthopaedic clinic and the results of tests performed elsewhere in the health care system. Faisal, who attended with a professional interpreter (electronically booked on the system), had previously had an in-depth interview and physical examination by specialists in a third-sector organisation; a letter summarising their thorough, culturally informed assessment was on his electronic record when I saw him – but it was, sadly, technically inaccessible to me last Friday.

Whilst multi-professional care is part of the business as usual of both general practice and hospital care, few who write on clinical method make explicit reference to a wider team, each member of which typically contributes partially but not exclusively to the care of the patient or to the information systems which (well or badly) support this activity. Yet if we broaden our conception of clinical method to embrace the wider socio-technical care network (i.e. networks of people and the technological infrastructure which links them across time and space), the model of clinical care becomes an order of magnitude more complex. Uncertainty becomes plural.

There is my own uncertainty about the evidence base, about the unfinished aspects of the patient's story and about the numerous interacting influences I need to take intuitive account of when making my here-and-now practical judgement of what to do next. There is also my uncertainty about what others in the team know and what they have already done (and *their* uncertainties about what *I* have done).

Then there is the uncertainty inherent in data. Is this data item reliable? Is it complete? Is it up to date? Is it technically accessible? Do I trust the person who entered it? Does the absence of a data item indicate that the patient is 'normal' in relation to this item? These questions about data are not unique to the shared electronic record. They also pertain to shared paper records, patient-held shared care notes, patient-recorded data (e.g. home blood pressure or peak flow readings), post-it notes, telephone messages, emails and so on – but the distributed electronic record makes the trustworthiness and accessibility of data a particularly prominent issue. Finally, there is uncertainty about whether a prompt set up by some other person at some other time and in some other place is relevant to the patient sitting in front of me in the here and now (a phenomenon termed time-place distanciation (Giddens 1984)) and whether I should (sometimes or always) disrupt the flow of today's consultation to respond to this interruption.

Given these complexities and interdependencies, it is perhaps small wonder that the leading cause of medical error is poor communication and collaboration between individuals and teams, including end-of-shift handovers, referral and discharge letters, real-time cross-referrals between members of acute teams, doctor-nurse communication in chronic disease management and transfer of prescriptions between physicians and pharmacists (Institute of Medicine 1999). It is often assumed that the solution to what has become known as the 'integration' problem is largely or wholly technological. In particular, many have speculated about a future electronic patient record which will be characterised by completeness, accuracy and extensive interoperability with other record systems (Institute of Medicine 2009). Data, it is assumed (or at least, implied), will be available at the touch of a button – at which point, uncertainty will become a thing of the past.

This framing of clinical care as wholly or mainly to do with data capture and retrieval suggests (wrongly) that knowledge about the patient can be accurately and completely recorded on the electronic record and passed as codified data items between professionals. 'Continuity of care' and 'integration of care' have become subtly redefined in technological rather than human terms. To explain why patients and staff alike so often experience multi-professional care in terms of *discontinuity* and *lack* of integration (and hence associated with greater rather than less uncertainty), we should remember the crucial role of tacit knowledge in clinical method:

> Direct, face-to-face human interaction comprises a rich, highly nuanced exchange of information; the wealth of verbal and non-verbal communication it includes is necessarily absent from written records, telephone interactions and subsequent memories of an interaction. The full range of tacit and explicit information about a patient's particular problem or illness is accessible only from within the clinical encounter. (Henry 2010, p. 293)

Technology-supported multi-professional care is a complex area of practice, the study of which owes much to an applied (and theoretically eclectic) field known as computer-supported cooperative work or CSCW (Berg 1998; Berg and Goorman 1999; Pratt et al. 2004). CSCW focuses not on the individual knower or computer user but on the wider network of people and technologies and the work that is spread in complex ways among them. Inter-professional collaborative work involves the sequential ordering and coordination of tasks and the management of the inter-dependencies of these tasks, which in turn requires both real-time processing of local information by individuals and an awareness of how everyone's contribution fits into the wider picture.

Shared electronic records tend to be seen as representing progress (e.g. greater accessibility, greater accuracy, searchability) from their paper-based predecessors. They can also (in theory) provide multiple views and framings of the data, hence can potentially tolerate (and overcome) the ambiguities inherent in inter-professional work and make the work of different professional groups more visible to others. In practice, however, this is rarely achieved, and the reality may be of 'clunky' inter-faces, missing data and a sense of fragmentation and mutual alienation rather than inter-professional co-operation (Stange 2009). Despite this well-described model-practice gap, humans are often very creative in developing ways to get the job done ('workarounds'), thereby overcoming inherent limitations of technologies and individual shortcomings of team members (Ash et al. 2004).

Some approaches to CSCW use the term 'distributed cognition' to depict knowledge and reasoning which are spread between people and technologies, perhaps across several departments or organisations. This model views people and computers as a linked set of information containers and processors, and implicitly views the key distinction between them as quantitative (e.g. computers have more memory and faster processing power). In this model, 'uncertainty' approximates to missing data items somewhere in the system.

More interesting for the purposes of this book are more nuanced approaches to CSCW whose starting point is the assumption that humans and computers are fundamentally different. The key accomplishment of the human team member is not in faithfully following a particular standardised routine (e.g. a shared protocol or computerized template) but in knowing the contingent detail of *when* (and when not) to follow that routine (Garfinkel 1967). This is what Garfinkel called 'ethnomethodology': 'the moment by moment management of contingent detail through sequential orderings' (Rawls 2008, p. 703). Only through effortful attention to situated detail can collaborative work occur, hence Garfinkel's definition of a group as people who are, at any moment in time, 'playing the same game'. A key dimension of this game-playing is trust, without which the continual production of meaningful, sequential action is impossible. The awkwardness between Faisal, myself and the interpreter (and in particular, her apparent interpretation of my silence as ignorance of which medication to prescribe for depression) illustrates how the three of us were playing 'different games' in this consultation.

Garfinkel influenced the seminal work of Lucy Suchman on situated action – that is, the subtle, contingent and context-dependent nature of action as humans use technologies collaboratively (Suchman 1987). Health care is a complex, nonroutine affair: contingencies are the rule, and the skill of professional practice is 'smoothly molding such continuous lapses of order into events to be handled with "standard operating procedures"' (Ash et al. 2004, p. 106). This essence of clinical work contrasts markedly with the assumption inbuilt into the design of many health care information systems – that much work is routine and therefore readily automated.

All this has crucial (but often poorly understood) implications for the management of uncertainty in clinical care. First, a data item (such as a coded diagnosis of depression) may be present on the electronic record and appear factual but still have much uncertainty associated with it. Who entered this code? On what grounds? Is the diagnosis still current? What does the absence of a code for depression mean? What does three separate codes for myocardial infarction in a patient's record mean – that the patient has had three heart attacks or that the quality control of data entry in the practice is poor?

Second, 'overcomplete' medical records may generate their own uncertainties through loss of overview (not seeing the wood for the trees) and information overload. Many of us remember as juniors sifting through dozens of pages of test results (paper or electronic) in a search for the one result that will change our management. In one extreme case, the introduction of a 'cut and paste' facility led to a junior doctor dumping an entire copy of a patient's hospital admission notes into the electronic discharge summary (Ash et al. 2004). Aisha's electronic record contained various imaging reports, some miscoded as 'letter from consultant', and numerous other items of correspondence, but no easily accessible overview of the extent or pace of deterioration over time.

Third, the collection and analysis of electronic record data for secondary uses such as audit, epidemiological research and surveillance of clinician performance is built on what is arguably an illusion – that it is only a matter of time before we will know exactly what is going on (e.g. what are the precise patterns of disease in this population? Who has been missed in each screening programme? Who are the 'poorly performing' general practitioners? and so on). In reality, there is a paradox: efforts to generate information (as in the Quality and Outcomes Framework in English general practice (Roland 2004)) may increase rather than decrease uncertainty. This is because (a) collecting and retrieving information both have an opportunity cost and divert activity from other, patient-facing work; (b) too much information leads to loss of overview at the policy level as well as the individual level; (c) incentivisation leads to gaming; and (d) information is rarely value neutral.

As Hari Tsoukas has put it in an article entitled *The Tyranny of Light* (Tsoukas 1997):

> The overabundance of information in late modernity makes the information society full of temptations. It tempts us into thinking that knowledge as information is objective and exists independently of human beings; that everything can be reduced into information; and that generating ever more amounts of information will increase the transparency of society and, thus, lead to the rational management of social problems. However… the information society is riddled with paradoxes that prevent it from satisfying the temptations it creates. More information may lead to less understanding; more information may undermine trust; and more information may make society less rationally governable. (p. 827)

The widespread notion that multi-professional care is best supported by the rationalist approach of standardised protocols, strictly delineated roles and an electronic record system that assures quality through coded entries, templates and pull-down menus, has been challenged by academics working in the field of complex adaptive systems (Lanham et al. 2009). These authors argue that when uncertainty is high (i.e. most of the time in primary health care), quality is not something that is achieved through careful planning and adherence to protocol but something that emerges through adaptive relationships, collective sense-making and on-the-job learning from one another. The implications of this are far-reaching and beyond the scope of this chapter but deserve further exploration by those researching the link between teamwork and the management of uncertainty.

Conclusion

In this chapter, I have begun to develop a new taxonomy (which is no doubt incomplete, but it will do for a Friday evening surgery and some ideas which others can take forward). I summarise this taxonomy below.

First, there is uncertainty *about the evidence* – the 'voice of medicine' dimension of the consultation, for which the key questions relate to the completeness, accuracy and relevance of research-based evidence and on the balance between potential benefits and potential harms. Second, there is uncertainty *about the patient's story* – the 'voice of the lifeworld' dimension, about which scholars of narrative medicine have offered much sound advice. Third, there is uncertainty about *what best to do* for a particular patient given a particular set of circumstances; this kind of uncertainty includes the philosophical question of how tacit knowledge informs clinical judgement. Finally, there are the many uncertainties (and associated threats to quality and safety) that inevitably arise when clinical care becomes a *collaborative endeavour* in which human-human, technology-human and technology-technology interactions all loom large.

Having artificially deconstructed uncertainty in clinical practice into four categories for analytic purposes, it is important to add that at a practical level, in the fast-moving and often down-and-dirty setting of front-line clinical work, uncertainty is a singular, shadowy and irrevocably fuzzy construct, not a multifaceted, tidy and well-defined one. Even when we try to be aware of uncertainty in the clinical consultation, it continually slips from our awareness.

It is for this reason, perhaps, that so many different groups from different countries (US, UK, Denmark, Sweden, Scotland, Canada) have independently arrived at a broadly similar way of addressing uncertainty in a general practice setting: the collective study of clinical practice through retrospective sense-making in groups. These examples differ substantially in the extent to which they view their work as grounded in particular academic traditions (e.g. in the psychodynamic focus of therapists such as Michel Balint (1957) and Carl Rogers (1951); the literary traditions of Michael Bakhtin (1981); the sociological perspective of Mike Bury and Arthur Frank (1995, 1998); the philosophical Aristotle's practical reasoning and Nicomachean ethics taken forward by Katherine Montgomery and Rita Charon (Charon and Montello 2002; Montgomery 2006); and my own work on combining evidence-based and narrative-based approaches to clinical decision-making (Greenhalgh 1999)), as primarily educational (with a focus on defining learning objectives and measuring performance) or as a 'branded' approach with a focus on structured steps to be taken by a facilitator to support the group process (e.g. with a proper noun, as in Sommers' Chapter on Practice Inquiry or Armson and MacVicar's on Practice-Based Small Group Learning).

I suspect, however, that despite the differences in form and style, the commonalities between the approaches described in this book are more noteworthy than their differences. I am confident that committed participation in any one of these approaches will help clinicians in their struggle to do the best for their patients despite the inherent uncertainty of primary care practice. And I am also convinced that no matter how long such groups go on meeting or how much any specific approach is refined, there will never be a fix for those problems and situations that most trouble us. The most we can do with those is muddle through while we continue to reflect in supportive environments.

References

Al-Dabbagh, S. A., & Al-Taee, W. G. (2005). Evaluation of a task-based community oriented teaching model in family medicine for undergraduate medical students in Iraq. *BMC Medical Education, 5*, 31.

Amant, F., Loibl, S., Neven, P., et al. (2012). Breast cancer in pregnancy. *Lancet, 379*(9815), 570–579. Epub 2012/02/14.

Ash, J. S., Berg, M., & Coiera, E. (2004). Some unintended consequences of information technology in health care: The nature of patient care information system-related errors. *Journal of the American Medical Informatics Association, 11*(2), 104–112.

Bakhtin, M. (1981). *The dialogic imagination: Four essays. Translated by Caryl Emerson and Michael Holquist*. Austin: University of Texas Press.

Balint, M. (1957). *The doctor, his patient and the illness*. London: Routledge.

Balint, E., & Norrell, J. (1983). *Six minutes for the patient: Interaction in general practice consultations*. London: Tavistock.

Benner, P. (1984). *From novice to expert: Excellence and power in clinical nursing practice*. Reading: Addison-Wessely.

Berandt, M. W., Mumford, J., Taylor, C., et al. (1982). Comparison of questionnaire and laboratory tests in the detection of excessive drinking and alcoholism. *Lancet, 6*(8267), 325–328.

Berg, M. (1998). Medical work and the computer-based patient record: A sociological perspective. *Methods of Information in Medicine, 37*(3), 294–301.

Berg, M., & Goorman, E. (1999). The contextual nature of medical information. *International Journal of Medical Informatics, 56*, 51–60.

Bourret, P., Keating, P., & Cambrosio, A. (2011). Regulating diagnosis in post-genomic medicine: Re-aligning clinical judgment? *Social Science Medicine, 73*, 816–824.

Braude, H. D. (2009). Clinical intuition versus ststistics: Different modes of tacit knowledge in clincial epidemiology and evidence-based medicine. *Theoretical Medicine and Bioethics, 30*(181), 198.

Bury, M. (1991). The sociology of chronic illness: A review of research and prospects. *Sociology of Health and Illness, 13*, 451–468.

Charon, R., & Montello, M. (2002). *Stories matter: The role of narrative in medical ethics*. London: Routledge.

Cipriani, A., La, F. T., Furukawa, T. A., et al. (2010). Sertraline versus other antidepressive agents for depression. *Cochrane Database System Review, 14*(4), CD006117.

Cox, K. (2001). Stories as case knowledge; case knowledge as stories. *Medical Education, 35*(9), 862–866.

Djubegovic, B., Guyatt, G. H., & Ashcroft, R. E. (2009). Epistemoloigcal enquiries in evidence-based medicine. *Cancer Control, 16*(2), 158–168.

Dreyfus, H. L., & Dreyfus, S. E. (1986). *Mind over machine: The power of human intuition and expertise in the era of the computer.* Oxford: Blackwells.

Eddy, D. M. (2005). Evidence-based medicine: A unified approach. *Health Affairs, 24*(1), 9–17.

Edwards, A., & Elwyn, G. (2010). *Evidence based patient choice* (2nd ed.). Oxford: Oxford University Press.

Engel, G. L. (1983). The biopsychosocial model and family medicine. *Journal of Family Practice, 16,* 409, 12, 13.

Frank, A. (1995). *The wounded storyteller: Body, illness, and ethics.* Chicago: University of Chicago Press.

Frank, A. (1998). Just listening: Narrative and deep illness. *Families, Systems and Health, 16,* 197–216.

Frankel, R. (2004). Relationship-centered care and the patient-physician relationship. *Journal of General Internal Medicine, 19*(11), 1163–1165.

Garfinkel, H. (1967). *Studies in ethnomethodology.* Engelwood Cliffs: Prentice-Hall.

Giddens, A. (1984). *The constitution of society: Outline of the theory of structure.* Berkeley: University of California Press.

Greenhalgh, T. (1999). Narrative based medicine: Narrative based medicine in an evidence based world. *British Medical Journal, 318*(7179), 323–325.

Greenhalgh, T. (2002). Intuition and evidence–uneasy bedfellows? *British Journal of General Practice, 52*(478), 395–400.

Greenhalgh, T. (2010). *How to read a paper: The basics of evidence based medicine* (4th ed.). London: BMJ.

Greenhalgh, T., & Hurwitz, B. (1999). Why study narrative? *British Medical Journal, 318,* 48–50.

Greenhalgh, T., Collard, A., Campbell-Richards, D., et al. (2011). Storylines of self-management: Narratives of people with diabetes from a multiethnic inner city population. *Journal of Health Services Research and Policy, 16*(1), 37–43.

Habermas, J. (1981). *The theory of communicative action.* Boston: Beacon.

Han, P. K., Klein, W. M., Lehman, T., et al. (2011a). Communication of uncertainty regarding individualized cancer risk estimates: Effects and influential factors. *Medical Decision Making, 31*(2), 354–366.

Han, P. K. J., Klein, W. M. P., & Arora, N. K. (2011b). Varieties of uncertainty in health care: A conceptual taxonomy. *Medical Decision Making, 31*(3), 828–838.

Heath, I. (1998). Following the story: Continuity of care in general practice. In T. Greenhalgh & B. Hurwitz (Eds.), *Narrative based medicine: Dialogue and discourse in clinical practice.* London: BMJ Publications.

Henry, S. (2010). Polanyi's tacit knowing and the relevance of epistemology to clinical medicine. *Journal of Evaluation in Clinical Practice, 16,* 292–297.

Hewitt, R. E. (2011). Biobanking: The foundation of personalized medicine. *Current Opinion in Oncology, 23*(1), 112–119.

Hinder, S., & Greenhalgh, T. (2012). "This does my head in". Ethnographic study of self-management by people with diabetes. *BMC Health Services Research, 12*(1), 83. Epub 2012/03/31.

Institute of Medicine. (1999). *To err is human: Building a safer healthcare system.* Washington, DC: Institute of Medicine.

Institute of Medicine. (2009). *Health and human sciences in the 21st century: Charting a new course for a healthier America.* New York: National Academies Press.

Kassirer, J. P., Kuipers, B. J., & Gorry, G. A. (1982). Toward a theory of clinical expertise. *The American Journal of Medicine, 73*(2), 251–259.

Kelly, M. P., & Moore, T. A. (2012). The judgement process in evidence-based medicine and health technology assessment. *Social Theory and Health, 10*, 1–19.

Kent, D. M., & Shah, N. D. (2012). Risk models and patient-centered evidence. *The Journal of the American Medical Association, 307*(15), 1585–1586.

Lanham, H. J., McDaniel, R. R., Jr., Crabtree, B. F., et al. (2009). How improving practice relationships among clinicians and nonclinicians can improve quality in primary care. *Joint Commission Journal on Quality and Patient Safety, 35*(7), 457–468.

Launer, J. (2002). *Narrative based primary care: A practical guide*. Oxford: Radcliffe.

Malterud, K. (2006). The social construction of clinical knowledge – the context of culture and discourse. *Journal of Evaluation in Clinical Practice, 12*, 248–256. Commentary on Tonelli, M. R. (2006). Integrating evidence into clinical practice: An alternative to evidence-based approaches. *Journal of Evaluation in Clinical Practice, 12*(3), 292–295.

Marinker, M. (1978). The chameleon, the judas goat, and the cuckoo. *The Journal of the Royal College of General Practitioners, 28*, 199–206.

Mattingly, C. (1998). *Healing dramas and clinical plots: The narrative structure of experience*. New York: Cambridge University Press.

McWhinney, I. R. (1986). *A textbook of family medicine* (1st ed.). Oxford: Oxford University Press.

Miles, A., & Loughlin, M. (2011). Models in the balance: Evidence-based medicine versus evidence-informed individualized care. *Journal of Evaluation in Clinical Practice, 17*(4), 531–536.

Mishler, E. G. (1984). *The discourse of medicine: Dialectics of medical interviews*. Norwood: Ablex.

Mol, A. (2008). *The logic of care: Health and the problem of patient choice*. London: Routledge.

Montgomery, K. (2006). *How doctors think: Clinical judgement and the practice of medicine*. Oxford: Oxford University Press.

Montgomery, K. (2009). Thinking about thinking: Implications for patient safety. *Healthcare Quality*, 12 Spec No Patient:e191–e4.

Moore, A. (2009). What is an NNT? Available in full text on http://www.medicine.ox.ac.uk/bandolier/painres/download/whatis/NNT.pdf. Bandolier. April 2009: 1264.

Murray, E., Jolly, B., & Modell, M. (1997). Can students learn clinical method in general practice? A randomised crossover trial based on objective structured clinical examinations. *British Medical Journal, 315*(7113), 920–923.

Noble, D., Mathur, R., Dent, T., et al. (2011). Risk models and scores for type 2 diabetes: Systematic review. *British Medical Journal, 343*, d7163.

Polanyi, M. (1962). *The tacit dimension*. New York: Anchor Day.

Pratt, W., Reddy, M. C., McDonald, D. W., et al. (2004). Incorporating ideas from computer-supported cooperative work. *Journal of Biomedical Informatics, 37*(2), 128–137.

Rawls, A. W. (2008). Harold Garfinkel, ethnomethodology and workplace studies. *Organization Studies, 29*(5), 701–732.

Reilly, B. M., & Evans, A. T. (2006). Translating clinical research into clinical practice: Impact of using prediction rules to make decisions. *Annals of Internal Medicine, 144*(3), 201–209.

Riessman, C. (2008). *Narrative analysis*. London: Sage.

Rogers, C. (1951). *Client-centered therapy: Its practice, implications and theory*. Philadelphia: Trans-Atlantic Publications.

Roland, M. (2004). Linking physicians' pay to the quality of care–a major experiment in the United Kingdom. *The New England Journal of Medicine, 351*(14), 1448–1454.

Sackett, D. L., Rosenberg, W. C., & Gray, J. A. M. (1996). Evidence based medicine: What it is and what it isn't. *British Medical Journal, 312*, 71–72.

Stange, K. (2009). The problem of fragmentation and the need for integrative solutions. *Annals of Family Medicine, 7*, 100–103.

Suchman, L. (1987). *Plans and situated actions: The problem of human-machine communication*. Cambridge: Cambridge University Press.

Swinglehurst, D., Roberts, C., & Greenhalgh, T. (2011). Opening up the 'black box' of the electronic patient record: A linguistic ethnographic study in general practice. *Communication and Medicine, 8*(1), 1–12.

Timmermans, S., & Angell, A. (2001). Evidence-based medicine, clinical uncertainty, and learning to doctor. *Journal of Health and Social Behavior, 42*(4), 342–359.

Tsoukas, H. (1997). The tyranny of light. The temptations and the paradoxes of the information society. *Futures, 29*, 827–843.

Chapter 3
Learning About Uncertainty in Professional Practice

Colin Coles

Introduction

In her chapter in this book, Trisha Greenhalgh (2012) cites the work of Kathryn Montgomery:

> Despite its own emphatic claims to the contrary, medicine is not a science at all – and nor, incidentally, is it an art. Medicine is a *practice*. (Montgomery 2006)

In this chapter, I will explore that notion of practice, particularly professional practice, especially in relation to dealing with uncertainty in general practice and the educational implications of that. This will inevitably lead on to some discussion about judgement and 'professional judgement' in particular, since this lies at the heart of dealing with uncertainty. I will explore what it is, what characterises it, why it is necessary for professional practice, what forms it takes, what knowledge underpins it, and ultimately how it develops naturally and can be developed educationally.

The focus of the chapter, then, is an educational one – how professionals learn to practise: examining critically what appears to work and why; what the constraints are that may prevent this happening; and what options educators have in helping clinicians deal with uncertainty. My aim is to generate discussion and to keep the conversation going – and to make some tentative recommendations.

I am conscious in writing this chapter of two audiences. One of these, practising clinicians, may or may not be interested in knowing more about educational theory and practice. Education may be self-evident to them: teaching is easy, so why

C. Coles (✉)
Faculty of Education, Health and Social Care, University of Winchester, UK
e-mail: Colin.Coles@winchester.ac.uk

L.S. Sommers and J. Launer (eds.), *Clinical Uncertainty in Primary Care: The Challenge of Collaborative Engagement*, DOI 10.1007/978-1-4614-6812-7_3,
© Springer Science+Business Media New York 2013

complicate it? Why indeed? I ask them to see the logic of my argument and hope that their natural intellectual capacity – as well perhaps as their curiosity – will carry them through this. The second readership will be my more natural colleagues: professional educators. Whilst some of what I write here will be familiar to many, some of it may not.

I have structured this chapter as follows: First, I explore the nature of practice, and of professional practice in particular, noting that uncertainty is normal, to be expected. Next, I show that professionals develop the general professional capacity of judgement to deal with this uncertainty, and that underpinning that judgement is the professional's 'practical wisdom'. I then turn to how professionals acquire such wisdom and describe four options that educationists have open to them. I comment on how these inform our understanding of ways in which health care practitioners can be helped to learn to deal with uncertainty.

My emphasis in this chapter will be on the uncertainties that are to be found not just in clinical practice but those that inevitably occur in the practice of education too. I will show that educators who strive to help clinicians deal with uncertainty have choices they can make and, in doing so, can make professional educational judgements themselves. In concluding, I suggest how these educators can develop ways of helping medical practitioners deal more effectively with the uncertainties they face in their clinical practice.

The Nature of Practice

It is generally accepted in the literature that practice is 'a more or less settled body of activities that is carried out to some distinctive end' (Fish and de Cossart 2007: 188). As Golby and Parrott (1999: 13) put it:

> The skills and techniques of a practice are not neutral instruments to be used to satisfy whatever desires a particular individual may happen to have. The way we see the world, what we try to achieve in it and how we go about trying to do so are not independent of one another. We see and behave as we do primarily because we act in accordance with a way of seeing and doing laid down by a tradition and because people who belong to that tradition see and behave in that way.

Carr (1995: 68/9) makes the same point when he says that:

> To 'practise' is always to act within a tradition, and it is only by submitting to its authority that practitioners can begin to acquire the practical knowledge and standards of excellence by means of which their own practical competence can be judged.

Physicians and educators both engage in their chosen practice when they collectively become members of a tradition of practice. This does not mean that such a tradition is static. Quite the reverse. By taking up membership of a tradition of practice, practitioners inevitably change that tradition, and so their wider practice moves forward by and through the very acts of practitioners practising within that tradition (Carr 1995: 69). Any practice is fashioned by its membership, that is, by how its members act. Practice, in this sense, is culturally, historically, and ultimately socially determined – and even (because of that) is vulnerable to ideological distortion (Carr 1995: 50).

Medicine, then, is best seen as a social practice and the quality of care best understood in the ways practitioners work together rather than in terms of an individual's capabilities (Lanham et al. 2011). Today's literature, apparently at odds with some of today's politics, tells us that context is everything (Regehr 2006).

Perhaps one reason why the social nature of practice is not always fully understood by the medical community is because most physicians, though not all, have been selected during their careers for their scientific interests. The medical community, generally (though by no means universally), thinks scientifically (Montgomery 2006), believing that there are right and wrong answers, and they may then not see medical practice as socially constructed.

What then can be said about professional practice? What makes a practice – and an individual practitioner – professional? Montgomery (2006) is clear that medicine is a moral practice: medical people intentionally engage in particular acts for the good of another person who is in need. The same is true of education. Whilst in medicine practitioners deal with the balance between sickness and health, in education, they deal with that of ignorance and wisdom. The medical person's duty of care is to the patient; the educationist's duty of care is to the learner. (Incidentally, this can mean a conflict of interest for the medical educator: whereas caring for patients may come before caring for learners, it does not replace it.)

Although medicine and education have distinctive specific aims, there is a point at which they meet since both share that same moral imperative, as Freidson notes:

> The idea of a profession refers to specialised work…[that] is esoteric, complex and discretionary in character: it requires theoretical knowledge, skill and judgement [of a particular kind] that ordinary people do not possess, do not wholly comprehend and cannot readily evaluate. Furthermore, the kind of work they do is believed to be especially important for the well-being of individuals or of society at large, having a value so special that money cannot serve as its sole measure; it is also Good Work. It is the capacity to perform that special kind of work which distinguishes those who are professional from most other workers. (Freidson 1994: 200)

Yet this moral imperative is not without its difficulties since people who are not practitioners do not always understand, let alone appreciate, what it means to practise as a professional. Gawande, a surgeon writing more for the public than his colleagues, reflects:

> Medicine is, I have found, a strange and in many ways disturbing business. The stakes are high, the liberties taken tremendous…We do so out of an abiding confidence in our know-how as a profession…We look for medicine to be an orderly field of knowledge and procedure. But it is not. It is an imperfect science, an enterprise of constantly changing knowledge, uncertain information, fallible individuals, and at the same time lives on the line. There is science in what we do, yes, but also habit, intuition and sometimes plain old guessing. The gap between what we know and what we aim for persists. And this gap complicates everything that we do…As pervasive as medicine has become in modern life, it remains hidden and often misunderstood. We have taken it to be both more perfect than it is and less extraordinary than it can be. (Gawande 2000:4, 7–8)

And Heath, writing as a general practitioner, says this:

> The mysterious secrets of…general practice seem to be poorly understood outside our discipline and, in the face of the current avalanche of change, there is an increasingly urgent need to explain ourselves…In doing so we tend to lose sight of those parts of our work which should not change because they are dealing with enduring aspects of the human experience of illness and disease. Unless we are able to make our specific contribution explicit, we will not be valued and we may be lost. (1995: 3–4)

In our present age, professionals appear to be under siege (Fish and Coles 1998: 3). We live in a world that values accountability, which policymakers have interpreted as best met through greater and tighter regulation. Yet, perhaps as a reaction to this, there are now calls for the reestablishment of trust in the relationship between professionals and those they serve (O'Neil 2002) – a relationship that is said to be 'fiduciary'. Alongside this, there is now the need for professionals more precisely to narrate what it means to be a professional practitioner (Fish and Coles 1998: 57; Coles 2006: 397). It seems that, in the face of being required to be accountable **for** their practice, professionals must give a clearer account **of** their practice.

To summarise, practitioners – both clinical and educational – are called upon by society to practise their profession in situations of great complexity, considerable uncertainty, and sometimes enormous paradox, where there is often the need for them, sometimes in the face of what members of the general public might think, to decide what is best for the good of an individual rather than what is right in some absolute sense (Tyreman 2000). On occasions, this might mean doing no more, and no less, than to watch and wait. Yet running throughout all this can be uncertainty as to what might be for the best. Of course, because of all that, there will be times when what the professional decides to do may not turn out to be for the best, and even (with hindsight) wrong. This raises the question as to whether this was because of some weakness or lack of ability on the part of the individual professional. The literature suggests that in the majority of cases it is not – rather that inevitably there is an inherent messiness about professional practice. Donald Schön (1984, 1987) captured this well of course when he characterised professional practices as being located in what he called 'the swampy lowlands'.

The Centrality of Judgement in Professional Practice

Above, I have shown that the literature strongly supports the view that professionals practise in situations of considerable uncertainty when they are asked by society to use their judgement for the good of those in need. That is both a factual statement (it is what professionals 'know' that they do), and it is also a 'values' statement (it is what professionals 'believe' to be the best thing to do). I have also shown that professional practice is a social phenomenon – practitioners may work alone on occasions but always do so in a social context and often alongside colleagues. Their collegial relationships with one another, and their professional relationships with those they serve, define their practice. In this way, professional practice is what happens when professionals practise.

I will not rehearse here the tensions that these statements generate within the evidence-based community, who appear to contend that there are right and wrong ways to practise, nor within the political community, who believe that there are ways that professionals ought to practise. That debate runs through other contributions to this book. Indeed, experienced medical and educational practitioners are only too aware that their decisions to act in a particular way may often occur without them being able to say with any precision why they came to this judgement, and so they often use terms such as intuition or 'gut feeling' to describe their actions (Atkinson and Claxton 2000; Dhaliwal 2010; Gawande 2002; Groopman 2007; Montgomery 2006; ten Cate 2006; Tripp 1993).

Rather, in this chapter, I explore different forms of evidence (Epstein 1999: 834) that come not from science – which offers only a particular kind of evidence – but from philosophy, history, and rational thought or to put it somewhat differently through 'a process of reasoning' (Carr 1995: 71). In Ancient Greece, Aristotle saw this most clearly: that it was helpful to characterise human action as either a 'making action' (which he called *poiesis*) which resulted in the creation of a specific product or artefact or a 'doing action' (which he called *praxis*). For him, these two forms of action were supported by different forms of knowing: *Poiesis* being underpinned by *techne* (which we would translate as 'technical knowledge') and *praxis* by *phronesis* (or 'practical wisdom').

The major difference for Aristotle between these two forms of action concerned the relationships between ends (what you were attempting to achieve) and means (the ways in which you might achieve these ends). For *poiesis* (the production of some object), both the end and the means were known in advance of the commencement of that action (as in a blueprint or plan). But with any 'doing action' (*praxis*), it was more helpful to assume that neither the ends nor the means could with any certainty be known in advance of that action commencing. On occasions, the ends only emerged as the means were being pursued – often to the surprise of the doer, as any doctor or teacher knows only too well. Not just this; with any 'doing action', both means and ends needed to be consistent with each other: you ought not to achieve even a worthy end by some unworthy means. Judgements concerning both means and ends involve moral considerations.

One implication of this is that if you observe someone engaged in *poiesis* – some action that results in someone making something – you can be pretty certain what they will do, how they will go about it, and what the outcome is likely to be. On the other hand, when you observe someone engaged in *praxis*, you cannot always predict what will happen or what the outcome might be. In fact, nothing that happens will come as a surprise. It will be obvious to professional practitioners that, in the light of Aristotle's reasoning, medicine and education are classic examples of *praxis*. It is worth noting at this point that in some modern European languages – German, for example – the contemporary word 'practice' translates as *praxis* and is understood within those cultures in the way Aristotle saw it. Put another way, uncertainty is an inevitable and entirely natural feature of professional practice. It is to be expected and hence needs to be anticipated.

This can be of some concern to newcomers to any professional practice (Lave and Wenger 1991). Understandably, they may be confused when they see their seniors acting differently in situations that appear entirely similar. They may even feel that uncertainty in their own practice is a sign of weakness or ineptitude on their part. Nothing could be further from the truth. Uncertainty is normal. The issue is not about learning how to eliminate it but how to deal with it, and certainly not learning how to deal with it once and for all, because every situation a practitioner encounters, however much it appears to be like other similar situations, will always be unique in certain ways.

As I noted earlier, other contributors to this book give many examples of uncertainty in medical practice. As an educationist, it is for me to do so from educational practice. Eisner's (2005: 5) comments about school teaching capture this well. I include them here as the principles underpinning these comments apply to education in all its forms:

> One of the important tasks of teaching is to be able to focus on the individual while attending to the larger classroom patterns of which the individual is a part. To complicate matters these patterns change over time. The good teacher…has to pay attention to several operations simultaneously…This process of shifting aims while doing the work at hand is what Dewey (1938) called 'flexible purposing'. Flexible purposing is opportunistic; it capitalizes on the emergent features appearing within a field of relationships. It is not rigidly attached to predefined aims when the possibility of better ones emerges. The kind of thinking that flexible purposing requires thrives best in an environment in which the rigid adherence to a plan is not a necessity. As experienced teachers well know, the surest road to hell in a classroom is to stick to the lesson plan no matter what.

There is an important further point, which has already been alluded to. Since professional practice is a social phenomenon, a professional judgement is best thought of as a collective one. Whilst it may appear that a professional, acting alone, is exercising his or her own judgement, that judgement cannot be assumed to be the isolated, individual judgement of that person for three reasons:

First, expert professional judgement will always take account of the needs of the person being served. In many cases, the professional will ask that person what he or she considers might in their view be the best course of action: What do they think ought to happen? What do they want now? This may strongly influence the judgement made.

Second, since professionals act within the traditions of their practice, and also within communities of practice, their judgement will inevitably be fashioned in part by those factors. In the primary care setting, where practitioners often see patients on their own, the practitioner's wise judgement often takes into account what his or her colleagues might have done in particular circumstances, as well as what the practice policy might be.

Third, certainly in more obvious social settings of health care, such as in a hospital ward and in primary care practices, collective judgements are commonly made (even if the individual is less than aware of doing this) when clinicians talk with their colleagues about the patients and situations they are encountering and how to deal with the uncertainties this raises. Professional judgement is inevitably collective judgement.

The argument so far is summarised in Box 3.1.

Box 3.1 Practice, Professional Practice, and Professional Judgement

Practice

- Doctors and educators are members of their respective 'traditions of practice', which they adopt and, in so doing, contribute to the ongoing development of those traditions.
- Practice (or what Aristotle called – and several European languages now call – *praxis*) is a form of 'doing' (rather than 'making') action which is inevitably (and so understandably) always characterised by uncertainty (including complexity and paradox).
- Human action is very different from the action of 'things' where cause and effect can most often be determined in advance and is often (though not universally) 'rule governed'.

Professional Practice

- *Professional practice (praxis)* is a social phenomenon.
- It is also moral action – for the good of another person in need.
- Uncertainty is normal, understandable, and to be expected in professional practice
- The ends, as well as the means for achieving the ends of professional practice, can never be fully determined in advance.
- Science helps us understand the action of things (largely to discover the rules that govern those actions), social science (which is very different from science) helps us understand human action, which may be governed by rules (often through political intervention), but humans are 'wilful' and can break the rules, often appropriately in particular circumstances. Understanding human action is best achieved by appreciating the nature of those situations when they break the rules rather than when they abide by them. That is also true when trying to understand how professionals deal with uncertainty.
- Professional *praxis* inevitably and necessarily involves rule breaking – professionalism begins when the rules no longer apply. Professional action where rules do apply (and there are some) is more akin to technical action (*poiesis*) than to *praxis* and requires *techne* (technical knowledge) rather than *phronesis* (practical wisdom).

Judgement

- Professionals break – or at least go beyond – the rules when they exercise judgement.
- There are several kinds of judgement that professionals make. One in particular ('deliberative judgement') involves moral action. This is the basis of professional *praxis*.

(continued)

Box 3.1 (continued)

- Since professional practice is a social phenomenon, professional judgement is most frequently a collective act – even when the practitioner is unaware of the influences on his or her judgements in a particular situation.
- Professionals cannot always explain the basis' on which they make some judgements.
- Because professional judgements are made in uncertain situations, some can turn out (in retrospect) to have been inappropriate or even wrong. That is a risk not so much for the professional but for society. This can cause difficulties both for – and misunderstandings between – professionals and society
- Since society can expect (and some politicians may demand) that professionals be 'accountable for' their actions, professionals themselves would do well to become more able explicitly to give a fuller 'account of' their judgements and why and how they make them.
- That is the educational challenge that professionals (and professional educators) face – how to help professional practitioners understand, appreciate, and articulate the nature of the judgements they have to make.

Types of Judgement

Professionals, then, make judgements which are not all the same. They vary with the context (Regehr 2006) in which those judgements are being made (Habermas 1972; Grundy 1987; Tripp 1993). At least four kinds of judgement have been identified (Fish and Coles 1998: 280–281):

Naive judgement. This arises when practitioners in a situation of uncertainty ask what they 'should' do next, that is by assuming that there is a single answer, which just needs to be found. This suggests that the practitioner may be aware that someone, somewhere, has said what should happen in such a situation, and this is the source of the solution to their problem. It is the question asked by the neophyte – the beginner: "I have a problem. What is the answer? Where can I find it? Who can tell me?"

Strategic judgement. This arises when practitioners ask what they 'might' do next. This suggests that these practitioners recognise that they have some choices but from a limited range of possibilities – not necessarily one right answer – and perhaps choices that have been assigned to them by others, perhaps as a published protocol or set of guidelines. Here, as with naive judgements, the practitioner is acting as a technical expert. Neither naive nor strategic judgements need be made by an experienced professional practitioner, but they are frequently made by artisans and technicians and by professionals developing their practice.

Reflective judgement. This arises when practitioners ask what they 'could' do next. This suggests that they recognise the complexity and uncertainty of the situation they are in and know what the options are – possibly recalling previous judgements they made in similar circumstances, though perhaps not fully recognising that all situations are different whatever the similarities may be. Here, the practitioner is a thinking (reflective) practitioner rather than a technician, aware perhaps of the theory (principles) underpinning the various choices available.

Deliberative judgement. This arises when practitioners ask what they 'ought' to do next. This is an ethical question and leads to a moral judgement. It involves professionals in deliberative reasoning, that is by going beyond not just the reflective thinking about their practice – as in 3 above – but by focusing on 'the problematic and contestable issues endemic to practising as a professional' (Fish and Coles 1998: 68). This involves 'meta' thinking. In taking this course of action, the practitioner is making meaning of both their practice and (importantly) the principles underpinning it, in relation to their own moral code and the system of values and the traditions of their practice. Perhaps more importantly for us here, they are going beyond the immediate situation to capture the more general learning to be gained from it in order to develop their practice further. Crucially, the practitioner is self-aware whilst making such a decision. He or she is exercising judgement; there is reflexivity here. Arguably, this is the only judgement of these four that is truly 'professional'.

Some writers argue that these four kinds of judgement are aligned in a developmental sequence – from novice to expert (Benner 1984; Dreyfus and Dreyfus 1985), as the professional's questions range from 'should' and 'might' through 'could' to 'ought'. The suggestion is that novices begin by using naive judgement, then proceed through experience to strategic and reflective judgement, and finally (though perhaps not inevitably) to deliberative judgement. This then raises the question as to how judgement is learnt, or possibly acquired, and to the broader question concerning how professionals learn to practise more generally and to deal with uncertainty more specifically.

Learning to Practise

Since practice is as we have seen a social phenomenon, professionals largely acquire the traditions of their practice through membership of their practice community, that is, when they belong to what is termed a 'community of practice' (Lave and Wenger 1991; Parboosingh 2002; Regehr and Mylopoulos 2008; Rushmer et al. 2004; Wenger 1999). However, professionals do not learn to practise unthinkingly through some kind of osmotic process, since, as a direct and natural consequence of being members of a community of practice, they engage in professional conversations with their colleagues within those communities:

> The practical knowledge made available through tradition is not mechanically or passively reproduced: it is constantly being reinterpreted and revised through dialogue and discussion about how to pursue the practical goods which constitute that tradition. *It is precisely because it embodies this process of critical reconstruction that a tradition evolves and changes rather than remains static or fixed.* (Carr 1995: 69 – author's emphasis)

This suggests that professionals learn from experience, but as with all human action, it is rather more complicated than that!

From some of the available evidence, it is clear that – certainly in the United Kingdom at least – the practice of experienced physicians is more 'economical' than that of less experienced physicians, for example, in terms of them requesting fewer follow-up appointments and completing more clinical episodes (Lota et al. 2011). But it is also clear that clinical error is more common in older physicians. In the UK, this has been shown particularly in general practice (see Wakeford 2011), and in the US, both in primary care and hospital medicine (see Choudhry et al. 2005). This is a finding that has proved controversial – to say the least! – within the medical community (Responses to Choudhry 2005). This suggests that acquiring experience and growing older are somewhat independent variables, and so the popular adage that 'wisdom comes with experience' is not always the case. Perhaps it is truer to say that the relationship between being wise and becoming older is a complex one.

How then is professional judgement – and its underpinning practical wisdom – developed? More particularly, what contribution can the study of education make to this debate?

Experienced educators are of course well aware that teaching is a complex and unpredictable matter, and in that regard, it shares many of the problems of uncertainty found in medical practice. Educators know, however, that there are options and that they have choices they can make. As we saw earlier, 'flexible purposing' in educational practice is essential – the relentless pursuit of some pre-planned educational objectives is at the very least unwise and may possibly result in miseducation (Pring 2000).

The seminal work of the UK educationist Lawrence Stenhouse (1975) identified three key educational options that are open to all experienced educators. Educators utilise these as and when appropriate, often without noticing, and almost certainly in most instances without them recognising that they are adopting educational theory. To Stenhouse's three options, I have added a fourth, reflecting more recent educational thinking, as shown in Table 3.1.

1. *Product option.* The term 'product' is used here to characterise education as a technical or mechanical act involving transmission of some knowledge and/or skill, and education of this kind is frequently described as delivery (Pring 2000: 24–26). Such an approach is best described as training, not least as the practitioners are acting largely technically, which, as noted earlier, Aristotle called *poiesis* requiring *techne*. The ends of such teaching (with its precise definition in advance of what are sometimes called learning objectives) are clear before the teaching begins, as are the means (the teaching methods, which are often formal) for achieving them. In this sense, training is indicated when some highly specific learning outcome is required, compared with education where the outcome is more open. Typically, when adopting the product option, the teacher is active, the learners largely passive, and lectures and demonstrations are the educational methods of choice. For some less expert educators, this is the default (possibly the only) form of education that they recognise – teaching is telling.

The literature on continuing medical education based on this option, however, is quite challenging in terms of its effects on changed clinical practice. The seminal work of Davis and his colleagues has consistently shown that what is sometimes called formal teaching has quite limited outcomes (Davis et al. 1995, 1999).

Table 3.1 Four contrasting educational options

	Product	Process	Research	In practice
Descriptive terms	Intentional/planned: linear	Intentional/planned: non-linear	Intentional: systematic enquiry	Non-formal/unplanned: natural
Educational method	Lecture	Small group work	Undertaking enquiries	Non-formal learning in situ
Who is involved?	Teachers often formally teaching passive learners about practice	Facilitators helping active/engaged learners (often in groups) to understand and develop their practice	Supervisor (critical friend or mentor) enabling usually individual learner to understand and develop his/her own practice	Learners learn with colleagues naturally in and through professional conversations in and about their everyday practice
What is the focus?	Specific skills and/or knowledge for specific circumstances	Exploration of uncertainty through case study, often with some formal (theory) input	Learners explore practical and theoretical issues within their own practice	Practitioners discuss with their colleagues issues/concerns regarding their own practice
Where/how does this take place?	Lecture room, lecture/demonstration	Seminar/coffee room, group work, some plenary input	Study, office, library, one to one	Workplace, coffee/lunch rooms, telephone, internet
Output (e.g. artefacts of learning)	Lecture notes (possibly further reading)	Written notes, case reports, (possibly further reading)	Case notes, related reading, (possibly published articles)	Often none, (possibly diary, notes)
Outcome (e.g. changed practice)	Variable (possibly none)	Increased understanding and insight, possibly changed practice	Increased understanding and insight, possibly changed practice	Changed practice, issues resolved or more fully understood, concerns shared
Support/resources required	Teaching facilities, teacher remuneration (or commitment), practitioner time out of practice	Facilitator remuneration (or commitment), facilities, practitioner time out of practice	Supervisor remuneration (or commitment), facilities, practitioner time out of practice	Learning culture, community of practice, valuing non-formal learning by all concerned (including managers) as part of everyday professional practice

Nevertheless, the product option is adopted especially in those situations where the actions of professionals can be determined in advance, need to be predictable, and above all must be clearly understood by others acting in the same circumstances. Examples of this in clinical practice are trauma management and resuscitation, where it is vital that health care practitioners act in unison and know what others are doing and why. Often, speed is of the essence, and quick decisions are necessary. Training is thought to work in such situations.

Even here, though, there may be uncertainty. Trauma care often involves triage and hence the need for wise clinical judgement, and it may not always go to plan, suggesting the need in such situations to adopt alternative strategies, possibly requiring 'flexible purposing'. Some resuscitation teams have reported (Hunter and Finney 2012: 37) what they call 'taking time out' at moments when their clinical interventions appear to be failing, where 'the whole team introduced themselves and focus was achieved in a moment,' suggesting the recreation (and the value), even in the heat of things, of a 'community of practice' (Wenger 1989). Such clinical situations may or may not include 'reflection "in" action' (Schön 1984) by individuals but can involve 'reflection "on" action' by the clinical team after the event, sometimes called debriefing and even 'wash-up'. In such circumstances, practitioners will be adopting, again probably without noticing, the next educational approach – the process option.

2. *Process option.* The term 'process' is used to characterise educational programmes where the learner is a more active participant than in the product option. The process option occurs where the need for 'flexible purposing' is perceived by the educator, that is where the ends of the educational encounter and the means for achieving them may be reasonably clear in advance but where the focus is allowed to be more open. This is typically seen educationally where group work is involved. The educator takes some responsibility for setting up the educational encounter but then acts as a facilitator of the learners' learning. In this way, the educational outcomes that are achieved may be unexpected, even creative, and perhaps different for each participant, though often within some predetermined parameters. In clinical practice, this option can be seen when physicians, possibly from the same practice, meet perhaps regularly, either in their own offices or clinics or on some neutral territory, with each of the participants perhaps presenting 'dilemma' cases from their own clinical practice, by sharing one another's clinical experience, with reviewing relevant literature such as clinically related guidelines, and by drawing implications for practice improvement. Group working is often facilitated either by an external educational expert, through leadership from a group member, or by rotating facilitation among the participants (Sommers et al. 2007).

The process option demonstrates clearly the huge value of group working when discussing the difficulties professionals experience in dealing with the uncertainties in their clinical practice. As such, it is within the long and greatly respected tradition of the work of Michael Balint (1890–1970 – see, e.g. Balint 1957). A strong feature here is that colleagues who meet together in their own location may develop a 'community of practice' (Wenger 1998) or, as some describe it, 'a learning organisation' (Davies and Nutley 2000; Isba and Boor 2011). Teaching, when seen as 'facilitation', suggests guidance rather than direction and a focus on managing the educational process rather than something being delivered by a subject expert. In clinical practice, group discussion is often very intentionally 'patient focused', and the method adopted frequently is called 'reflective practice' (Mann et al. 2009), an educational approach which was identified in North America in the early part of the twentieth century by John Dewey (1916) and developed in more recent times by Donald Schön in his seminal work on 'the reflective practitioner' (1984, 1987).

The major limitations of the process option largely concern the time needed for participation – often requiring participants to take time out of their clinical work – and in maintaining the motivation and commitment of the participants – such as regular attendance at meetings. In addition, the quality of facilitation is likely to vary, and facilitator motivation and commitment, and possibly remuneration, may also be issues. In addition, there may or may not be any discernible output (e.g. in terms of any written records kept by participants or 'personal development plans') nor any formal input (e.g. the presentation of theoretical constructs that might be considered relevant such as the nature of practice, professional judgement, and practical wisdom). Similarly, process-based initiatives are often less concerned with the degree to which participants' clinical practice actually changes, or any clinical gain for patients noted, in the light of their participation, at least within the relatively short timescales that some groups are able to devote to this kind of work. Changed behaviour can take time.

Nevertheless, participation by a clinician who has never engaged in such discussions may itself be regarded as changed behaviour, and where this involves enhanced understanding of their problems, increased personal esteem, and perhaps improved communication with their professional colleagues, this can be the precursor for changed clinical practice which has been associated with improved clinical gain (Lanham et al. 2009; Leykum et al. 2011).

3. *Research option*. Whilst the term 'research' may conjure up notions of scientific experimentation, it is used here more generally to mean 'any systematic, critical, and self-critical enquiry which aims to contribute to the advancement of knowledge' (Pring 2000: 7). In helping practitioners to understand their practice more fully – and hence further develop their practice by engaging in some form of enquiry into that practice (Fish and Twinn 1997) – it is the advancement of the practitioner's 'own' knowledge that such an enquiry contributes towards, and is sometimes called, 'insider practitioner research' (Fish and Coles 1998: 308–313). This option is often used more on a one-to-one basis with the teacher, acting as a supervisor, mentor, or 'critical friend' (Driessen et al. 2011) who is enabling the learner (who might be a colleague or student) to explore his or her own understanding of a relevant topic or some aspect of their practice.

An example taken from Fish and Coles' book *Developing Professional Judgement* (1998: 126–138) demonstrates this. There, a palliative care physician reflects on a difficult case of a patient who recently died, where he felt greatly troubled because of a conversation with the patient's GP, during which he had offered some specialist advice in this particular case, which the GP appeared to resent. Through his reflection, the palliative care physician came to recognise that whilst it was, in his words, relatively easy to be generous to one's patients and relatives, it was more difficult in some situations to be generous to one's colleagues, and he wistfully added, even more difficult to be generous to oneself. In conclusion, he recognised the importance of inter-professional generosity, and this reflection prompted him to change his unit's practice so as to engage GPs much more fully in clinical collaboration by instituting combined educational sessions with them regarding difficult-to-resolve cases. This example shows not just that the palliative care physician changed his practice but that, in doing so, this changed clinical practice much more widely.

Another example from the same source shows how a review of a critical incident can lead to development of professional practice even more generally through the practitioner's reference to related literature. Rosemary Richardson (in Fish and Coles 1998: 77–125), for example, concludes that her engagement in researching her own practice:

> ...has reinforced my belief (my personal theory) that we should...encourage students to discuss and to write about practice issues which then lead [them] to the exploration of relevant theory-in-the-literature. (1998: 97)

Similar examples of this are seen in the work of de Cossart and Fish (2005) and Fish and de Cossart (2008).

Whilst the research approach is similar to the process option described above, there are some significant differences. Reflection (which is the basis of the process option) can be limited to 'the critical consideration of one's practice and one's thinking during it' (Fish and Coles 1998: 68). It is important to recognise, then, that the educational focus of the research option involves practitioners 'researching' (not simply reflecting on) their practice. Here, the emphasis is on deliberation, which is 'another term for practical reasoning...[used specifically] to focus on the problematic and contestable issues endemic to practising as a professional' (Fish and Coles 1998: 68). The research option, then, takes the practitioner further and deeper into understanding their practice than the process option.

The research option also differs from the process option as it 'intentionally' involves input from the literature on professional practice generally and output in terms of written records of the practitioners' deliberations (for further examples of reflective writing, see Fish and de Cossart 2007). In this regard, the research option is largely consistent with the related literature:

> ...learning is driven by needs and is characterised by a dynamic and emergent personal learning plan with explicit goals, protected time for reflection and study, mentoring or peer support, and perhaps a written learning log or record of achievement. (Fraser and Greenhalgh 2001: 802)

In addition, the research option most often engages the practitioner in writing an account of their deliberations. In this way, practitioners becoming involved with researching their practice are likely to be more engaged than those involved with either the product or the process option. They probably come to this work more conscious of what is involved and what might come from it.

Nevertheless, as with the process option, perhaps the greatest constraint of the research option is the time involved, which medical practitioners must take either from their clinical work or their personal lives. Similarly too, it requires commitment by participants to reading new material, often of an academic nature, and more particularly engaging in narrative writing (Greenhalgh and Hurwitz 1998) which is very different from the scientific writing with which many clinicians are perhaps more familiar and which some clinicians find difficult to undertake. Also, questions concerning practice change and clinical gain are often not fully answered.

There is, though, a larger and perhaps more significant concern about educational programmes based on the process and even the research approach: They often involve participants who engage in them voluntarily, and the effectiveness of these programmes is almost entirely dependent on learners assessing (and being aware of) their own learning needs, often referred to as 'self-assessment', the cognitive model behind which has been strongly challenged (Regehr and Eva 2006).

Developing this further, Regehr and Mylopoulos (2008: 19) argue that much continuing medical education is based on four highly questionable assumptions: that professionals naturally reflect on their performance for the purposes of highlighting their own weakness or gaps, that professionals self-assess their own weakness when they do try to look for them, that professionals try to redress weaknesses through learning when they do identify them, and that professionals effectively incorporate knowledge acquired in educational settings into practice.

Regehr and Mylopoulos conclude that the continuing medical education community needs to shift its perspective from a focus on what might be called 'intentional' educational activities to a focus on understanding:

> …how professional learning not only arises from practice, but actually occurs *in practice* and is informed by practice…by focusing research efforts on further understanding and developing this form of learning *in practice*. (2008: 22 author's emphasis)

Their conclusions rehearse many of Davis' groups' earlier findings (Davis et al. 1995, 1999) that changes in health professionals' practice that are associated with improved health care are more likely to result from informal (unintentional) rather than formal (intentional) educational activities. It is this shift of focus away from 'intentional' education to understanding learning in practice that underpins the fourth option.

4. *In-practice option.* This option is not so much adopted; it simply happens *in situ* (Fleming 2011). The rationale is this: All human action is based on some form of learning. Watching a child at play reveals quite dramatically the learning that is occurring. Any 'interventions', for example when a parent offers some help, perhaps by showing the child 'what to do' or even by simply reading the child a story, can be thought of as a form of 'teaching' (facilitated learning), which might have occurred in this example because the parent noticed (assessed) that the child was encountering some difficulty or chose (made the judgement) to read a story at a level that the parent recognised (perhaps 'unconsciously') to be appropriate to the child's development and interest.

Put in educational terms, this everyday example reveals that the teacher (parent) had assessed (come to a view of) the progress or level of the learner (child) and chosen how to proceed for the good of the learner. As such, in this example, teaching, learning, and assessment were all present – but they happened quite naturally, without any of those present realising (and almost certainly without them recognising) that education was occurring or that educational options were being chosen. Nothing educational was happening intentionally.

Doctors' learning too is very much embedded in their everyday clinical work with their 'most relevant learning activities related to patient care rather than motivated by competence improvement goals' (van de Wiel et al. 2011: 81). They learn most from the patient cases they encounter through often informal discussion with colleagues about dilemmas they have concerning how to deal most effectively with difficult cases. Uncertainty is dealt with naturally in and through normal everyday communicative encounters between practitioners.

This is entirely consistent with the theoretical principles I presented earlier about how professional practice develops with the 'critical reconstruction of practice', involving 'dialogue and discussion' (Carr 1995: 69) within 'communities of practice' (Wenger 1999), and reflects the seminal work of Michael Eraut in the UK on what he calls 'non-formal learning in the workplace', which has consistently shown that doctors' learning is largely 'implicit and reactive' (Eraut 2000, 2004, 2007).

Doctors, then, appear to acquire the capacity to practise medicine largely through 'situated learning' (Lave and Wenger 1991). Such learning is relevant and timely in that it happens as and when it is required and most urgently needed. Eraut further suggests (2007: 419) that the quantity and quality of such learning can be enhanced by increasing opportunities for consulting with and working alongside others in teams or temporary groups and adds:

> Managers have a major influence on workplace learning and culture that extends far beyond their job descriptions. Their role is to develop a culture of mutual support and learning, not to provide all the support themselves. They need to share this role with experienced workers, and this implies some form of distributed leadership. This role should be given much greater priority in management development programmes, incorporated into qualifications for managers and supervisors, and included in the appraisal of all managers. (Eraut 2007: 420)

In-practice learning, then, depends on there being appropriate opportunities for learning in the workplace, particularly in the 'busyness' of clinical practice, where clinical need understandably most often trumps educational need.

Perhaps, also, a limiting factor of in-practice learning concerns the mindset of the learner, which experienced educators know only too well can be variable, by encouraging learners to pursue the educational potential in every working moment. There may be need here for educating the learner in some way if non-formal learning is to be universally effective.

Clearly, too, it depends on what we might call the educational culture of the practice setting. In this regard, a study by Coles and Mountford (1999) found that trainee doctors' clinical placements in hospitals were most highly rated when those placements were characterised by them as having three features: 'community' (a sense of belonging), 'collegiality' (being seen as a colleague), and 'criticality' (being able to discuss openly and honestly the practice they were observing and engaging in). It was clear that these characteristics were established and maintained by key people within those placements, not least in terms of the values they held regarding the importance of education and the contribution that trainee doctors could make to the clinical load. Moreover, highly rated clinical placements were also perceived by trainees to offer the highest quality clinical care to patients. Similar observations have been made in the primary care setting (see, e.g. Lanham et al. 2009; Leykum et al. 2011; Frankford et al. 2000; Parboosingh 2002; and Rushmer et al. 2003).

It is clear from this that the prevailing culture within the practice setting and the interpersonal relationships between the staff (Knaus et al. 1986; Lanham et al. 2009) may well be a crucial factor in determining whether or not learning occurs naturally in the workplace and whether health care is improved. This culture may well be determined as much by managers and administrators – and maybe politicians and policy makers (see Tomlinson 2005) – as by the clinical professionals more directly involved.

Since learning in practice is non-formal, it is unlikely that practitioners will record the learning that is occurring – and indeed, it may be unnatural to expect or even to ask them to do so, as this might break the continuity of their clinical practice and even distort their perception of what they are learning. This is particularly so where the knowledge involved is 'tacit' (Polanyi 1966) and as such not recoverable:

> Although expert diagnosticians…can indicate their clues and formulate their maxims, they know many more things than they can tell, knowing them only in practice, as instrumental particulars, and not explicitly, as objects. The knowledge of such particulars is therefore ineffable, and the pondering of a judgement in terms of such particulars is an ineffable process of thought. (Polanyi 1962: 88)

Whilst some kind of output regarding learning may be welcomed, or even required, by regulatory authorities as a record that some form of learning activity has been engaged in, particularly where this record (or some summary of it) is submitted for accreditation or revalidation, it is at present unclear that to do this represents educational progress (Driessen et al. 2011). Educators frequently believe that it is more important to evaluate the quality of some educational action by considering not the amount that is learnt but how much it helps learners to make sense of things, to understand matters further, or to give a clearer and more fruitful way of conceiving the problem and its possible solutions. Does it, for example, lead the learners to ask further questions, to open further lines of enquiry, to engage more fruitfully with the experience confronting them? (Pring 2000: 13). Moreover, such important educational outcomes may not become evident in the short term. At what point does one evaluate whether important learning has occurred? At the end of the session, which may be far too soon? A week later, which may also be too early? Or ten years later, by which time it may well have happened, but when and by what other means? Cause and effect – in this case, some high-quality teaching that leads to some related learning – is never straightforward in education. Even those who regulate professionals may not fully appreciate the complexities of what professional practice actually entails and how becoming a professional practitioner can best be achieved educationally or within what timescale.

Conclusions: Towards a Policy for Educating for Uncertainty

In the previous section, I argued that educators involved in helping clinicians deal with uncertainty have options. They are in a position to choose to focus their efforts in a particular way – most probably determined more by their values than their understanding of any educational theory, whether as intentional educational activity or by supporting non-formal learning in practice.

An implication here could be seen as being that there is a right (and hence wrong) way of going about this. Nothing could be further from the truth. The four options I have discussed are not independent of one another. There is no either/or here. Educators mix and match their options, as do clinicians of course. Whilst an educational programme might be underpinned by the process option, a need might arise for some formal input (utilising the product option) or participants might explore their reflections further by undertaking some insider practitioner research utilising the research option. Educators – both those who formulate educational activities and those who participate in them – make judgements about which option to choose in particular circumstances. Table 3.1 shows the range of options open to the educator. It does not show how to choose between them in uncertain educational situations. That requires educational practical wisdom, which needs to be developed (see Box 3.2).

Box 3.2 Educating for Uncertainty

Educational Options

- Product: education as something that can be 'delivered'
- Process: the learner is an active participant in a process managed by the teacher
- Research: any systematic, critical, and self-critical enquiry which aims to contribute to the advancement of the practitioner's knowledge
- In-practice: the education that happens naturally and unintentionally in and through the practitioner's practice

Learning to Practise

- Occurs through both intentional and natural educational actions.
- Education may or may not bring about desired effects.
- Educators involved in this may need to choose alternative actions.
- In doing so, they exercise professional educational judgements.
- These are underpinned by 'practical wisdom'.
- This is acquired in the same ways as with clinicians.

(continued)

Box 3.2 (continued)

Educating the Educators

- This is essential if education for uncertainty is to be effective.
- It fundamentally concerns helping educators develop their professional educational judgement.
- This occurs through an appreciation by all concerned of the educational options open to the people engaged in educating educators.

An Iteration of Educational Action

- Understand what helps in-practice learning to work (and not work)
- Identify practitioners' development needs in and through their practice
- Identify ways in which 'intentional' educational actions can support those developmental needs
- Facilitate the translation of what is learnt 'intentionally' into people's practice
- Continue to support this iteration

The effectiveness of educational activities (not least in helping doctors cope with the uncertainties of their clinical practice) depends, then, on the effectiveness of the professional judgements made by the educators involved – on the wisdom behind the options they choose. And this is dependent on the development of those educators' professional judgements. As Stenhouse wisely put it:

> there can be no educational development without [educator] development. (1975: 73)

The development of educators' professional judgements is predicated on precisely the same issues as those involved in the development of medical practitioners' clinical judgements (Fish and Coles 1998). Fundamentally, this will require educators to deliberate on their practice and is best brought about through an appreciation of the contributions made by the educational options shown in Table 3.1 and described above, whilst recognising that no one option will bring about this development, only some appropriate combination.

Finally, is there some way of establishing a robust and evidential policy for the continuing education of practitioners regarding the uncertainties of their practice? Regehr and Mylopoulos conclude that:

> by understanding and accepting the limits of human abilities and propensities to self-identify and redress areas of weakness, we may be able to reposition and effectively improve the value of formal [that is 'intentional'] continuing education activities. (2008: 19)

Eraut similarly argues that formal learning 'contributes most when it is both relevant and well-timed, [but] still needs further workplace learning before it can be used to best effect'. (2007: 419)

Both of these contributions to the debate suggest a clear relationship between in-practice (that is naturally occurring) and intentional (that is planned) educational activities in the education of clinicians regarding helping and enabling them to deal with the uncertainties in their practice. So how might this happen? Some kind of iteration between in-practice and intentional educational action appears indicated, perhaps as follows:

First, it would be best initially to focus on the non-formal learning that, inevitably, is occurring in the everyday setting of clinical practice. Understanding how this happens naturally and what factors are associated with its effectiveness (and those that constrain it) is a useful starting point. Then, in-practice learning needs to be developed and enhanced. Through this, practitioners ought to be able to identify areas for their further development. Hopefully, though by no means inevitably, this identification will be through self-assessment of practitioners regarding their own practice resulting from their everyday interactions with their colleagues, though on occasions, it may be through others coming to a view of practitioners' needing some development.

Through identifying development needs by understanding more fully the contribution and constraints of in-practice learning, forms of intentional educational activities can then be introduced specifically to target those identified needs in the ways that the work of both Regehr and Mylopoulos and of Eraut suggests above. Clearly from the evidence presented earlier, time within practitioners' everyday practice must be made available for this intentional development to occur, and this is a managerial matter. Those who oversee workforce decisions and the configuration of clinical services have to value professional development and the need for protected time for this to occur. The nature of the educational activities themselves needs to relate (and be relevant) to the developmental needs of the practitioners participating in these events, and (from the evidence presented in the literature) needs to focus on clinical practice by practitioners not just reflecting on 'the thinking that got us into this fix' (Schön 1987:28), but 'to focus on the problematic and contestable issues endemic to practising as a professional' (Fish and Coles 1998: 68).

This, though exemplary, is not enough in itself. Eraut reminds us that what he calls formal learning 'still needs further workplace learning before it can be used to best effect' (2007: 419). As Stenhouse puts it, learning must be 'translated into practice' (1975:4). Note here the word 'translated'. Stenhouse did not say that knowledge acquired in one setting (formal education) is to be 'applied to' practice; rather that it is to be 'translated into practice'. The word 'translated' is significant here. Knowledge and knowing, like practice and practising, are essentially contextual (Regehr 2006).

And the development of professional practice does not end even there. This iterative process between in-practice and 'intentional' education is, and must continue to be, ongoing and never ending. It must be valued and supported by all concerned, which means it being acknowledged and resourced. The challenge to both educational and clinical practitioners – as well as to their managers – is to keep the conversation going.

References

Atkinson, T., & Claxton, G. (2000). *The intuitive practitioner*. London: OUP.

Balint, M. (1957). *The doctor, his patient and the illness*. London: Pitman Medical.

Benner, P. (1984). *From novice to expert: Excellence and power in clinical nursing practice*. Menlo Park: Addison-Wesley.

Carr, W. (1995). *For education: Towards critical educational inquiry*. Buckingham: Open University Press.

Choudhry, N. K., Fletcher, R. H., & Soumerai, S. B. (2005). Systematic review: The relationship between clinical experience and quality of health care. *Annals of Internal Medicine, 142*, 260–273.

Coles, C. (2006). Uncertainty in a world of regulation. *Advances in Psychiatric Treatment, 12*, 397–403.

Coles, C., & Mountford, B. (1999). Supporting education in a clinical environment: Report of an enquiry into the characteristics of acclaimed educational units in the Wessex. Winchester: Deanery, Wessex Deanery for Postgraduate Medical and Dental Education.

Davies, H. T., & Nutley, S. M. (2000). Developing learning organisations in the new NHS. *British Medical Journal, 320*, 998–1001.

Davis, D. A., Thomson, M. A., Oxman, A. D., et al. (1995). Changing physician performance: A systematic review of the effect on continuing medical education strategies. *The Journal of the American Medical Association, 274*(9), 700–706.

Davis, D. A., O'Brien, M. A. T., Freemantle, N., et al. (1999). Impact of formal continuing medical education: Do conferences, workshops, rounds, and other traditional continuing medical education activities change physician behaviour or health care outcomes? *The Journal of the American Medical Association, 282*, 867–874.

Dewey, J. (1916). *Democracy and education*. New York: The Free Press.

Dhaliwal, G. (2010). Going with your gut. *Journal of General Internal Medicine, 26*(2), 107–109.

Dreyfus, H., & Dreyfus, S. (1985). *Mind over machine: The power of human intuition and expertise in the era of the computer*. New York: Free Press.

Driessen, E., Overeem, K., & van Tartwijk, J. (2011). Learning from practice: Mentoring, feedback and portfolios. In T. Dornan, K. Mann, A. Scherpbier, & J. Spencer (Eds.), *Medical education: Theory and practice* (pp. 211–227). Edinburgh: Churchill Livingstone.

Eisner, W. (2005). What can education learn from the arts about the practice of education? The Encyclopaedia of informal education. www.infed.org/biblio/einsner-arts-and-the-practice-of-education.htm.

Eraut, M. (2000). Non-formal learning and tacit knowledge in professional work. *The British Journal of Educational Psychology, 70*, 113–136.

Eraut, M. (2004). Informal learning in the workplace. *Studies in Continuing Education, 26*(2), 247–273.

Eraut, M. (2007). Learning from other people in the workplace. *Oxford Review of Education, 33*(4), 403–422.

Fish, D., & Coles, C. (1998). *Developing professional judgement in health care: Learning through the critical appreciation of practice*. London: Butterworth Heinemann.

Fish, D., & de Cossart, L. (2007). *Developing the wise doctor*. London: Royal Society of Medicine.

Fish, D., & Twinn, S. (1997). *Quality clinical supervision: Principled approaches to practice*. London: Butterworth Heinemann.

Frankford, D. M., Patterson, M. A., & Konrad, T. R. (2000). Transforming practice organizations to foster lifelong learning and commitment to medical professionalism. *Academic Medicine, 75*(7), 708–717. July.

Fraser, S. W., & Greenhalgh, T. (2001). Coping with complexity: Educating for capability. *British Medical Journal, 323*, 799–803.

Freidson, E. (1994). *Professionalism reborn: Theory, prophecy and policy*. Cambridge: Polity Press.

Gawande, A. (2002). *Complications: A surgeon's notes on an imperfect science*. London: Profile Books.

Golby, M., & Parrott, A. (1999). *Educational research and educational practice*. Exeter: Fair Way.

Greenhalgh, T., & Hurwitz, B. (Eds.). (1998). *Narrative based medicine*. London: BMJ Books.

Groopman, J. (2007). *How doctors think*. Boston: Houghton Mifflin.

Grundy, S. (1987). *Curriculum: Product or praxis?* Brighton: Falmer Press.

Habermas, J. (1972). *Knowledge and human interest*. London: Heinemann.

Heath, I. (1995). *The mystery of general practice*. London: The Nuffield Provincial Hospitals Trust.

Hunter, D. N., & Finney, S. J. (2012). Follow surgical checklists, especially in a crisis. *British Medical Journal, 343*, 37.

Isba, R., & Boor, K. (2011). Creating a learning environment. In T. Dornan, K. Mann, A. Scherpbier, & J. Spencer (Eds.), *Medical education: Theory and practice* (pp. 99–114). Edinburgh: Churchill Livingstone.

Knaus, W. A., Draper, E. A., Wagner, D. P., et al. (1986). An evaluation of outcome from intensive care in major medical centres. *Annals of Internal Medicine, 104*, 410–418.

Lanham, H., Reuben, R., McDaniel, R., et al. (2009). How improving practice relationships among clinicians and non-clinicians can improve quality in primary care. *Joint Commission on Accreditation of Healthcare Organizations, 35*(9), 457–466.

Lave, J., & Wenger, E. (1991). *Situated learning: Legitimate peripheral participation*. Cambridge: Cambridge University Press.

Leykum, L., Palmer, R., Lanham, H., et al. (2011). Reciprocal learning and chronic care model implementation in primary care: Results from a new scale of learning in primary care. *BMC Health Services Research, 11*, 44.

Lota, A., Sutton, R., & Francis, D. P. (2011). When is a 'free' registrar not free? *British Medical Journal, 343*, 1332–1333.

Mann, K., Gordon, J. J., & KacLeod, A. M. (2009). Reflection and reflective practice in health professions' education: A systematic review of the literature in the health professions. *Advances in Health Sciences Education: Theory and Practice, 14*, 595–621.

Montgomery, K. (2006). *How doctors think: Clinical judgement and the practice of medicine*. Oxford: Oxford University Press.

O'Neil, O. (2002). *A question of trust*. Cambridge: Cambridge University Press.

Parboosingh, J. T. (2002). Physician communities of practice: Where learning and practice are inseparable. *The Journal of Continuing Education in the Health Professions, 22*(4), 230–236. Fall.

Polanyi, M. (1962). *Personal knowledge*. Chicago: The University of Chicago Press.

Polanyi, M. (1966). *The tacit dimension*. London: Routledge/Kegan Paul.

Pring, R. (2000). *Philosophy of educational research*. London: Continuum.

Regehr, G. (2006). The persistent myth of stability: On the chronic underestimation of the role of context in behaviour. *Journal of General Internal Medicine*, 554–5 (editorial).

Regehr, G., & Eva, K. W. (2006). Self-assessment, self-direction, and the self-regulating professional. *Clinical Orthopaedics and Related Research, 449*, 34–38.

Regehr, G., & Mylopoulos, M. (2008). Maintaining competence in the field: Learning about practice, through practice, in practice. *Journal of Continuing Education Health Professions, 28*, 19–23.

Rushmer, R., Kelly, D., Lough, M., et al. (2004). Introducing the learning practice – II. Becoming a learning practice. *Journal of Evaluation in Clinical Practice, 10*(3), 387–398.

Schön, D. A. (1988). Coaching reflective teaching. In P. P. Grimmett & G. L. Erickson (Eds.), *Reflection in teacher education* (pp. 19–29). New York: Teachers College Columbia University.

Schön, D. A. (1984). *The reflective practitioner*. Basic Books, New York.

Schön, D. A. (1987). *Educating the reflective practitioner*. Basic Books, New York.

Sommers, L. S., Morgan, L., Johnson, L., et al. (2007). Practice inquiry: Clinical uncertainty as a focus for small-group learning and practice improvement. *Journal of General Internal Medicine, 22,* 246–252.

Stenhouse, L. (1975). *An introduction to curriculum research and development.* London: Heinemann.

Ten Cate, O. (2006). Trust, competence, and the supervisor's role in postgraduate medical training. *British Medical Journal, 333,* 748–751.

Tomlinson, S. (2005). *Education in a post-welfare society.* Maidenhead: Open University Press.

Tripp, D. (1993). *Critical incidents in teaching: Developing professional judgement.* London/New York: Routledge.

Tyreman, S. (2000). Promoting critical thinking in health care: Phronesis and criticality. *Medicine, Health Care, and Philosophy, 3,* 117–124.

van de Wiel, M. W. J., Van den Bossche, P., Janssen, S., et al. (2011). Exploring deliberate practice in medicine: How do physicians learn in the workplace? *Advances in Health Science Education, 16,* 81–95.

Wakeford, R. (2011). Who gets struck off? *British Medical Journal, 343,* 1325–1327.

Wenger, E. (1999). *Communities of practice: Learning, meaning and identity.* Cambridge: Cambridge University Press.

Part II
The Challenge of Engagement

Chapter 4
Balint Groups and Peer Supervision

Henry Jablonski, Dorte Kjeldmand, and John Salinsky

Introduction

Michael Balint (1896–1970) was a psychoanalyst and psychiatrist from Hungary who worked at the Tavistock Clinic in London from the late 1940s to the 1960s. He was always interested in the work of GPs (his father had been a GP in Budapest), and together with his wife Enid Balint, he started a series of small group seminars for GPs interested in 'the psychological aspect' of their work.

General practice was in a depressed state in the 1950s. With all the developments in high-technology medicine, the hospitals seemed to have taken over all the interesting patients. Meanwhile, the GP was left with large numbers of people with confusing symptoms which did not add up to any diagnosis to be found in the textbooks. Many patients were also depressed or anxious, but psychiatrists seemed unable to help. The GPs who joined the first Balint groups were desperate for advice but surprised by what was on offer. Instead of being told what they should do next, they were invited to explore and to tolerate uncertainty. In particular, the Balints were

H. Jablonski (✉)
President of the International Balint Federation; President of the Swedish Association of Medical psychology (Swedish Society of Medicine), Psychiatrist and psychoanalyst in private practice, Kvarngatan 2, Stockholm 11847, Sweden
e-mail: drhj@jablonski.se

D. Kjeldmand
Department of Public Health and Caring Sciences,
Section for Health Services Research, University of Uppsala, Sweden.

Eksjö Primary Care Center, 57581 Eksjö, Sweden
e-mail: kjeldmand@gmail.com

J. Salinsky
Ellis Practice, The Welford Centre, 113 Chalkhill Road, Wembley HA9 9FX, UK
e-mail: JVSalinsky@aol.com

L.S. Sommers and J. Launer (eds.), *Clinical Uncertainty in Primary Care: The Challenge of Collaborative Engagement*, DOI 10.1007/978-1-4614-6812-7_4,
© Springer Science+Business Media New York 2013

interested in the relationship between doctor and patient; the feelings that doctor and patient developed for each other and the many ways in which these emotions could affect the clinical outcome. This work was described in Michael Balint's very influential book, *The Doctor, His Patient and the Illness* (Balint 1957).

Today, Balint groups are available for medical students, postgraduate trainees in general practice and psychiatry and occasionally in other specialties, and for established GPs. The basic principles and the format remain much the same as in Balint's day. Group members are invited to present patients who are causing them concern or uncertainty. These presentations are given without notes and often on the spur of the moment without preparation. They are listened to without interruption. The group leader will then invite everyone to discuss the story they have heard. In some groups, the leader will ask for questions of fact to be disposed of first, after which the presenting doctor pushes her chair back few centimetres and listens, without taking part, for 15 or 20 minutes, before rejoining the discussion. In other groups, the presenting doctor contributes throughout, but the leader tries to protect her from too much interrogation. The idea is for the other group members to reflect on what they have heard, and the feelings that the story has evoked in themselves. The advantage of having the presenter sit back for a while is that the other group members can no longer ask her questions and have to use their own ideas and imagination. However, those group leaders who have not adopted this style feel that the presenter's temporary absence from the group impairs the development of the 'parallel process' in which the presenter mirrors the patient and the group reflects the doctor's reaction.

The leader may contribute from time to keep the discussion focused on the particular doctor and patient rather than going off into generalisations (such as 'these patients are best referred for cognitive therapy'). He may offer occasional insights of his own, but on the whole, he keeps these to himself, encouraging the group members to do the work. The session may end inconclusively; uncertainty is explored but not banished. The group is concerned more with 'what is going on' than with looking for a solution. The presenting doctor will go on thinking about the patient and the discussion, and the next consultation will usually be different as a result.

The Balint Group in Action: Four Examples

The following brief examples show Balint groups at work in different circumstances. All are based on real discussions but fictionalised for anonymity.

The Group Begins

Four out the eight group members announce that they would like to present a case, a couple of them adding 'It is not urgent, it can wait', another one sighing, 'All my surgery today has been a bloody case'.

Leader: (inquiring about the urgency of each case, including checking with those who have a case but say it can wait till next time, and considering when was the last time the prospect presenters had the opportunity) 'OK, so I think Jonathan will start, then Leila and if there is time, Holly, and if not, your case will be on next meeting's agenda, if you still wish. Is that all right? Please, Jonathan.'

Jonathan: 'I really do not know where to start, this will be a bit confused...I saw this patient two days ago, and I really cannot get him out of my mind. Hmm, where to start?'

Leader: 'That is all right, just tell us the story as it comes to you now. If we need clarifications we'll ask you later.'

The leader and group members wait and listen attentively while Jonathan presents. Sometimes, the presenter will end up formulating the problem he/she is facing; more rarely the presenter will declare, 'I am completely at loss.'

Jonathan has finished. The leader now invites questions from the group *but on factual matters only*. For example, was this the first consultation? How old did you say he was? Is he at work now? Did he see any other doctor prior to consulting with you? If it is a newly started group, almost certainly an eager group member will ask the presenter a question like, 'Did you have the feeling this patient was pushing you?' or 'did you consider an autoimmune disease as a cause of his muscular pains?' If that happens, the group leader will intervene: 'That is a very interesting question. I think we should keep it in mind for the discussion to come. But, for now, if there are no more factual questions about this case, why don't you sit back, Jonathan, and have a rest from talking. Just listen and let the group do the work on your case. We'll invite you back in a while.' And, turning to the others he says, 'So what are our thoughts on this case?'

The group reflects and speculates on the case from many angles: the patient's agenda, his medical record and his life; diagnostic considerations; the doctor's reactions and management; the thoughts and emotions arising in group members as they listened to the case being presented etc. At times, group members identify with the patient, at times with their colleague; at times they draw parallels from their own personal and professional perspective. In some aspects, the group reaches a consensus; in others, their views on the case are quite divergent. The group leader may be silent or pick up on some of these consensuses or divergences or ask some of the group members whose viewpoints are undisclosed or are half-spoken to elaborate a little more, or he may point out that a certain issue has been allowed to die or, in his view, seems entirely missing.

Jonathan, after a while, is invited to join the discussion: 'Well, thank you, I actually had, during the consultation, the same thought as you, Alice, and you, Peter, but it got lost, so I will have to check on it next time. Now, what you pointed out, Sol, never occurred to me, but it strikes me as very relevant. I just wonder how it would be possible to bring this up with my patient.'

Leader: "So would you like us to have a go for a few minutes at considering how to do this?"

Jonathan: "Yes, that would be interesting!"

Leader: "Move back again, and we shall see!"

There is a renewed group discussion after which Jonathan is invited back again.

Jonathan: 'Hmm, interesting that you have so many different approaches. I need to think about how to deal with it. I don't think I can be as confronting as you, Sol, but I definitely feel I cannot let this matter slip away if I am going to remain this patient's GP. Now I see things more clearly. I'll think about it. Maybe I'll see a way that I feel is me. If not I'll probably play it by ear at the next consultation. Thanks a lot for your comments.'

Leader: 'And thank you. OK, Leila, now it's you. Please.'

A Group for GP Trainees

Sarah, the presenting doctor, told her group about an encounter which had upset her and made her feel uneasy about her performance. The patient was a woman of 44 with a history of facial acne. She wanted a repeat of her antibiotic which she had been taking for 5 years to prevent the spots coming back. There was no trace of acne on her face. Sarah had been reluctant to prescribe because the acne was cured and there seemed no need. She also warned the patient about the possible adverse effects of continuing the treatment indefinitely. The patient was insistent. The doctor persisted in trying to convince her. The patient said, 'Have you ever had skin problems on your face?' The doctor told the group that she had had acne as a teenager, but her skin was now clear. She had not wanted to disclose her personal experience.

The consultation turned into a battle. The doctor refused to prescribe. The patient left angrily. The doctor felt that her youth, female gender (and unblemished skin) had made the patient all the more angry (and envious?) Would an older male doctor have got on better, she wondered?

The group approved of Sarah's clinical correctness and her firm stand. At the same time, they felt uneasy about the patient. Would she see another doctor and get the antibiotic? Why was it so important to her? Why this dread of acne returning? It was St Valentine's Day. Did she want to look her best for her husband (or someone else)? The group leader encouraged them to explore their own feelings as doctors and imagine what the patient might have been going through. It proved difficult to feel any empathy for the patient. But Sarah, the doctor, said that she felt much better after the discussion. She was very curious about whether the patient would make another attempt to get her prescription, perhaps from another doctor in the practice.

An Experienced Physician and an Unexplained Pain

The presenting doctor is a middle-aged, experienced internist who became a GP specialist after several years at the medical department of a city hospital. He has worked as a GP for about 5 years. He reports on a male middle-aged single patient: an engineer who comes frequently complaining about a great variety of symptoms. He has been to quite a few doctors and is very concerned. He has been on a wide range of medication for many years; he has hypertension which seems a bit volatile but not severe. Does it really require medication? Anyway, the effects of his medication are difficult to establish. It is unclear if he is actually taking the drugs as prescribed. But when his medicines are reviewed, he gets apprehensive and reluctant at the thought of discontinuing any of them or even reducing the dose. The presenter read out the long list of drugs to the group. He perceives his patient as demanding and anxious. But he feels sympathy for this man, who is apparently struggling on with his life in spite of his discomforts. It seems that he carries on with his work conscientiously and he is very rarely on the sick list. He has been referred for many tests and examinations by previous doctors, but the presenter can sense there has been something erratic, a bit desperate about the handling of this patient. Our doctor has taken great care to go through his previous medical history and present complaints. He feels exhausted: he has done everything possible to clarify the problem and rule out anything dangerous, but the patient keeps complaining. For the past 6 months, the main issue has been stomach pains. And that is really strange because he has investigated him so carefully and everything seems normal.

The group discussion covers a wide range including medical concerns, the personality and medical history of this patient, his anxieties, his life and work situation, what he is doing to the doctor and what his relations to previous doctors might have been. Appreciative comments are expressed on how well the doctor is caring for his patient. The group tries to define the boundaries of the doctor-patient relationship. Can the patient feel reasonable held by the contact with his doctor and at the GP centre and feel reasonably cared for? Or will he run to the emergency room? Or consult with other specialists?

The presenting doctor appreciates the comments, recognises this is a difficult case and that he will have to work out some kind of deal with his patient lest he be suffocated by him. 'But,' he adds, 'There is something strange about his stomach symptoms. They are not like his ordinary poly-symptomatic complaints, which I think I managed to calm him down about. But I checked him so carefully. It's strange.' There is a long silence. Finally, a member says: 'Could his somewhat outdated and odd anti-hypertensive medication hydralazine have anything to do with it? It seems really odd that he is still on it. But I suppose the patient has kept his doctors busy with other matters.' The presenting doctor is stunned. As an experienced internist, how could he have avoided thinking about that as a possibility? The group and the presenter agree that the doctor-patient interaction has partially clouded the doctor's mind. The other colleagues feel that they would have functioned on a far lower level in the face of such a massive anxious onslaught from this lonely patient. After all, he seems more at ease now. They all express sincere respect for the doctor's persistence in being concerned with the stomach pains as something alien from the other/obsessive symptoms that the patient is presenting.

A Well-Established Group and a Long-Established Patient

This group of established GPs had been meeting with the same leader for 4 years. Dr B presented Gloria, a woman of 60 who had been his patient for 30 years. She had always been emotionally volatile, usually friendly and ingratiating but sometimes flying into rages when she felt she had been snubbed or ignored. On one occasion, she had shouted at the receptionist and had been on the brink of expulsion from the practice by the senior partners. Dr B, then a junior partner, had calmed her down and pleaded for her to be given another chance. Ever since then, he had been her hero. His feelings towards her were ambivalent. He liked her friendly attitude and admired her determination in bringing up her young son after his father deserted them. On the other hand, she made many demands on him for letters to the authorities, for prescriptions of doubtful value and for frequent appointments. Among many other complaints, she was suffering from osteoarthritis and had a painful knee following an unsuccessful joint replacement.

In a recent consultation, Gloria had been tearful and distressed because she had been told that her knee would require further surgery. She feared that she would be confined to a wheelchair or perhaps lose her leg altogether. She wanted to phone her son so that he could give Dr B a detailed account of the consultation, as she was too upset. She also wanted several idiosyncratic prescriptions that had to be written out by hand and obtained from a particular chemist who stocked them. Finally, she wanted Dr B to write to the director of social services to ask if she could have more help at home in view of her disability. All in a 10-minutes consultation!

Dr B, though sympathetic at first, found himself increasingly irritated. He refused to speak to the son and said that the letter would have to be postponed. He told her that the special prescriptions were useless. Gloria subsided and looked very meek and contrite. Dr B immediately felt that he had been very cruel. This had happened before and he had had to be especially kind to her at the next consultation. H wondered why Gloria had such powerful effects on him and what he could do to keep calm.

What follows is a much-abbreviated version of the group discussion.

The discussion started with a few questions about Gloria's past history and home situation. Then Dr B was asked to sit back for a while. Some group members were very sympathetic to the doctor and said they would have felt just as angry with her in his position. One doctor said that Dr B should be more strict with her and not allow her to manipulate him. The group leader asked how it might feel to be in Gloria's position. A group member said she felt very sorry for Gloria. She must feel very helpless and needs to be more in control of her life. Another marvelled at the 30-year relationship and said that it was like a marriage! They were quarrelling like an old couple who could not live with or without each other. (This provoked laughter in the group and a wry smile from Dr B.) Another doctor responded by saying she had probably had fantasies about marrying him ever since he came to her rescue 30 years earlier. He had probably been too indulgent to her as he was such a nice man.

The leader then pointed out that Dr B had been disturbed when he found himself being not very nice to Gloria. What was this all about? Someone said, perhaps she enjoys it when he is cruel. Dr B came back in again and thanked his colleagues for their thoughts. He was beginning to realise what a complex relationship he had with Gloria. Did he want to go on seeing her, someone asked? Dr B thought for a moment and then said, yes he did. But he would have to try not to be cruel. If she really enjoyed it that only made matters worse! He thought he would have to try and be more firm with her but in a kindly way, without giving way to his irritation. The leader commented that perhaps they should all remember that Dr B was not in fact married to Gloria but was her GP.

Basic Principles and Practice in Balint Group Work

Having seen some examples of groups in action, we are now in a position to look at the basic principles underpinning the Balint group work.

Ground rules. As in any other small group, the members are asked to agree to certain ground rules:

1. Confidentiality must be maintained within the group about the patients discussed and also any personal disclosures by group members.
2. Group members listen to and respect everyone's contribution.
3. No unwanted personal questioning. People are free to talk about themselves and ways in which the patient's history reminds them of their own difficulties, but only if they wish to do so.

Learning to listen. One of Balint's main aims was to teach GPs to listen to their patients in depth, in a way that was different from medical 'history taking'. He wanted the doctors to tune into some of the patients' thoughts that were underneath the surface, perhaps mentioned very briefly or barely hinted at. At the same time, he wanted them to listen to the similar processes going on in their own minds, in response to the patients. Group leaders can teach this by example in the way that they listen to their group members.

The group as a safe space. The group should be a friendly space where everyone feels safe to talk about their work, including aspects of which they don't feel particularly proud. Uncertainty troubles everyone in the group and there is no shame in admitting it. Group members can disagree, but point scoring and destructive criticism is very rare in a group that is functioning well and would be firmly discouraged by a good leader. (See below: role of the group leader.)

Group continuity. It is important, wherever possible, for the group to consist of the same people with the same leaders, meeting regularly over a period of time which may extend to several years. As the members get to know each other better, they come to trust each more, and the work can reach greater depths of understanding. Where this is not possible, something of the kind can be achieved in a weekend or workshop or weekend in which the group meets several times a day for several days and members also live in the same accommodation. This intensive atmosphere enables trust and depth to develop more quickly over a short period.

The doctor-patient relationship. With its roots in psychoanalysis, as well as general practice, the central focus of the Balint work is on the doctor-patient relationship and especially on its often-hidden emotional content. Many of us find that our relationships with the patient can provoke more anxiety, uncertainty and difficulty in being a clinically effective doctor than any deficiency in our medical knowledge. Although medical uncertainties over diagnosis and treatment can also be greatly helped by small group discussion, the Balint group does not on the whole deal with these problems.

Learning about other styles of practice. Despite the prevalence of guidelines, doctor still bring a lot of individuality to the way they practice and relate to their patients. The Balint group provides an opportunity to learn about different approaches used by other group members. This is not only interesting but may offer a way of modifying one's approach to patients which may be useful and enlightening.

Follow-ups. The Balint group encourages and thrives on following up initial presentations. A follow-up gives the group an opportunity to see how the doctor's approach has changed as a result of the initial discussion. If there is a series of reports over a year or more, the group can watch the evolution of the doctor-patient relationship and hopefully observe that both have benefited.

Learning about 'blind spots' and 'typical presentations'. As the group continues and develops, it will become clear that each doctor has his or her own 'blind spots' or areas of particular difficulty. One doctor may have a horror of drug or alcohol dependency, another may find difficulty with patients with boundary issues, or a particular diagnosis, such as cancer or heart failure, may arouse undue uncertainty. Other group members will notice that Dr A is telling yet another case history that is 'typical' for him. This may be noted in a friendly or even humorous way. Someone may say 'this one sounds like another of your patients who won't listen to your advice, Jim!' Some patients may remind a doctor of her own personal difficulties. If she is able to gain some insight into why she finds these patients upsetting, she may be able to make some changes. This is what Michael Balint described as 'a limited though considerable change in personality'. However, it would be inappropriate for other doctors in the group to press this kind of interpretation without the presenting doctor's clear consent, as the following exchange shows:

'Does this lady remind you of anyone in your family, Jim?'

'No, I don't think so.'

The idea will not usually then be pursued. But after the group is over, Jim might begin to wonder if there was some truth in it.

Tolerating uncertainty. The purpose of the group is not to solve the case, desirable though this might be. The focus is not so much on 'what the doctor should do next' in the way of medical diagnosis or treatment but on 'what is going on between this doctor and this patient and what does it mean'. So the discussion often ends inconclusively, which some members at first find frustrating. But there is always the follow-up to look forward to!

Uncertainty

This section looks more closely at uncertainty, its sources, and how Balint groups can help doctors to live with it.

Both the Doctor and the Patient Can Experience Uncertainty

Few GPs would deny that the concerned states of our patients, to a larger or smaller extent, also have an impact on us as doctors. At times, the impact is obvious, but more often, we are affected in a more insidious way. In fact, 'mentally contagious phenomena' in clinical practice seem unavoidable in the doctor-patient relationship. What importance should we attribute to these quite ubiquitous influences? And how do we, as doctors, affect our patients with our personal styles, the different ways in which we try to maintain our 'comfort zone' in the surgery? (Jablonski 2010). Relationship is indeed a powerful ingredient of health care. The doctor's interaction with his patients can be looked upon as a drug in its own right, producing a feeling of safety and hope, reducing uncertainty and anxiety in the patients (Balint 1957). But it also has side effects – adverse reactions, poor compliance. The Balint work is about inquiring into the vast area of these issues to the benefit of practice.

Uncertainty and the Doctor-Patient Relationship

The GP is expected to provide his patients with medical expertise and good medical judgement. But at the same time, many of our patients are insecure and worried when they consult us. They wish to have their concerns and anxieties about their condition reflected in the face and eyes of the doctor. At the end of the consultation, the patients will, hopefully, feel that they have been understood and adequately examined and treated. The human response of the doctor plays an important part in reassuring them that examination procedures, treatment schedules and prescriptions have been well considered. But to many patients, the way the doctor relates goes beyond that. A majority of patients wish, and are better off with, a doctor who is willing to engage in an ongoing therapeutic relationship and take continuing personal responsibility for their health in the widest sense. For some patients, it is crucial.

Many doctors find this responsibility too open-ended and limitless. They find it hard to reconcile with other responsibilities to the community, the practice, the health service and not least, their families and themselves. What do these patients want? How far should I go in being their advocate when their demands begin to seem unreasonable? Is this really part of my brief as a GP? The emotions experienced by the GP are complex and contradictory; they include uncertainty, bewilderment, fascination, fatigue and numbness. The Balint perspective attempts to provide a pragmatic way in which these problems can be acknowledged as a challenge to the clinically–committed practitioner rather than being 'swept under the carpet'.

Sources of Uncertainty

Typical sources of uncertainty include the following:

• *Medical inexperience and mistakes.* Doctors, especially at the beginning of their careers, are often uncertain about their diagnostic skills and their medical knowledge in general. They are afraid of missing serious illness among the many symptoms of a non-life-threatening nature which are the bread and butter of general practice. When something does go wrong, such as a missed diagnosis, the doctor may be emotionally ill–equipped to admit his mistake, to apologise and to restore a good relationship with the patient. If the relationship has been a good one before the mistake and the doctor is perceived as caring and accepting of responsibility, the relationship can continue. There will be much that a doctor can do to help and be with a patient with cancer even if he has been slow to make the initial diagnosis.

• *Problems in the workplace and the health care system.* Doctors may feel insecure in their position in the practice if there is conflict and lack of harmony and good relationships within the team. This may make it difficult to ask for advice from colleagues or to enlist help in managing patients with complex problems. The doctor may feel depressed and uncertain where to go for help. Also, the changes of the health system framework and the great global changes – demographically, politically and culturally – affect GP work and the doctor-patient relationship. They challenge and may complicate further the doctor-patient communication, which must still remain central in health care, to provide meaningful and efficient medical support for the ordinary citizen. How do doctors handle the conflict between protecting the patient against authorities and protecting public welfare values from individual excessive demands? How are doctor-patient relations affected by cultural differences? How do we cope with the complexity of an individual patient? Do the drugs available today combined with the workload tempt the doctor to prescribe a more or less standardised treatment programme to his patients? How can we maintain and develop a holistic approach to our patients, given that our resources are limited?

• *Unwelcome requests from patients.* Patients in general practice are less submissive than in secondary care, where the panoply of teams of white-coated professionals and the array of high-technology equipment can have a chastening effect on individual assertiveness. Primary care patients frequently make the doctor feel he is being asked to behave in an unprofessional or even an unethical way. At the same time, he may feel that he is being unkind and obstructive when the patient pleads for what he wants. Requests that make the doctor feel uncertain and uncomfortable include those for the following:

Sickness certificates, especially if the patient seems fit to work or has not even seen a doctor. The doctor, coming from a different social milieu, may have no idea of the importance of the disastrous effect of the sudden deprival of sickness benefit when there is no other source of income.

Inappropriate prescriptions. These may be clinically ineffective, harmful to the patient, likely to encourage drug dependence, too expensive or harmful to the community (encouraging bacterial drug resistance). But they seem vitally important to the patient.

Letters of advocacy which patients hope may help them to acquire a home, to receive increased welfare payments, a better education for their children, to avoid a court appearance or a custodial sentence, a better settlement of an insurance claim and so on.

Inappropriate referrals or requests for expensive investigations. ('I need a whole body scan.')

- *Patients behaving badly* may cause extreme discomfort and uncertainty. On the one hand, they may be intrusive, overfamiliar, flirtatious or, worst of all, 'manipulative'. They may bring gifts or send greeting cards. Their praise may be fulsome and embarrassing. They may want long consultations with multiple problems. They may want to come every week with the consequent risk of dependency on the doctor. On the other hand, they may be confusing and contradictory, dissatisfied, disrespectful, scornful, threatening or aggressive. They may even tell lies.

How Can the Balint Group Help?

Many of these uncertainties can be addressed as ethical dilemmas and this approach is very helpful in managing uncertainty. The Balint group offers the additional benefit of exploring and untangling the emotional conflicts associated with wanting to show kindness and empathy to the patient while 'doing the right thing' and being a good professional. The aim of the group is not to come up with a definitive solution but to explore the interplay between one doctor and one patient, with the aim of reaching a better understanding of the emotional undercurrents that can prevent a solution being reached. The discussion will move back and forth, considering what it might be like to be first the doctor in the case and then the patient. The presenting doctor will often find herself reproducing some of the patient's behaviour, thus bringing the patient into the group for all to see. Although we are trained to cultivate and show empathy, there are some patients with whom this can be quite difficult. Some patients (notably drug addicts) make the doctor feel 'I could never be like that.' The Balint group leader may say 'what would it be like to be in this patient's shoes?' Some of those shoes look so ugly and uncomfortable that we are reluctant even to try them on. But once we have struggled into them, we may think, 'that's why she is in so much pain.'

Intuition

The Balint group may also help doctors to confirm and develop their clinical intuition and sensitivity. As important as such qualities are for clinical work, they may nevertheless cause uncertainty and doubt in the doctor as they may be difficult to account for. A Balint group facilitates a discussion on such aspects. It may encourage doctors not to see their sensitivity as opposed to rational judgement, but complementary – one of several 'tools' in clinical practice. There have been attempts to formulate intuition in GP work in several different kinds of terminology:

1. *The flash technique* (Balint and Norell 1973) encouraging pivotal/transformative encounters between the GP and the patient.

'The flash' and the 'flash technique' were described and discussed at length in *'Six Minutes for the Patient'* (Balint and Norell 1973). It was observed that there were moments of mutual understanding between doctor and patient which occurred suddenly, briefly and with great intensity – just like a flash of lightning. The impression was 'not that the doctor did something but that something happened'. The technique, if it was a technique, was simply for the doctor to be able to free himself from trying to find out what was going on and merely open himself to the patient's feelings and his own evoked responses. It was perhaps an example of Keats's 'Negative Capability' rather than a technique as such. In later years, Enid tended to play down the importance of the flash. It came to be regarded as a relatively rare event, although the free-floating attention which allowed flashes to happen is still well worth cultivating.

2. *Bodily empathy* (Rudebeck 1992) refers to the GP's bodily response to the patient, to be used for assessment of and communication with the patient.

Carl Edvard Rudebeck drew our attention to the difficulties doctors have in sharing their patients' experience of bodily symptoms. We know a lot about anatomy, he pointed out, but our introduction to the body is via the corpse in the dissecting room. And yet we inhabit the same living bodies as our patients. Most of the time, our bodies go on unobtrusively supporting and enabling our activities. We don't need to think about how essential their functioning is to life and contentment. But a palpitation in the chest reminds us that our hearts will one day stop beating, a trivial eye symptom suggests the possibility of blindness and a tingle in a limb may be the first warning of paralysis. Only when a symptom erupts are we reminded that the organ in question could one day give out. Rudebeck argues persuasively that we need to be aware of how a patient experiences a symptom and its existential threats.

3. *Countertransference reactions*

'Transference' is a term coined by Freud to describe the way a patient's childhood feelings about parents and other important figures may be imprinted on the analyst. Similarly, 'countertransference' describes the feelings evoked in the analyst by the patient (Racker 1968). The analyst needs to be aware of these phenomena and so does the GP, as Balint pointed out. Only, in this context, he preferred to avoid the technical language of psychoanalysis and simply talks about 'the doctor-patient relationship'. Balint implicitly encouraged his GPs to study their own reactions but seems never to have talked about 'the way the patient makes you feel'. Present-day group leaders are more explicit in inviting their group members to examine the emotions, positive and negative, induced by the patient's mood and personality.

Living with Uncertainty

Most Balint group sessions end without an agreed solution to the case. Indeed, if there is a neat conclusion, the group leader may feel uncertain about whether the really important issues have been addressed rather than 'pushed under the carpet'. Medical education rightly makes use of scientific method and the assessment of evidence to give us sound basis as possible for our diagnostic and therapeutic decisions. But human life remains uncertain and individuals are all different. In primary care, there is more uncertainty because illnesses are at an early stage, undifferentiated and often combined with other illnesses and unexplained symptoms. Fortunately, our role is not always to achieve certainty. As Marinker (1994) has put it:

> The diagnostic task of the specialist is to reduce uncertainty, to explore possibility and to marginalise error. The diagnostic task of the GP, on the other hand, is to accept uncertainty, to explore probability and to marginalise danger.

We are more likely to be able to marginalise danger if we can live with ongoing uncertainty, while continuing to be alert for signs of danger. This means listening to the patient and respecting his thoughts and feelings even if we don't believe that he has an undiagnosed, dangerous illness.

We have to live with uncertainty but its better if we can explore it together rather than face it in isolation.

The Role of the Group Leader

The most effective group leaders say very little but are able to provide, by their presence, the necessary conditions for the group to function well.

Timekeeping

The leader's first responsibility is to keep an eye on the time. Most groups last for an hour to an hour and a half, although in Germany, they may go on for two hours. In the UK and the US, it is customary to accommodate two cases in 90 minutes, each given equal time. There may also be time for brief follow-up reports. In groups where the presenting doctor 'sits out' after her presentation, the leader needs to make sure that she is brought back in plenty of time to contribute further to the discussion.

Making the Group a Safe Place

The group members need to feel that it is safe to say anything they want so long as it is not offensive to the rest of the group and does not breach confidentiality to patients by making their identity too obvious. Everyone should be listened to attentively and their ideas treated with respect.

People are free to disagree with each other but this should be done politely. Attempts to interrogate another member in an intrusive way about his personal life and its connection with the case will be firmly discouraged by the leader so that members feel protected from abuse. The leader can model good listening in the way that he gives his full attention to the initial presentation without interruption.

Other kinds of case discussion, such as the hospital grand round, may expose the doctors to scathing criticism and aggressive questioning that puts them on the defensive. It is important, in a Balint group, to be able to talk about things that have gone wrong and actions that do not show the presenter acting always with courage and wisdom. Everyone is aware of their own similar inadequacies and failures. Everyone 'has been there.'

While he listens to the discussion, the leader will be looking round the group to check out everyone's welfare. Someone may be trying to speak but is unable to get a word in. If so, the leader will make a space for her. Someone else may be talking too much and the leader may have to ask him diplomatically to give others a chance. Someone may be personally affected by the patient's story and be on the verge of tears. A good leader will spot this and care for the group member. This can be done in several ways. Recognising a group member is in pain may be enough. In a group that is functioning well, other members will be supportive too. Sometimes, the painful effects point at something central about the case presented. In a group with a lot of mutual trust, the discussion can continue incorporating the pain of a member and yet protecting him. The leader will decide if there is a need to offer more support (perhaps after the session has finished).

The Doctor-Patient Relationship

The group leader's main function in guiding the group's work is to keep reminding them about the doctor-patient relationship. To start with, and particularly in groups for beginners, the discussion will include medical matters and suggestions for solving the problem simply, such as prescribing or referring. The group may drift into generalisations ('the trouble with these patients is that they are manipulative') rather than exploring what went on in these particular encounters. The leader's job is to steer the group back to the doctor-patient relationship whenever it strays too far or for too long. He/she does this mainly by putting open questions to the group as a whole. 'How does this patient make us feel? What is it like to be in Dr A's position?' If there is a lot of sympathy for the doctor and the patient is in danger of being lost, the leader may bring the patient back into the room by saying something like: 'I guess this patient must have been feeling very frightened. What would it be like to be in his position?' A good leader will intervene to challenge a prevailing mood of cynicism and dislike for the patient.

Michael and Enid Balint observed that the doctor's feelings and behaviour in the group often reflected those of the patient and were a valuable diagnostic instrument. Sometimes, the whole group will catch the patient's mood through the presenter and, for example, feel depressed. The leader may point this out to the group but only as a general observation. It is helpful to include herself as a member of the group: 'the group has gone very quiet now; I wonder if we are all feeling depressed…'

The leader may have a definite view of what the case is all about, but he/she will do better, on the whole, to keep it to herself and let the group do the work. She will not draw attention to herself by producing a clever 'interpretation', but brief suggestions pointing out underlying psychological factors that the group may be missing can be very helpful. On the other hand, the group may come up with a metaphor that neatly symbolises the interaction (e.g. 'this patient is like a little stray dog looking for a home'), and the leader may refer to this as a way of crystallising the group's discoveries.

In many ways, two leaders are better than one as they can complement each other. There are no fixed roles, but one leader may see things going on in the group that her colleague has not spotted. If one leader's attempt to refocus the group has failed, the other may come to her assistance. It is also helpful for a group leader to have a partner to discuss the session with afterwards. (The training of leaders is discussed below.)

The Benefits of Balint Groups

What might doctors gain from being in a Balint group? To begin with, they have a chance to 'unburden themselves' and share their experiences with a group of sympathetic colleagues who have all been in similar situations. There is considerable relief from being able to 'talk freely' about ones difficulties (and uncertainties). The doctor is also able to hear about many 'different' *approaches* to the patients presented and to compare them with his own. To this extent, the Balint group is probably not very different from any other ongoing reflective small group.

However, as the Balint group develops, under the leader's guidance, the doctors will begin to risk *feelings of identification and empathy* with a wider range of patients, including those who previously evoked revulsion or contempt. They will feel *better equipped to deal with feelings* of sadness or anxiety which come from the patient and carry a share of their unhappiness without collapsing under the strain. They will learn to consider and reflect on these *emotions aroused by the patient* in themselves and then withdraw to a safe distance to make decisions rather than getting enmeshed with the patient. Each member will be aware of the group as an inner resource. When they see a presented patient again, they will *remember the group discussion* and draw strength from the support they have received. Box 4.1 gives some examples of the typical kinds of cases that doctors bring to Balint groups.

Box 4.1 Typical Presentations

What kind of cases do doctors bring to a Balint group?
A patient the doctor has known for many years
Someone who makes the doctor feel helpless
Someone the doctor dislikes or fears
Someone with many symptoms and no clear diagnosis
A patient who makes unreasonable or 'inappropriate' demands
Someone who makes the doctor feel ill-used
A patient dependent on drugs or alcohol
A patient too dependent on the doctor
Someone who makes the doctor feel 'stuck'
Seductive or 'manipulative' patient
Patients who fall in love with the doctor
Doctors who become over-involved with their patient
Patients who bring gifts and seem to expect something in return
Patients in whom a major diagnosis has been missed
Difficulty in differentiating major organic illness from functional symptoms
A dying patient
Conflict with secondary care colleagues
Relationship problems in the workplace
Patients with marital and family problems
Suspected child abuse

Hopefully, as time goes on, there will be *greater insight* into blind spots, denials and over-identification with particular patients who remind the doctor of a part of himself he would rather ignore. For example, a doctor may become more self-aware about situations that make him feel excited or angry. All this should lead to *greater work satisfaction* and *avoidance of burnout*. The evidence for these beneficial effects will be considered in the next chapter.

Setting Up a Balint Group

The original seminars in the 1950s were advertised, and GPs who were interested were invited to apply to join a new group. They were interviewed by Balint to see if they were 'suitable'. He wanted to assure himself that applicants were able to learn from what the group had to offer and also to make sure that they were not seeking psychological treatment for themselves. This was never the purpose of the groups. Towards the end of his life, Balint also started a group for medical students at University College, London. There have also been groups for doctors in other specialties and other professionals dealing with human relationships such as teachers, lawyers, clergy, counsellors and social workers.

Nowadays, a Balint group for GPs may function in one of a number of different contexts:

1. Groups for established doctors set up independently of any institution.
2. Workplace groups (some of which may include several neighbouring centres).
3. Groups set up as part of a GP or family medicine teaching programme, using the university or medical school premises. These are for either GP trainees (residents) or students.

Independent Groups

Many doctors joining a Balint group often say they have reached a stage where they feel a need to compensate for something missing in their medical training. They miss a sincere professional exchange on their clinical practice. They are troubled by the uncertainties of medical practice and aware that this has at least partly to do with relationships with patients. Younger doctors (in their 30s) often add that they are concerned that in 10–15 years, they will end up in a kind of petrified state that they have observed in some older colleagues.

These doctors are mature and experienced enough to have some awareness of shortcomings and frustrations in various clinical situations; they are curious enough and have the moral courage to explore what they are feeling and thinking and how they are acting professionally. Prospective Balint group members are expected to involve themselves with each other in a respectful and empathetic way. These qualities will not necessarily manifest from the beginning; they may take some time to emerge. But the 'embryo' must be there from the start. By interviewing prospective group members, as Michael Balint did, a leader may diminish the uncertainty and dropout frequency. But that is not possible if a leader is contracted by a group and he has had no or little influence on the group formation process.

How do these groups start? Two or three doctors in a neighbourhood may discuss the idea. One or more of them may have been to weekend workshops or experienced a Balint group during their training. They will make enquiries to see if a viable number for an ongoing group can be assembled. They will then need to find a leader or leaders. They may approach their national Balint Society who will know of trained leaders in their area. Alternatively, a local psychiatrist or other mental health professional may be invited to lead the group. These prospective leaders will need to get some Balint group experience and leadership training if they do not already have it. If the group can have two leaders, that is usually even better.

A mental health professional and a GP with Balint experience make a good combination. The GP with his knowledge of primary care provides street credibility and anchors the leadership in day-to-day reality, while the psychologist or psychotherapist can provide useful insights from his more specialised training and practice. Whatever their background, both leaders need specific Balint group training and they need to get on well as colleagues. Leaders may be paid a fee collectively by their group members, or outside funding may be available. In the UK, GP leaders often give their services unpaid.

Independent groups, once successfully launched, may continue to meet usually fortnightly for a number of years with either a constant membership or a gradual turnover. Some are known to have lasted for decades!

Groups in Training Programmes and Other Institutions

These were started in the UK by some of the Balints' early group members who found themselves in charge of the first vocational training schemes for general practice in the 1970s and 1980s. Small-group work was recommended by the Royal College of Physicians as part of the curriculum, and if the course organiser had been an enthusiastic Balint group member, then the group was conducted as a Balint group. These groups continue in a minority of UK training programmes, and a substantial number of others have small groups working along similar lines, although not referred to as Balint groups.

In the US, Balint groups began to appear in family medicine teaching departments in the 1980s, and following the formation of the American Balint Society in 1991, they spread quickly across the country. By the 1990s, they were present in about half of the country's 450 teaching programmes (Johnson et al. 2001). The group leaders are drawn from the teaching faculty and usually consist of a family physician and a behavioural scientist (psychologist).There are similar groups for trainee family doctors in European countries. The impetus for starting a Balint group in a teaching institution may come from the head of the training program or an enthusiast in the faculty.

Workplace Groups

In Sweden, for example, the director of a clinic or department may recognise the need for a professional development group, such as a Balint group. The initiative may come from 'above' or more often from the 'clinical factory floor'. In the latter situation, the nucleus of the group has already formed. It is a matter of getting the project sanctioned and possibly recruiting more members and a leader. When the initiative comes from the management of the centre, a meeting is held to give information about the Balint method, which ideally is done by the prospective leader and the management jointly, allowing for all obstacles to be discussed simultaneously. Then people can sign up for the group. Complicating motives for joining the group may be an open or hidden need for personal psychotherapy, as Michael Balint realised. Balint group work might occasionally highlight such a need. As long as the framework is kept and the group member does not invade the group with

---

Box 4.2 The Head of a Centre Wishes to Join a Balint Group

A Balint leader was invited to lead a group of seven or eight specialist GPs working at the same centre. In the first session, the GP director of the centre said he would participate as an observer to see how the work was running, but he would not present cases himself. The group members tacitly agreed, but the group leader immediately felt that this was an impossible situation. The director was putting himself in both a controlling and a self-protective position that would be likely to hamper the group work considerably. The leader said he would have to think carefully what that meant for the group work. The first session was quite tranquil, although the director made a couple of distinct policy remarks. At the next meeting, 2 weeks later, the leader explained that members of a Balint group must take part on an equal and open basis; otherwise, the group would not fulfil its purpose. If that was not acceptable, the leader would not be able to continue working with the group. The director decided to leave. Within 2 weeks, he had also left the centre for another position. One of the members of the group was appointed as the new director of the centre. She continued participating in the group, contributed and was open about herself, just like all the other colleagues at the work place.

---

personal issues, this does not have to be a problem. For trainee doctors, the Balint group is regarded as beneficial, even vital, for all and there is no question of excluding trainees because of any personal psychological problems, provided that the functioning of the group is not disrupted.

The head of a centre may wish to join the group himself and a genuine wish to share clinical experiences and difficulties on an equal basis with his colleagues, or, more worryingly, in order to exercise a controlling influence. An example of the difficulty this may cause appears in Box 4.2.

How Are Balint Group Leaders Trained?

The biggest obstacle to setting up a new Balint group is the availability of trained group leaders. The technique is very specific and it is not enough to be a qualified mental health professional if one has no Balint group experience. Originally, potential leaders served as group members for several years, absorbing leadership skills by osmosis and by discussion of each session afterwards with the leader-tutor. However, it is not always possible to find a group in which to learn in this slow but thorough way. More formal training is provided by Balint Societies in various European countries including France, Germany, Belgium, Sweden and the UK. The US has a very successful program of intensive leader-training courses which has

Box 4.3 History and Development of Balint Groups

1950s Michael and Enid Balint start leading groups for GPs in London. Other groups start with psychoanalyst leaders from the Tavistock Clinic.

1957 publication of Michael Balint's book, *The Doctor, His Patient and the Illness*.

1960s Change in emphasis from long interviews to the study of ordinary GP consultations. The Balints travel widely, demonstrating their method in other countries.

1969 First national Balints Society forms in France. Other countries soon follow.

1970 Death of Michael Balint. British Balint Society forms with annual publication of a journal.

1970s Balint groups begin in Scandinavia and Eastern Europe.

1972 First International Balint Congress held in London attended by 800 doctors. (Hopkins, 1972) Since then, 17 world congresses have been held. The 18th will be held in Heidelberg in 2013.

1974 First groups with GP leaders start in UK, mainly in GP training schemes.

1974 Formation of the International Balint Federation. International Congresses held in a different country every few years.

1980s Formation of more Balint Societies in Europe.

1991 Formation of the American Balint Society in the US.

1990s Rapid spread of groups for residents in family medicine training programmes. Intensive group leader-training courses start in the US.

1994 Death of Enid Balint.

1997 International guidelines for group leader accreditation agreed.

2000s Growth of Balint groups for medical students.

2011 First international conference to study group leadership development. Balint Societies starts in Australia, New Zealand, Austria, Bulgaria and other countries. Balint groups are active in China. International Federation has 25 member countries (2011)

been running since 1991. These courses provide Balint groups, supervised by tutors in which the leadership is rotated round the group members, giving everybody a turn. Each session is followed by 45 minutes of feedback and discussion of the leadership. After completing six of these courses, an applicant is encouraged to lead a group of his own with feedback to a supervisor for a period of 2 years. If he has then reached the required standard, he is accredited as a group leader by the American Balint Society. The UK Balint Society has a similar though more modest scheme with leader training weekends and supervision at a regular group leaders' workshop Box 4.3.

References

Balint, M. (1957). *The doctor, his patient and the illness*. London: Pitman. Millennium edition 2000. Edinburgh: Churchill Livingstone.

Balint, E., & Norell, J. S. (1973). *Six minutes for the patient: Interactions in general practice consultation*. London: Tavistock.

Hopkins, P. (1972). *Patient-centred medicine*. London: Regional Doctor Publications.

Jablonski, H. (2010). Meeting with the patient: Between fascination and routine, certainty and doubt – How do doctors cope and develop emotionally and cognitively? (pp. 185–6). *Primary care*. Muttenz: Swiss Medical Publishers.

Johnson, A. H., Brock, C. D., Hamadeh, G., et al. (2001). The current status of Balint groups in US family practice residencies: A 10-year follow-up study, 1990–2000. *Family Medicine, 33*(9), 672–7.

Marinker, M. (1994). *The End of Physicians*. Bayliss lecture. London: Royal College of General Practitioners.

Racker, H. (1968). *Transference and countertransference*. New York: International University Press.

Rudebeck, C. E. (1992). The general practitioner and the dialogue of clinical practice and symptoms. *Scandinavian Journal of Primary Health Care*, Supplement 1, 1–87.

Chapter 5
Research on Balint Groups

Dorte Kjeldmand, Henry Jablonski, and John Salinsky

Introduction

Do doctors, and their patients for that matter, benefit from conversations in small groups about clinical cases? Doctors are paid for curing patients, their time is expensive, and, in many countries, there is a shortage of GPs. Whether small groups are called Balint groups or have other names and work in different ways, we need solid evidence if we want doctors to spend time sitting there, telling stories to each other. Heads of teaching institutions want to know if it is educationally effective and health care organizers and authorities need to know whether groups are just as or even more efficient as other methods for Continuing Professional Education (CPE) and if there are other advantages such as working environment benefits. The GPs themselves need to know whether they should choose to join a group that will take precious time on a continuing basis, and may also have some anxiety about opening up to colleagues about uncertainty and shortcomings. They may also benefit from knowledge about the different kinds of groups available so they can choose the

D. Kjeldmand (✉)
Department of Public Health and Caring Sciences,
Section for Health Services Research, University of Uppsala, Sweden

Eksjö Primary Care Center, 57581 Eksjö, Sweden
e-mail: kjeldmand@gmail.com

H. Jablonski
President of the International Balint Federation; President of the Swedish Association of Medical psychology (Swedish Society of Medicine), Psychiatrist and psychoanalyst in private practice, Kvarngatan 2, Stockholm 11847, Sweden
e-mail: drhj@jablonski.se

J. Salinsky
Ellis Practice, The Welford Centre, 113 Chalkhill Road, Wembley HA9 9FX, UK
e-mail: JVSalinsky@aol.com

L.S. Sommers and J. Launer (eds.), *Clinical Uncertainty in Primary Care: The Challenge of Collaborative Engagement*, DOI 10.1007/978-1-4614-6812-7_5,
© Springer Science+Business Media New York 2013

method that may suit them best. What are the goals and results from each method and for how long should groups go on? That may depend on whether the purpose is educational or maintenance of the doctor's mental well-being during a long working life. Do Balint-trained doctors last longer?

Perhaps the most important reason to do research on case-based discussion peer groups for doctors is to discover whether they ultimately benefit the patients. They are the people who lend their stories to be told in the groups, and whose doctor is not available when meeting with the group. They have a right to know what is going on and to be assured that this activity is worthwhile and ethically justified. However, as we show, the question of patient benefit is the most difficult one to investigate directly.

Who should carry out this research? The people who are engaged in a process they believe in will most often be the ones with the incentive to "prove" that their method is the best and applicable in all contexts. Hence they will have the motivation and stamina as devoted prophets to work hard, but may also be blind to negative findings in the studies. The qualitative approach is essential, as is a critique from co-workers who have no personal experience of the Balint method and can see it simply as a pedagogical intervention. It is necessary to invite other scientific professions into the work of researching our activity if it is to gain credibility outside our own circle of consensus. Anthropologists, work environment scientists, and other professions can certainly make an important contribution to our research. We need to combine the energy of committed enthusiasts with that of skeptical outsiders if research is to be credible.

In what follows we survey the field of Balint research under the following headings:

- Balint groups as a form of research
- Challenges for Balint research
- Balint's *A Study of Doctors*
- Some recent research
- *The Doctor, the Task and the Group*

Balint Groups as a Form of Research

One perspective on Balint groups is to see the groups themselves as a form of research. This was Michael Balint's own view. In his introductory chapter to *The Doctor, His Patient and the Illness* (Balint 1964) he described his seminars with GPs as "a mixture of research and training." He had an idea that GPs were doing more good for their patients than was generally realized by specialists and that this was achieved through their relationships with their patients. As well as training GPs in psychotherapeutic skills, he wanted the group to be an instrument of research into the way GPs and patients reacted to each other emotionally. In a way, he was like an ethnographer exploring an unfamiliar culture by living with the people he wished to study. The work of the group was thus an early form of qualitative research into health care. It is important to bear in mind that there were no books on consultation "technique" and no teaching of communication skills for doctors at the time Michael Balint developed his groups. The early group members took up the idea of research with enthusiasm. After a period of improving their listening skills, a number of groups agreed to focus on presenting cases that they hoped would illuminate a particular problem area of general practice.

To do this it was important to document the presentations and to follow up each case at intervals to get some idea of the outcome. A research group would need a verbatim record on audiotape of the proceedings of every session, and these would be transcribed and circulated to members. When the group was fully in research mode, the first part of a session might be devoted to a discussion of the previous week's transcript. This would include drawing out themes that could be seen as illuminating and meaningful. After gathering and discussing material for a number of years, one or more of the group members, sometimes including the leader, would write up the research and draw some conclusions. Among the topics studied were asthma, night calls, repeat prescriptions, and sexual discord in marriage. A number of these projects were published as monographs but all are, sadly, out of print.

Other research groups looked more broadly at the nature and consequences of doctor–patient interactions in ordinary brief consultations. Initially Balint had insisted that, before presenting a patient, the doctors should conduct a long interview of an hour or more with the patient outside surgery hours. These interviews produced spectacular results and enabled the doctor to know the patient as a person, perhaps for the first time. However, the group members became concerned about their responsibility to all their other patients who were not getting the benefit of long interviews. As a result of this groundswell of discontent, Balint had a change of mind and asked the doctors to present patients seen only in normal GP consultations. This resulted in a book with the celebrated title of *Six Minutes for the Patient* (Balint and Norell 1973). After that, the long interview became exceptional rather than mandatory.

There was also a good deal of curiosity about what might be happening in brief but highly charged general practice encounters which were seen as changing the course of the relationship, and perhaps, even improving the patient's health. In *Six Minutes for the Patient* this was described as "the flash", a rapid and dramatic moment of mutual illumination and insight (see also Chapter 4). The only problem was that flashes were relatively rare and difficult to generate. Subsequent research groups (Elder and Samuel 1987; Balint et al. 1993) preferred to study "moments of change" which were less sensational, but perhaps more productive in the longer term.

A later group (Salinsky and Sackin 2000) chose cases in which the doctors felt that their personal defenses had inhibited them, unnecessarily, from empathizing with the patient. This group, whose members had worked together in various combinations for many years, were able to disclose more about the way their personal experiences resonated with those of their "problem" patients.

Michael and Enid Balint wanted to know what was really going on in general practice between the doctor and the patient. Did a significant ongoing relationship help patients to regain physical and mental health? If, as they believed, the doctor himself or herself was the most powerful medicine available in general practice, what was the correct dose? How often should it be given? And what were the adverse effects to beware of? They also wanted to know how a GP might best be trained to understand and use this relationship-medicine. Which members of their seminars were likely to benefit and was it possible to predict and discourage those who were unlikely to benefit? Their endpoint or outcome for "benefit" was the "limited though considerable change in personality" which showed, to their satisfaction and those of their colleagues, that a doctor was now more aware of her own and her patients' feelings and could make therapeutic use of this awareness. These days, we would probably express this in the one word "empathy" or a phrase such as "emotional intelligence."

Challenges for Balint Research

The Balints' pupils and their successors have always believed very strongly that Balint groups could make a powerful contribution to medical education if only they were allowed to enter the academy and be part of the curriculum. We believe that membership of a Balint group can provide benefits at all levels: for students, post-graduate trainees (especially in general practice and psychiatry) and as part of continuing education for established physicians, to which the heads of medical schools and the postgraduate deans and tutors reply, "Where is your evidence for these beneficial effects?"

A Balint doctor might reply by saying, "Look what Balint training has done for me! I enjoy my work much more, I listen to my patients with empathy, and they feel better cared for. Surely it can do the same for others." The Dean shakes his head and with an ironic smile says, "I am afraid that is not good enough. Putting your groups in my curriculum would cost a lot of money and I would need to be able to justify it to my provider organization in terms of objective scientific results. Where are your controlled trials? Without them your personal stories are no more than anecdotes." The same question will be asked by the senior doctors and managers of a family doctor practice who want to know whether the investment of time and money needed to provide a continuing Balint group can be justified by evidence from research.

The problem for Balint doctors, then, is that no one else is sufficiently motivated to do this research and they will have to do it themselves. They face two problems. The first, as we have already mentioned, is that they find it difficult to be objective because they are so committed to their cause. They will happily look for the answer to the question, "Is Balint training effective?" But they will want and expect the answer to be a resounding "Yes." Otherwise, in the event of negative results, they would have to say, "Very well then, the method has not been shown to be effective; I will give up Balint and try something else." This would be hard to do because positive personal experience is very convincing, even if others call it anecdotal.

The second problem is that research on Balint has enormous difficulties that it shares with all research in the social and psychological sciences, among which we would include education. These apply particularly to quantitative research and so we consider this first.

Quantitative research is about outcomes and numbers and comparisons. Researchers want to know if there is a significant difference in the study group compared with a control group. To demonstrate significance they need sufficient numbers to ring a statistical bell. And they need to have a precise endpoint (or outcome) to measure in order to compare the two. In a trial of a new medication, for example, for diabetes, it is easy to assemble a control group who differ from the study group only in that they are receiving a placebo instead of the drug being tested. But when the new medicine is a human being, things get more complicated. In choosing outcome measures, we would want to look at the possible ways in which a patient might benefit from having a Balint-trained physician looking after him.

Conceivably, the Balint doctor's patients might live longer, be less prone to chronic disease, lead happier and more fulfilled lives, or simply cope better with adversity. All these may have been influenced by the Balint doctor's special qualities; but in the course of the patient's life she will have been subjected to many other influences, good and bad, including contact with a variety of other doctors and health professionals. These confounding factors have made research on patient outcome of Balint groups more or less untenable and we know of no published studies. It may be relevant here to mention that there is a considerable amount of literature on the effect of the patient-centered approach in health care. The largest project was done by Huygen et al. who demonstrated hard effects on the patients' health status related to the working styles of their general practitioners (Huygen et al. 1992).

Because of these problems, quantitative Balint research has usually looked at doctor outcomes. Positive outcomes for the Balint-trained physician would include a greater degree of empathy, psychological effectiveness, tolerance, patience, and lack of burnout. These and other aspects of the "limited though considerable change in personality" can be quantified by giving the subjects carefully designed questionnaires with numerical scales. Perhaps Balint doctors use their psychological skills to such great effect that they have less need of other resources. Do they prescribe fewer drugs, refer fewer patients to specialists, and request fewer investigations than other doctors? Such outcomes would greatly appeal to heads of departments eager to save money.

Whatever the outcomes used, the quantitative researcher will gather the results in the form of numbers which will be happily carried away to present to the statistical adviser. The adviser may not be impressed by the findings. Do Balint doctors have higher mean scores than the control group? Well, perhaps they do, but might some of them have achieved these without their specific Balint training? Perhaps they chose to go into a program that they knew had Balint groups because they were more psychologically minded and empathetic to begin with. Testing them before and after the Balint training makes it possible to detect change, but may mean that the project extends over several years. And still there are confounding factors lurking in the undergrowth. Perhaps the control group had other ways of improving their psychological skills and will produce equally good scores without passing through a Balint group.

Another major difficulty is that there are relatively few Balint groups, each with only a small group of members who may enter and leave the group quite frequently. This means that the methodological obstacles to doing Balint group research are huge and the possibility of making any kind of controlled study or even a before-and-after study is small. One main problem is locating groups, because there is no system for registration of Balint groups. As described in Chapter 4, Balint groups emerge rather chaotically here and there and most of them disappear after some time without a trace. There are many Balint groups for established GPs whose existence is known only to their participants and leaders. If they are not affiliated with a national Balint Society, with accredited leaders, it may be impossible to tell whether they are really "true" Balint groups as we understand them.

As even the mainstream groups at any given moment are few, it is also difficult to carry out a study with enough statistical power to compare methods, for example, Balint versus other methods or Balint versus no training. The researcher may find that the group doesn't keep still long enough for its attributes to be accurately counted. So the number of people studied in each project will be small, often in single figures. If this is the case, the statistician's verdict is likely to be disappointing. A way of increasing statistical power is to use meta-analysis in which the results of many studies are combined so that the total numbers may become more meaningful. There are probably enough Balint studies (although they are of variable quality) to make this worth a try, but to our knowledge, no such meta-analysis has yet been attempted.

For all the reasons we have outlined, nearly all research ever carried out into Balint groups has been qualitative. Qualitative studies are not concerned with numbers. The researchers are interested in what goes on in a particular group: what happens and how it happens. The researcher may be allowed to sit in on the group sessions to make her observations. She may also interview the leaders, individual members, or the group as a whole. She will be looking for recurrent themes or threads that will shed light on what the group does and does not do for its members. She is looking for meaning, not statistical significance. The study by Ruth Pinder et al. (2006) is a good example. And, as we have already mentioned, the Balint groups that studied themselves in the early days were also carrying out a kind of qualitative research. Qualitative studies are probably more worthwhile in terms of eliciting meaning, even though they are less likely to convince the heads of academic departments.

A Study of Doctors by Michael Balint et al.

This leads us to the first major research study led by Michael and Enid Balint and two other Balint group leaders, *A Study of Doctors*. This was the report of the first 13 years of seminars with GPs at the Tavistock Clinic (Balint et al. 1966), an extensive evaluation of the activity of Balint groups, at that time called "seminars for general practitioners," from 1952 at the Tavistock Clinic. Balint kept a register for every seminar showing the attendance of each participant, and the participants also kept a recording of their training. When a GP left, Balint would add a brief description, especially of the participant's responses to the experiences in the group and the presumed reason for leaving.

He and his colleagues discovered that there were a large number of "early leavers"; more than half of group members dropped out before the end of the first year. This led to the initiation of the so-called "mutual selection interviews" whose purpose was to make sure that the applicants understood the scope and method of the group work and could be expected to benefit from participation in it. This measure was successful in that the number of early leavers and doctors with little progress diminished considerably. The authors made a classification system by which the participants were rated according to their progress in the groups and their reasons for leaving. The highest level a participant could reach, according to the ranking system, was "F: definite changes of substantial quality," described as follows. It defines what Balint himself regarded as the goal of successful training:

> He can contribute to and learn from the seminar; what he learns he applies in his practice and the result is brought back to the seminar for further work. He becomes more flexible in the seminar and more versatile with his patients. As his understanding of his cases increases he develops new skills in handling them which he applies consciously and deliberately. His understanding comes to include a sense of what is relevant in his ideas and observation; his remarks therefore are more appropriate and meaningful. He can learn more from the patient than from the seminar and can notice some of his mistakes and can then recover from them.

Half of the participants reached the two highest levels, E and F, indicating that definite changes were achieved, but in addition to these, one-quarter seemed to have:

> increased their understanding of the cases discussed, and some liberating of knowledge which perhaps they already had but which was unavailable to them previously. In their cases this slight increase in understanding is shown rather in feeling more at ease with their patients and in toleration of them than in their deliberately applying it when considering what to do.

Balint studied the time factor and found that, in order to reach a rating of F, most doctors needed considerable time. The critical period seemed to be the third year. Roughly one quarter of the doctors who could commit themselves enough to stay longer than 3 years developed so much that they were rated F. Nowadays, we tend to assume that a Balint group will benefit almost everyone to some extent and the use of mutual selection interviews is rare. Some of the more recent studies seem to confirm that some doctors greatly appreciate and benefit from the group experience, whereas others do not and tend to leave early. *A Study of Doctors* also suggested that there is an intermediate group of doctors for whom the results, although not dramatic, are definitely worthwhile.

Some Recent Research

We now look at some of the more recent studies that have taken place and try to assess their usefulness. Because of the methodological problems discussed above, most research has been done with groups lasting only 6 months or a year and consisting of interns or residents in closed settings. When looking at these studies, we need to bear in mind that it takes time for doctors to change as a result of being in a Balint group. The groups need to continue for a number of years. Balint thought that 2 years were needed for the group members gradually to develop the necessary sense of security to allow for "the limited though considerable" change in their personality described above.

Musham and Brock (1994) tested and interviewed frequent ($n=9$) and infrequent ($n=7$) Balint group-attending residents and found that intuition scores were higher among the frequent attendees. The residents who participated on a regular basis in Balint groups during their residency perceived this training as helpful in understanding themselves in relationships with their patients. They expressed the belief that Balint training had a direct and beneficial effect on developing empathetic skills and becoming more versatile with a broader repertoire of patient-specific responses. However, the interviews gave the impression that there are two sorts of residents: those who benefit from and thrive and develop quickly in Balint groups and those who do not, and the proportion of each is about 50%. They also questioned whether the latter could be hurt by attending and not feeling successful in the group. In this study the numbers were small and although the results favored Balint, there were no pretest scores. As often happens, the qualitative (interview) results were more interesting and revealed that different doctors may respond to the group experience in very different ways.

Johnson et al. (2003) did extensive psychological testing of family practice residents in order to detect differences between residents who continued Balint groups for 2 years and those who chose to finish after 6 months. The 2-year attendees were more intuitive and this had statistical significance, but no other significant differences were found. Again, we are left unsure about whether the long-term attendees were more receptive to the method in the first place.

Turner and Malm (2004) compared a group of family doctor residents ($n=6$) who participated for 9 months in a Balint group, with other residents ($n=8$) who did not participate. The Balint group participants significantly improved their abilities in behavioral medicine, as measured by the Psychological Medicine Inventory, compared to the control group. However, the numbers are very small and as far as we know, the study has not been repeated on a larger scale.

Cataldo et al. (2005) studied empathy and physician satisfaction after graduation from a family residency program in which the physicians could choose to continue in a Balint group for the whole 2-year program, or only for the first 6-month mandatory period. They found that the 113 prolonged attendees had a similar mean empathy score to the 69 nonattendees. There was also no difference in overall work satisfaction, but the Balint attendees were more likely than the nonattendees to say that they would choose the same specialty if they could choose again, thus, they seemed more satisfied with their choice of family medicine as a specialty. However, it is possible that their choice of family medicine was more secure to begin with and hence they valued the group more highly.

Margalit et al. (2005) evaluated two teaching programs that, among other things, aimed at improving GPs' knowledge of the biopsychosocial approach, their patient-centered attitudes, and professional self-esteem. Both programs consisted of different learning methods over a period of 12 weeks. The first was a "didactic" program and the second was "interactive" and included Balint groups. There were 22 GPs who participated in each program after randomization and their knowledge, intentions, and attitudes were evaluated before and 6 months after the end of the program, by questionnaires. Both groups showed improvement, but in the interactive group the learners' professional self-esteem and intentions improved significantly more than in the didactic group. It is difficult to know whether this improvement had to do with the Balint group sessions; 12 weeks of Balint activity is probably not enough to make a lasting impact.

An Occasional Paper from the Royal College of General Practitioners presented a study by Ruth Pinder et al. (2006) exploring how Balint's work influences general practice education in the United Kingdom today. The authors took an ethnographic approach in a qualitative study of groups of young doctors in a vocational training scheme in London to see what use the members made of the experience. They found that the group work was often what one could call "Balint lite" (our interpretation), meaning not too challenging. It was used as a container for difficult feelings that the participants experienced during their assignments. They could offload these feelings in the group and get some sympathy and support. The group was an integral part of the training; members were not volunteers. The leaders were aware of this and tried not to push too hard. But the members felt they were in a dependent position to the leaders and each other, making safety an issue. They also felt that there was a clear tendency to search for consensus, which differs from the traditional Balint group approach. Yet the overall findings in the study were that the Balint group experience was beneficial in many ways. Self-knowledge could be gained, and the group enabled them to exchange ideas and feelings with colleagues, while at the same time, it provided a great opportunity for the young doctors to catch some sense and meaning in the world of primary health care.

Student Balint groups were studied by Torppa et al. (2008) in Finland. This was a qualitative study including two student groups with nine participants over 15 sessions. They found that the student groups discussed cases related to a wider range of problems than did groups for qualified doctors. The discussions often touched upon professional growth and future professional identity. They identified five triggers for presentations: witnessing injustice, value conflict, difficult human relations, incurable patients, and role confusion originating from the three contexts: patient encounters, confusing experiences in medical education, and tension between privacy and profession. Four main discussion themes were identified: feelings related to patients, building professional identity, negative role models, and co-operation with other medical professionals. These findings are very much in line with the findings of Risör, who made an extensive observation study with an anthropological perspective with interns in Denmark (Risör 2010). Their problems with uncertainty are considerable, but of a more global and contextual nature related to their being newcomers and guests in the hospital. Their problems are more often related to finding their place in the ward and with co-workers, rather than related to patients, which is different from the problems of experienced and established GPs.

This informs our view that Balint groups for students and very young doctors, although they may be very useful to the members, differ substantially from those for established GPs who have ongoing patient relationships and responsibilities. This opinion is in line with Michael Balint, writing: "… one of my earliest discoveries, that without the pressure of constant and on-going therapeutic responsibility, our method proved, as a rule, unsuccessful" (Balint et al. 1966, p. 34). However, he did modify this view in later life and started a group for students at University College Hospital in the 1960s.

Some interesting studies on leadership techniques have also been published, providing important information if we want to standardize the methods used in the groups we study (Johnson et al. 2004; Merenstein and Chillag 1999).

Thus far we have looked together at a range of research by others, primarily about residents and medical students. We have also tried to do so from an "impersonal" perspective. In the next section, Dorte Kjeldmand describes the three studies she carried out as parts of her Ph.D. thesis (Kjeldmand 2006) with her tutors Inger K. Holmström and Urban Rosenqvist on established GPs attending Balint groups, and she writes in the first person. This highlights the close connection between research in Balint groups and the personal experiences and commitment that often informs such research.

The Doctor, the Task and the Group

Dorte Kjeldmand writes: I am a GP, a Balint group leader (and member) and a researcher. My own Balint group membership has been a strong and important experience, which I want to share with as many colleagues as possible. In what follows I not only describe some research methods that are applicable to small groups, but also offer some reflections on the predicaments involved in doing research on activities to which you feel strongly attached and whose advantages you do not really doubt. This was my own point of departure and my journey was long and to some extent painful. The researcher's reflective process is essential to rigor in all research and Kirsti Malterud (2001) gave me important inspiration. According to Malterud, the researcher's declaration of preconceptions is mandatory. Hence I start by telling my "Balint-story."

I held the preconception that Balint groups are beneficial and that was my incentive to start my research. This view has become modified to some extent during the research process, as I have found that Balint groups are most often effective, but can sometimes have problems. Being a GP and Balint group leader made access to the informants easy for me in my research, and the interviews had more of the character of collegial dialogues than formal interviews. The informants shared in a very creditable way their experiences from their professional lives as general practitioners and Balint group leaders, including difficulties, worries, and mishaps. But, on the other hand, our shared experiences led to the risk of common blind spots and preconceptions preventing a full illumination of the subject. I asked for clarifications, examples, and negative aspects in an attempt to face up to this problem. I worked together with critical researchers who did not share my experiences and during the whole process I exposed my research to the scrutiny of other researchers from other professions.

Researchers try to say something objective about the topic of their study, but this does not always give you the "real-feel." So before I go into research (designs and outcomes), I describe here my own workplace-based Balint group back home in the provincial town of Eksjö, with 13,000 inhabitants in a rural part of southern Sweden.

The group started in 1993, has been working ever since, and is still going strong. It is situated at a primary health care center employing 10 specialist GPs, most of them working part-time, and between two and five interns and residents. I initiated the group myself after reading Balint's book, *The Doctor, His Patient and the Illness* (Balint 1964) as a young GP. I immediately understood that this was a method that would work for me and my colleagues. They accepted the idea and we knew of a psychiatrist who had been involved in the first Balint groups in Sweden in the 1970s. She agreed to be our group leader and to meet with us every 3 weeks, and so we started out. We met no hindrance from the management, and the nursing staff accepted that we should be left in peace when the group was meeting. These circumstances have been stable and the number of times we have been disturbed is negligible.

At the beginning we were four GPs and gradually we included the young, newly qualified specialists. For some time, we tried to include the residents, but had to stop because of their inability to attend regularly as a result of their commitments in other clinics. A more serious problem that made us decide not to include them was the presence of their tutors in the group. We found it necessary to allow the tutors free space to admit their own weaknesses and uncertainties without being inhibited by the presence of their pupils. Also, it could be difficult for the tutor not to judge the resident's contributions to the discussions. The residents now have a reflection group together with those from the adjacent health care centers, which I lead in my role as director of studies.

Gradually I took over the leadership of the group after having completed a 2-year education in Balint group leadership. The group meets for 2 hours every 4 weeks and the attendance is good, with everyone attending if they are at work. We work according to the traditional Balint method, although it is untraditional in that the leader is also a group member. When I want to present a case, one of the other seniors will take over the leadership. In one session we usually manage two new cases and some follow-up reports.

The members of our group have quite close professional relationships and some of us are personally close as well. It makes our group different from the original Balint model and many contemporary nonworkplace Balint groups where members almost never meet outside the group. What does that imply? I would answer: mostly advantages. The disadvantages are that discussions may not go so deeply into matters touching on private life. We have a married couple in the group and have found that some measures are necessary to handle that. When one of them knows that he or she will present a case, the partner will be asked to stay away from that particular meeting. But on the other hand, the trust that has developed throughout the years allows members sometimes to reveal very difficult situations where they have acted as doctors in quite questionable ways, and are painfully aware of it. And the trust emanating from the group work has created an open and egalitarian atmosphere at our center that affects everyone in every setting: doctors, nurses, and receptionists.

This applies particularly to the ideology of patient-centeredness that is inherent in the Balint group method. The group work helps us to implement this better in our clinical practice. Another advantage is the awareness of our colleagues' condition. Everybody is able to keep an eye on how the others are doing; we can observe whether they are showing signs of burnout or other hardship and, in that case, help to share the burden. It could be considered a disadvantage that the patient who is presented in the group is often known to other members, even though names are never mentioned. But it is also valuable for the doctor to learn that others may have very different experiences of the same patient. These intimate relations emphasize the need for confidentiality.

My perspective has been affected by the shared experience in our group over many years. To give an idea of how we work, Boxes 5.1 and 5.2 show examples of cases from our group with appropriate changes of details for confidentiality reasons.

Box 5.1 First Case

Harold:	I have had this old woman on my list for ages. She came to this town many years ago after having divorced her husband. She has three daughters. She smokes and has lung problems. She had breast cancer 5 or 10 years ago, and when she was at the hospital, the consultant called me because she was completely hysterical and asked me to come and talk to her. I did that and she calmed down. But the patient claims that, since this hospitalization, she has had a hospital anxiety and she refuses all kinds of investigations. At the same time she comes often with lots of different complaints: cough, bowel problems, weight loss, dizziness. She continues smoking, but has now moved to an apartment in a shelter for old people. Our contact is often by telephone because she is too weak to go out. In the last few weeks, her breathing problems have increased, and I wondered if they were caused by heart failure. It might be

(continued)

Box 5.1 (continued)

	metastases as well, or smoker's lungs. I wanted to hospital-ize her, but she refused. Probably, she is afraid of what they will find. Yesterday I made a home visit. She was really in a bad state and too weak to resist, so I sent her to the hos-pital. I feel a bit bad about that.
Leader:	You will remember that Harold has brought up this woman in the group many times before. Any questions to Harold? OK, we will let him stay out of the discussion for a while and listen in peace. What kind of feelings do you get from Harold's story?
Jim:	I think this is difficult, when you may miss a serious dis-ease because the patient refuses investigations and you don't know what will happen afterwards. Maybe the rela-tives will file a complaint against you for negligence. I feel afraid of that.
Sally:	Yes, and I wonder what the daughters say, whether Harold has contact with them. Maybe the patient does not want him to.
	(The group discusses this for a while.)
Dorothy:	I wonder what Harold feels about having tricked the patient into going into the hospital. He took advantage of her weakness, and it is comfortable for him to have her there and not having to care for her for a while.
	(Harold sighs, but remains silent.)
Mary (smiling):	Yes, it is convenient for him, but on the other hand, she has been evading the truth and it will be much easier for him to help her afterwards. So I guess he felt he still acted in the best interest of his patient.
Dorothy:	I recognize Harold's sadness from some of my own patient relationships, when they get old and sick, and you sort of feel really sad, as if they were real relatives and you don't want them to die, you are so close to them. The strange thing is that they may be some of the worst patients you ever had, but you mourn them really badly.
Leader:	Let's get Harold into the discussion now.

Harold confirms the feelings of uncertainty concerning the risk of miscon-duct, and that he in fact had had contact with one daughter; he put mild pres-sure on the patient who then gave him permission. He did feel badly about having taken advantage of the patient's weakness to get her admitted, but he knew he had to. It is true, she has always been quite burdensome but he always felt very close to her.

(continued)

Box 5.1 (continued)

The group talks for a while about these longstanding doctor–patient relationships that are sometimes on the edge of what is good for the doctor. How much of the doctor's time may one patient take up? They talk about this patient's loneliness and weakness, and how important the doctor had become. He may very well be the patient's only friend: how this fact makes it possible even for the patient to accept being sent to the hospital by Harold and nobody else. Maybe this hospitalization will be a good experience for the patient and it will be easier to go on in the future, as it broke up a treatment stalemate that was dangerous for the patient. It also brought in one of the daughters, thus diminishing the loneliness of the patient and the doctor's feeling that he was the only person in the world in this patient's life.

Box 5.2 Second Case

Leader:	Who's got a case?
Sally:	I have this young woman, I don't know if I'm doing right. I'm worried.
Leader:	Tell us!
Sally:	She's about 25, has two young kids and a husband. I'm not sure if he's OK; he's weird too. The woman is always complaining about pains, here and there, and minor illnesses and she wants sick leave all the time. I can't get really close to her, so I'm never certain if it is right to let her be off work or not. I mean, maybe she needs it in order to cope with the kids and her life, and the work is a bit heavy: she is a shop assistant. But maybe it is all wrong; maybe I just collaborate in a process which will end up in long sick leave and real disability and unemployment. And the kids, I don't know how they are doing, and the father's role in all this. I don't think I get any contact with him; he's so weird when he's here with the wife. (She falls silent.)
Leader:	Do tell us a bit more!
Sally:	I feel sorry for her, and sometimes also irritated. And very uncertain if I'm doing the right thing. I may destroy her life. And I'm afraid about the kids. (A heavy atmosphere settles in the group and everybody is quiet for a moment, contemplating the case and the worried colleague.)

(continued)

Box 5.2 (continued)

Leader:	Well, this feels heavy. Before the group starts working, does anybody want to ask Sally anything?
Jim:	Is she really ill?
Sally:	It's difficult to know. She acts strangely, sometimes as if she's very unwell, and sometimes all smiling, even when she says she is in pain.
Leader:	All right, we will let Sally sit a bit back for some time and the group can work on Jim's question. What does it feel like?
	(The group then talks for some time about how difficult it may be to understand how this patient really feels and what she wants from Sally, or what she is using the doctor for. The issue of sick-leave certificates is always a hot topic for GPs and their frustration is obvious. They discuss the risk of pacifying the patient by putting her on the sick-list and the uneasy feeling it gives to use this tool, whether it is a weapon for or against the patient. They also talk about the kids. Are they in trouble? Should the doctor react? This responsibility weighs heavily on the GPs' mind, highlighting the conflict of breaking the confidentiality by reporting to the social authorities on behalf of the children.)
	Then Harold says: I am quite certain that I know this patient.
Sally nods:	Yes I have seen in her card that she visited you sometimes with the kids.
Harold:	And with her mother, the kids' grandmother. She is my patient and has been for many years. And her mother too!
	(The group laughs and it suddenly feels easier.)
Harold:	I recognize the behavior Sally describes. Her mother was just the same and also the grandmother. And I have also seen how the patient and her mother behave together with the kids, and it felt right. Maybe it is not so bad after all.
Sally:	So it may be a way of living that runs in the family?
Dorothy:	And maybe it is not so important what you do in detail; the patient has learned how to live from her mother and grandmother.
Harold:	But I think she needs Sally anyway. To help her cope now and then.
Sally:	Then maybe I can be a bit more laid back. I guess that I cannot change her way, when it is inherited like that. But as long as she comes to me I can keep an eye on her and the kids. That may be a meaningful role for me.

In the research I carried out with my tutors, we made use of both quantitative and qualitative methods and studied both participants' and leaders' experiences. But the major difference from previous research is that the settings we chose were classic Balint groups in real life featuring ordinary GP specialists with long-term membership in the groups. The groups were spread over a large area of Sweden and had started in the ordinary way as described above. GPs gather around a leader and start a Balint group that goes on as long as practical circumstances allow it, and the members are sufficiently satisfied to be willing to spend time and money on it.

First Study: "Balint Training Makes GPs Thrive Better in Their Jobs"

In our first study, we set out to see whether experienced GPs participating in Balint groups differed from other GPs with regard to satisfaction with their work situation and their perceived competence in handling patients with psychosomatic problems (Kjeldmand et al. 2004). The members of existing Balint groups in the region of southeast Sweden were included together with a group of general practitioners from the same region with similar conditions, used as a reference group. An existing questionnaire was modified to fit the purpose of the study. There were 26 Balint group members with at least 1 year of Balint group experience who were recruited for the study. An equal number were recruited for the reference group. They were chosen intentionally to get a group resembling the study group concerning the size of workplace, rural/urban situation, and ordinary working conditions, meaning not too many vacancies and a similar management system (all participants were public employees). The physicians in the reference group never had any possibility of joining a Balint group.

We adapted an existing questionnaire from a working environment study previously performed in the area and used 30 of the items. We added six questions about psychosomatic issues and 13 about the doctor-patient relationship. The final questionnaire consisted of 49 questions in eight categories: *workload* (three questions), feeling of *control* of the working situation (11 questions), *satisfaction* and stimulation regarding work (six questions), estimation of the *quality* of one's own work (four questions), *co-operation* and support (five questions), ongoing *training* and education (four questions), work-related *health* (10 questions), and treating and dealing with *psychosomatic* patients (six questions). (The terms in italics are used later as labels for the various categories.)

The participants responded to each item in the questionnaire by rating their responses on a 10-point visual analogue scale (VAS) where 0=least favorable, and 10=most favorable. Differences between the groups' means were assessed with Student's *t*-test for unpaired data.

Of the 52 general practitioners allocated to the study, 41 responded: 20 Balint group participants and 21 in the reference group. We could validate the reference group by comparing their answers to the 30 borrowed items with the results from

Fig. 5.1 The mean results of the answers categorized in groups of the physicians with more than 1.5 years in a Balint group compared to the reference group, showing the results of the *t*-tests (* $p < 0.05$; ** $p < 0.01$; *** $p < 0.001$)

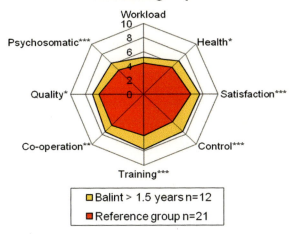

previous working environment studies, and it was considered representative of GPs in the region. The Balint group participants were split into two subgroups depending on the duration of their participation; physicians with more than 1.5 years in a Balint group were labeled experienced Balint group participants ($n = 12$).

The experienced Balint group participants had significantly higher scores than the reference physicians in all categories except *workload,* predominantly concerning a feeling of *control* in the working situation, *satisfaction*, and dealing with *psychosomatic* patients (see Fig. 5.1). Two specific items of interest where experienced Balint group participants scored significantly higher ($p < 0.005$) than the reference groups were: "Do you sometimes refer patients or take 'unnecessary' tests in order to terminate the consultation?" (indicating the doctor's frustration in the encounter), and "Do you have to deal with patients that do not 'belong' in the health care system?" (indicating the doctor's uncertainty about the patient's reason for coming).

The means of the total results of the Balint group participants with long and short experience and the reference group are displayed in Fig. 5.2.

Second Study: "Balint Groups for General Practitioners: A Qualitative Study. A Means to Increase Job Satisfaction and Prevent Burnout?"

In our following study, we interviewed nine GPs who participated in six different Balint groups (Kjeldmand and Holmström 2008). They made up a varied sample for gender (four women, five men), age (43–60 years), professional experience, and geographical setting. They participated in six different Balint groups led by six different

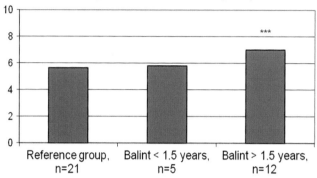

Fig. 5.2 Mean total results of all the questions answered on the VAS scale, 0 least favorable, 10 most favorable, showing improvement, not significant in a short time, but clearly significant after long participation in Balint group (*** $p<0.001$)

leaders. They had permanent employment and at least 3 years experience as specialized general practitioners. Their Balint group experience varied from 3 to 15 years (mean 8 years). The interviews were analyzed using a phenomenological method. As in our first study, we also wanted to investigate the effect of Balint participation from a working environment perspective, in addition to the effect on the physicians' experienced achievements in the relationships with their patients. Much bad feeling and exhaustion reported by physicians in primary health care arises from the burden of frustration and feeling of responsibility for the patients' health, which is multiplied by the complex uncertainty of the wide range of problems presented to the GPs.

In the interviews with the GPs, we found some quite amazing reports about the ways they had found to carry them through the hardships of their work. They described the Balint group as a safe and stable place to which they could bring their troubles and uncertainties. Gradually, they increased their understanding of what went on in their consultations with the patients and how they managed to exert more control. They felt they had learned to steer safely between the Scylla and Charybdis of doctoring: cynicism and, on the other hand, emotional over-involvement in the patients' suffering. This happened through a process in which they increased their competence in the meetings, enhanced their professional identity, and found a sense of security, which increased through parallel processes between the GP and the group and the GP and the patients. In the Balint group, they created a base of endurance and satisfaction enabling them to rediscover the joy of being physicians. Many Balint members told us how the atmosphere in the consultation room changes the moment the thought rises in the GP's mind: "This is difficult, but I can take it to the Balint group," or "I wonder what the Balint group would have said about this?" One GP said, "When it gets really hard in a meeting with a patient, I can imagine having the Balint group in the room with me, and then I feel much safer, and I can do what I need to do."

Third Study: "Difficulties in Balint Groups: A Qualitative Study of Leaders' Experiences"

This enthusiasm had to be scrutinized critically as no method is so good that it is without drawbacks, and we wondered if there could be people who were hurt in Balint groups. The mere fact that Balint groups are so few might be an indication of this, or at least that there are some difficulties in managing the activity. To explore this question we interviewed eight Balint group leaders from five countries, the United States, Israel, Sweden, Denmark, and the United Kingdom, about their experiences of Balint group leadership, specifically focusing on difficulties and problems in the groups (Kjeldmand and Holmström 2010). We asked them to tell the stories of the "dropouts" they had had.

Three categories of difficulties emerged from the analysis:

The individual participant: Individual GPs had their own needs, vulnerabilities, and defenses. Everybody is part of a complex psychosocial system that in many ways interferes with Balint group participation. These range from practicalities such as the place of residence and working hours of the spouse, to more or less severe personal problems, disabilities, or psychological vulnerabilities. In times of turbulence in the participant's own life, such as illness or other traumas, the personal vulnerability to issues arising in the group was increased. Issues of members' cultural background were mentioned that could have both positive and negative implications. It was also clear that people dropped out because they simply did not like the method; they did not think that the method satisfied their needs and were looking for other ways of learning. They would often ask for more practical advice and instructions.

The group and the leader: Leaders acknowledged their central role as the keeper of boundaries and rules, of which confidentiality was one of the most important, while creating a safe environment in which the members could talk freely. Leaders tried to balance their interventions, but sometimes somebody was hurt. The Balint group was shown to be as susceptible to the same subversions as other groups, and stories of rivalry, hidden agendas, and scapegoats were told. Hierarchical relations could lie behind these events. Sometimes members simply did not like each other. No leader practiced "mutual selection interviews."

The surroundings: The environment greatly affected a group and its ability to exist and work. Society's economic, cultural, and political state together with the biomedical health care paradigm constituted a rather hostile setting, against which the Balint group had to fight. Often, GPs ended their participation because of lack of time and had no incentive in their work situation or staff management that pushed them to continue. Some leaders who had obligatory Balint group for residents experienced difficulties with the processes in the groups, particularly when there were conflicts in the relationship between the resident and the faculty.

These findings correspond well with theories on small groups as complex systems as presented by Arrow et al. (2000) and Girard's (1986) theories on the scapegoat process.

This is only a brief account of the studies that I successfully submitted for my Ph.D. thesis. The results speak for themselves but three points are worth emphasizing. First, the doctors in the quantitative study were drawn from different regions of Sweden and those in the reference group had not had the possibility of joining a Balint group, thus enhancing the rigor of the results. Next, there is clear evidence to support the idea that doctors vary a good deal in their capacity to benefit from a Balint group. In addition, it does seem from our research that qualitative studies give a more accurate picture of how and why group participation is beneficial for some doctors.

Conclusion

From this short survey of 60 years research on the Balint group method and its effects, one can cautiously summarize the likely benefits of group participation for at least some of the participants (and some more than others). A group provides a space for physicians where, together, they can explore their relationships with individual patients. The safe and stable milieu enables them to be open about their uncertainty and doubts. By trying to understand their own emotions they can better understand what goes on in their encounters with patients, especially those with ill-defined conditions. These situations often lead to inappropriate referrals and tests, but Balint-trained doctors may resist this to a higher degree. They develop a better control of what goes on in the consultation, leading to a better work environment.

In the Balint group, both young and old doctors search for and often find the core of primary care and this leads to greater professional self-esteem and joy in work. The Balint group helps to unburden the doctors of bad feelings and troublesome experiences that might lead to burnout; in the group's collegial atmosphere, the doctor can find comfort and tolerance. This may be even more efficient in workplace groups where this atmosphere may spread outside the group both in time and space, to include the other professionals on the team. Balint groups have been shown to offer receptive members a better capacity to tolerate uncertainty and an increased ability to empathize with patients.

But the challenge to researchers in the future is to discover whether the doctor's participation in a Balint group has a measurable effect on their patients. Do the patients experience any difference? Do they get healthier? Are their lives more fulfilled? Are Balint groups better than other groups? Or is it the case that doctors have different individual needs for education and professional maintenance?

The problems inherent in Balint studies are also experienced by those trying to draw valid conclusions from research on psychological and psychodynamic therapies, social studies, and educational methods. They all involve individual human differences that resist being firmly assigned to different categories. The same difficulties would apply to studies on other forms of case discussion in small groups, such as the ones described in other chapters of this book. Although all these groups have slightly different aims and theoretical backgrounds, it may be that they have more in common than we think.

There is now a widely held view in psychotherapy that the theoretical orientation of the therapist is less important than his or her personal and professional qualities (Hubble et al. 1999). It may be that all case discussion groups have the same power to enhance personal and professional growth through the strengths that they share. They all provide a feeling of community and shared experience; a friendly space where members can talk freely about their work, including voicing their doubts and fears; an opportunity to learn from one's peers; and the knowledge that the group will continue for a period of years. Some group members will thrive on this kind of education, some will find it moderately useful, and others will find it of little use and reject it. Nevertheless, there may be a majority coalition of those for whom it is significantly helpful. Perhaps if small group enthusiasts of different persuasions could set aside their concern with theoretical differences and concentrate on what they have in common, more meaningful research might follow.

References

Arrow, H., McGrath, J., & Berdahl, J. (2000). *Small groups as complex systems*. London: Sage.

Balint, M. (1964). *The doctor, his patient and the illness* (2nd ed.). London: Pitman Medical.

Balint, E., & Norell, J. S. (Eds.). (1973). *Six minutes for the patient: Interactions in general practice consultations*. London: Tavistock Publications.

Balint, M., Balint, E., Gosling, R., et al. (1966). *A study of doctors*. London: Tavistock Publications.

Balint, E., Courtenay, M., Elder, E., et al. (1993). *The doctor, the patient and the Balint group revisited*. London/New York: Routledge.

Cataldo, K. P., Peeden, K., Geesey, M. E., et al. (2005). Association between Balint training and physician empathy and work satisfaction. *Family Medicine, 37*(5), 328–31.

Elder, A., & Samuel, O. (Eds.). (1987). *While I'm here, doctor*. London: Tavistock/Routledge.

Girard, R. (1986). *The scapegoat*. Baltimore: The John Hopkins University Press.

Hubble, M. A., Duncan, B. L., & Miller, S. D. (Eds.). (1999). *The heart and soul of change: What works in psychotherapy*. Washington, DC: American Psychological Association.

Huygen, F. J. A., et al. (1992). Relationship between the working styles of general practitioners and the health status of their patients. *The British Journal of General Practice: The Journal of the Royal College of General Practitioners, 42*, 141–144.

Johnson, A. H., Brock, C. D., & Hueston, W. J. (2003). Resident physicians who continue Balint training: A longitudinal study 1982–1999. *Family Medicine, 35*(6), 428–433.

Johnson, A. H., Nease, D. E., Jr., Milberg, L. C., et al. (2004). Essential characteristics of effective Balint group leadership. *Family Medicine, 36*(4), 253–259.

Kjeldmand, D. (2006). Thesis: *The doctor, the task and the group, Balint groups as a means of developing new understanding in the physician-patient relationship*. Department of Public Health and Caring Science, Section of Health Services Research, Uppsala University, Sweden.

Kjeldmand, D., & Holmström, I. (2008). Balint groups for general practitioners – A qualitative study. A means to increase job satisfaction and prevent burnout? *Annals of Family Medicine, 6*, 138–145.

Kjeldmand, D., & Holmström, I. (2010). Difficulties in Balint groups: A qualitative study of leaders' experiences. *The British Journal of General Practice: The Journal of the Royal College of General Practitioners, 60*, 808–14.

Kjeldmand, D., Holmström, I., & Rosenqvist, U. (2004). Balint training makes GPs thrive better in their job. *Patient Education and Counseling, 55*, 230–35.

Malterud, K. (2001). Qualitative research: Standards, challenges, and guidelines. *Lancet, 358,* 483–488.

Margalit, A., Glick, S., Benbassat, J., et al. (2005). Promoting a biopsychosocial orientation in family practice: Effect of two teaching programs on the knowledge and attitudes of practicing primary care physicians. *Medical Techcher (Stuttgart), 27,* 613–618.

Merenstein, J. H., & Chillag, K. (1999). Balint seminar leaders: What do they do? *Family Medicine, 31,* 182–186.

Musham, C., & Brock, C. D. (1994). Family practice residents' perspective on Balint group training: In-depth interviews with frequent and infrequent attenders. *Family Medicine, 26,* 382–386.

Pinder, R., McKee, A., Sackin, P., et al. (2006). Talking about my patient: The Balint approach in GP education. *Occasional Paper, Royal College of General Practitioners, 87,* 1–32.

Risör T. (2010). *Why don't we take a look at the patient? An anthropological analysis of how doctors become doctors.* Ph.D. dissertation, Faculty of Health Sciences, Aarhus University.

Salinsky, J., & Sackin, P. (2000). *What are you feeling, doctor?* Abingdon: Radcliffe Medical Press.

Torppa, M. A., Makkonen, E., Mårtenson, C., et al. (2008). A qualitative analysis of student Balint groups in medical education: Contexts and triggers of case presentations and discussion themes. *Patient Education and Counseling, 72,* 5–11.

Turner, A. L., & Malm, R. L. (2004). A preliminary investigation of Balint and non-Balint behavioural medicine training. *Family Medicine, 36,* 114–7.

Chapter 6
The Thistle and the Maple Leaf: Practice-Based Small-Group Learning in Canada and Scotland

Heather Armson and Ronald MacVicar

Introduction

Family physicians work in a complex practice environment that requires the practitioner to balance patient-centred care with evidence-based practice. Uncertainty is inherent in this as research evidence is neither generally directed at primary care issues nor straightforward to apply in the multidimensional practice environment. It is rare that clinical decisions about diagnosis or treatment can be made with absolute certainty.

Continuing medical education (CME) has traditionally been focused primarily on the dissemination of new research information, but new information is only helpful to patients to the extent that it can be applied to clinical practice. 'For practicing physicians, knowing is simply a prelude to applying that knowledge to patient management problems' (Premi 1994). Unfortunately, traditional approaches to CME including didactic large-group sessions have been shown to be ineffective in changing physician practice. New approaches are needed that incorporate interactive strategies that have been shown to change behaviour including reflection on practice, discussion of evidence in the context of actual patient cases with peers, feedback on performance, opportunities to practise newly learned skills and a focus on integration of new knowledge into the practice environment (Davis et al. 1999).

H. Armson (✉)
Department of Family Medicine, University of Calgary, 2685 36 St NE,
Calgary T1Y 5S3, AB, Canada
e-mail: armson@ucalgary.ca

R. MacVicar
NHS Education for Scotland, Centre for Health Science, Old Perth Road,
Inverness IV2 3JH, United Kingdom
e-mail: ronald.macvicar@nes.scot.nhs.uk

L.S. Sommers and J. Launer (eds.), *Clinical Uncertainty in Primary Care: The Challenge of Collaborative Engagement*, DOI 10.1007/978-1-4614-6812-7_6,
© Springer Science+Business Media New York 2013

Box 6.1 An Overview of PBSGL

Key Components of the PBSGL Programme

- The process – a facilitated small-group discussion focused on:

  - Practice reflection
  - Identification of gaps between current practice and best practice
  - Strategies to enhance change in practice
  - Commitment to practice change

- Trained peer facilitators who:

  - Are chosen by their group
  - Are trained in a 1-day workshop conducted by experienced facilitator trainers
  - Play a vital role in the enduring success of PBSGL

- The content – evidence-based educational modules that:

  - Present specific representative patient cases that stimulate participants in the small groups to reflect on similar cases from their own practices.
  - Summarise relevant best available evidence relevant to primary care practice.
  - Promote application of scientific knowledge to the specific patient problems members encounter in their practices, resulting in improved patient care.

- The development and sustenance of a community of practice that

  - Is consistent with educational theory
  - Is borne out by the function and longevity of groups

The Practice-Based Small-Group Learning (PBSGL) programme is an example of a successful international programme that is focused on facilitating discussions between peers who understand the context in which patient care is practised. This enables a focus on real problems in practice and the challenge of integrating evidence-based care with the uncertain problems with which patients present. This chapter will explore the development of the programme, the theoretical underpinnings and the lessons learned in the process.

Practice-based learning is derived from problem-based learning and represents an attempt to drive learning into day-to-day practice (MacVicar 2003; Armson et al. 2007). It is based upon a peer-facilitated small-group learning format where groups meet to discuss practice issues supported by evidence-based educational modules. PBSGL involves a delicate balance between two equally important elements: the evidence-based content and the process within the peer-facilitated small group (Box 6.1).

The Small Groups

PBSGL groups have approximately the same format wherever the programme takes place. Groups of four to ten family physicians self-select to form a peer-learning group. Groups usually meet in their own communities for 1½–2 hours, once or twice a month. There is no standard model for group formation. Some groups form around a group practice or clinic facility allowing learning to be shared and change in practice managed within a single organisation. Other small groups form amongst friends or acquaintances with the advantage that differing experiences and viewpoints can be brought to the discussion from a variety of perspectives and organisations. Although the most prevalent model is one of family physicians learning together, many groups include other health professions, mainly, but not exclusively, nurses and nurse practitioners including some groups made up solely from these practitioners. Although new groups continually form and existing groups reconfigure, many groups have met together for many years (see Fig. 6.1).

The facilitator will address common group issues at the start of the first group meeting including ground rules and expectations for group function. This discussion includes outlining the process role of the facilitator and the importance of reflection, including the completion of the practice reflection tool (PR-CTC). The facilitator will also explain how modules are developed and organised with a discussion on how the group will choose modules to be covered during their sessions. The importance of reading the modules before the meeting will be emphasised by the facilitator to enable reflection prior to the meeting to include identification of the participants' own cases that are relevant. Finally, a process for covering topics for which a module has not yet been developed is also explored.

Case-based discussion, using the educational modules, facilitates active reflection on clinical practice. Pivotal to this reflective process is the discussion of participants' own patient cases and practice challenges. Group discussion encourages members to share their experiences and to consider strategies to implement changes in practice and how barriers to those practice changes may be addressed.

Trained Facilitators

Each group includes a trained peer facilitator chosen by the group. The facilitator is trained in a 1-day workshop conducted by experienced facilitator trainers. The workshop provides the new facilitator with individual opportunities to lead a small

Fig. 6.1 Participant time in Canadian PBSGL programme (2010)

Time in PBSGL Programme	Percentage of members
<1 year	12%
1-5 years	24%
6-10 years	26%
>10 years	38%

group using the PBSGL modules and with feedback around managing group process issues.

The facilitator is one of the key elements of the programme that plays a vital role in the enduring success of PBSGL. The role of the facilitator is to develop an atmosphere that encourages participants to identify their learning needs, to examine their current practice and to explore the application of new knowledge into practice. Although the facilitators are not content experts, they are 'practice experts' familiar with issues common to their peers in the group. The effectiveness of the learning group depends on the willingness of participants to identify, acknowledge and share gaps between current practice and best practice including errors that may result from these gaps. These candid discussions will only occur if a safe environment has been developed by the facilitator.

Facilitators are trained to link the discussion to participants' practice. References to cases and challenges are interspersed throughout the meeting starting from the group discussion of the practice gaps at the beginning of the meeting. Subsequently, after cases are read, participants are encouraged to articulate the commonality between the cases presented in the module and those in their practices. These discussions usually serve to focus participants on their learning needs as they relate to actual practice cases or specific identified challenges.

Educational Modules

Each PBSGL meeting is focused on a specific topic with an evidence-based educational module providing the substrate for discussion. The modules are built around an identified gap in current practice. Each group collectively decides on a topic for discussion from a list of available modules based on member interest, patient challenges or identified learning needs. For each module, groups are encouraged to compare the learning objectives presented in the module to their own learning needs. Each member is expected to have read the information section of the module prior to the meeting, thereby preventing discussion from being content focused rather than practice focused. They typically require at least 90 minutes to complete. Some modules may require more than one session depending on the needs and interests of the group.

Sample modules can be viewed on http://www.gpcpd.nes.scot.nhs.uk/pbsgl or http://www.fmpe.org. Each module follows a consistent format that consists of six elements:

1. *Introduction.* The introduction is not 'just' an introduction to the topic; rather, it is the all-important foundation for the subsequent content of the module and the group discussion, leading to a desired change in practice. The introduction attempts to engage the learner and present the topic as relevant to him or her by explicitly identifying the gap between current practice and best or better practice. The introduction also outlines the objectives for the module. Great care and much time are taken in the module production process on the introduction.

2. *Case materials and stimulus questions.* The cases are authentic practice cases. Together with the stimulus questions that follow each case, they are provided to highlight the gap in practice described in the introduction. The cases are not primarily provided as a substrate for problem-solving by the group, although in the absence of group members being able to draw on their own cases, this may be the result. Rather the aim is to use the provided cases as a scaffold or stimulus for members to draw on their own experiences of similar cases, to ensure that the discussion and the resulting learning is based in practice rather than an abstract problem-solving exercise.

3. *Information section.* The information section is not a thorough systematic review of the topic; rather, it represents a distillation of the best evidence, available at the time of writing relevant to the module topic. The focus is on providing information to bridge the gap identified in the introduction. Emphasis is placed on issues that are of particular relevance to primary care and referencing with levels of evidence related to best practice recommendations are made explicit.

4. *Case commentaries.* The commentaries are linked to the cases presented in the module but are not 'the answers'. Rather they present one possible approach to the presented cases and serve to illustrate practical ways of applying the information presented in the information section.

5. *References.* The source material that supports the information section is made explicit by a full reference list.

6. *Appendices.* Appropriate practical tools to support change in practice are provided as appendices, including algorithms, chart aids, patient information leaflets and guides to resources.

Extracts from a single module 'Hypothyroidism in Adults' are used throughout the next part of this chapter to illustrate the content, structure and use of the modules.

At the conclusion of each group meeting, a Practice Reflection/Commitment to Change (PR-CTC) tool (see Fig. 6.2) is used to guide members to reflect on the discussion and explicitly to commit to changing practice or reinforcing current practice. The main purpose of the tool is as a structured tool for promoting reflection on the topic and for identifying plans for practice change. A secondary purpose is to capture data important for the group, including the module discussed, date and length of meeting, module rating and any unanswered questions.

Within the group, members endeavour to identify specific barriers to these proposed changes and to formulate implementation strategies to facilitate desired changes. Groups that are based within practice communities may choose to develop consensus on the desired changes and the strategies that are required to facilitate their implementation. More often, however, group members will develop individual plans for change as they reflect on their own needs that have been clarified throughout the group discussion.

Often the facilitator will document statements within several of the boxes in the commitment-to-change component of the PR-CTC tool (see Fig. 6.2) depending on the responses to the particular topic, its relevance to their practice and their

We <u>will change</u> our current practice in the following way: ->	The barrier(s) that we are anticipating include the following:
We are <u>considering</u> making the following changes to our current practice? ->	What would enable us to change our current practice?
These current practice(s) were confirmed: ->	What supports my current practice?
We are <u>not convinced</u> there is a need to change our current practice because:	

Fig. 6.2 The commitment-to-change section of the PR-CTC instrument

readiness to commit to making a change in practice. The role of the facilitator in this discussion is to ensure that all participants consider the impact of the preceding discussion in the context of their individual practices and look for ways to implement the insights generated by the meeting. Once commitments are made, the facilitator encourages further discussion about barriers to and enablers for the identified change(s) using the experience of the group as a whole to generate strategies to enhance the likelihood of implementation.

Ideally a date is set to review the PR-CTC, usually after 3–4 months, often at the beginning of a subsequent meeting. During this review, the group members' experiences are discussed, focusing on successful implementation of proposed practice changes or barriers that prevented successful change. The group is encouraged to explore further specific practice changes, and an implementation plan is developed.

A Glimpse into a PBSGL Meeting

Content and process are brought together in the PBSGL meeting. At each meeting the facilitator initiates the discussion about the current topic by presenting the practice gap identified by the module authors and enquiring as to the validity of the identified gap for the group members. As an illustration, the introduction to the 'Hypothyroidism in Adults' module produced in 2010 is reproduced in Box 6.2.

> **Box 6.2** Hypothyroidism Module
>
> **Introduction**
>
> Hypothyroidism is one of the most common endocrine disorders in primary care. Its management may seem less than straightforward, particularly in pregnancy or when symptoms persist despite appropriate treatment. The good news is that most patients can be successfully treated when a tailored, evidence-based approach is readily at hand.
>
> **Practice Challenges**
>
> - Investigations: For patients presenting with vague symptoms suggestive of possible hypothyroidism, which investigations are appropriate and why?
> - Treatment: What is the optimal approach to medication?
> - Monitoring: How (and how frequently) should patients be monitored?
> - Hypothyroidism in pregnancy: What is the best management approach?
>
> **This Module Is Intended to Help You**
>
> - Clarify the investigations for hypothyroidism;
> - Provide an overview of pharmacotherapy;
> - Highlight the recommendations for ongoing monitoring;
> - Review the management of hypothyroidism in pregnancy.

Additional goals for the group session based on additional gaps are often established at this point. Facilitators will often 'check in' with the group to see if anything in the module was confusing or surprising and needs to be clarified. Examples from groups' feedback on the 'Hypothyroidism in Adults' module include:

> None of the group was aware of the real detriment to both mother and baby in early pregnancy if the mother was hypothyroid.

> Highlighted areas such as temporary thyroiditis that naturally resolved that most of us had forgotten about.

> With changing GP roles in ante-natal care we need to ensure with our colleague midwives that management of hypothyroidism in pregnancy is optimal.

Typically, the group will decide which patient case to discuss first, and often one member will read the first case out loud to focus the attention of the group. The facilitator will check to ensure this is a representative case and enquire whether there are other nuances or issues that need to be addressed. This is often the time that a member of the group identifies a case of their own that is similar to the one selected. The discussion around the case is aided by the use of the stimulus questions provided in the module or by other questions the facilitator feels are relevant to meet the learning needs of the group. To illustrate, one case from the 'Hypothyroidism in Adults' module is reproduced in Box 6.3.

Box 6.3 Case Material from 'Hypothyroidism in Adults' Module

Mary K, female, 61 years old.

Part 1. Mary is a woman in excellent health. She has no chronic illnesses and takes only a multivitamin and a calcium supplement on a regular basis. She sees you with complaints of weight gain and constipation. She denies other symptoms.

What would be your approach to assessment?

Part 2. On further questioning, Mary remembers that she has had a persistent feeling of fullness in her neck but no local pain. Her physical examination revealed dry coarse skin and delayed relaxation phase of the deep tendon reflexes. Her thyroid feels normal in size, is non-tender and there were no lumps. Her thyroid-stimulating hormone level was 10 mU/L (normal 0.4–3.0 mU/L).

Would you consider additional investigations and if so, why?

Part 3. Follow-up results are as follows:

T4: 10.9 pmol/L (normal: 10–22 pmol/L)
TSH: 10.2 mU/L (normal: 0.4–3.0 mU/L)
Antithyroid peroxidase antibodies: 78 kIU/L (normal: 0–60 kIU/L),
Antithyroid globulin: 90 kIU/L (normal: 0–60 kIU/L)
ESR: 12.

What would be your approach now?

The facilitator is trained to centre the discussion on current practice, with a focus on identifying gaps, the knowledge needed to bridge those gaps, and discussion of strategies and barriers to implementing new knowledge into practice.

As the discussion proceeds, reference is made, as appropriate, to the numbered points in the information section as well as to the appendices and tables that comprise the module. Throughout the meeting, the facilitator focuses the discussion on the information needed to address the clinical issues and encourages the group to make the connection between the case under discussion and cases that occur in their practice setting. To illustrate, extracts from the information section of the 'Hypothyroidism in Adults' module is presented in Box 6.4.

Box 6.4 Extracts from the Information Section of the 'Hypothyroidism in Adults' Module

The Information Section in this module is organised into 35 numbered paragraphs, three tables and one figure in six sections. To illustrate, the first numbered paragraph in each section is copied below

(continued)

Box 6.4 (continued)

Background

1. Prevalence of overt hypothyroidism ranges from 0.1% to 5% (even higher in select populations like the elderly). It is 5–8 times more common in women than in men, and seen more frequently in women with a small body size both at birth and during childhood.

Symptoms and Signs

7. The clinical presentation of hypothyroidism varies with the individual. 'Classical' signs and symptoms may include:

- Fatigue and weakness
- Cold intolerance
- Weight gain
- Constipation
- Dry skin, brittle nails, coarse hair
- Periorbital oedema that obscures the curve of the malar bone
- Enlargement of tongue
- Depression
- Memory, cognitive and sleep disturbances
- Menstrual irregularities, infertility

Screening

9. Although some guidelines recommend routine screening for hypothyroidism, most evidence-based sources indicate that there is *insufficient* evidence that 'treatment improves clinically important outcomes in adults with screen-detected thyroid disease.' Routine testing of thyroid function is *not* recommended in asymptomatic adults. It is recommended that 'clinicians maintain a high index of suspicion' and investigate at-risk patients with vague symptoms which could be related to thyroid dysfunction.

Diagnosis

10. TSH and T4 are the recommended initial tests for suspected primary hypothyroidism. [Level III, Expert Opinion]

(a) TSH has a high sensitivity (98%) and specificity (92%) for confirming thyroid disease.
(b) TSH is a poor indicator of the clinical severity of hypothyroidism. Some patients with low levels of thyroid hormones may have mild symptoms; others with less pronounced biochemical results may be more symptomatic.

(continued)

Box 6.4 (continued)

(c) In addition, different TSH assays use antibodies that recognise different epitopes of TSH and different forms of TSH are present in the circulation. As a consequence, it is difficult to reach agreement about a single common value for the upper reference limit of TSH.

(d) Consultation with a specialist to interpret TSH results may be indicated for patients taking certain medications that can alter thyroid function.

(e) It is the responsibility of the requesting physician to provide clinical information to guide the laboratory in the selection of the most appropriate TFT but if clinical details are not available that allow the identification of the above categories of patient, then it may be prudent for laboratories to measure serum TSH and FT4 on all specimens rather than embark on a first-line serum TSH testing strategy followed by a cascade to include FT4 and FT3 if indicated.

Management (Includes Subsections on Thyroxine Replacement Therapy, Monitoring and Persistent Symptoms: What to Do?)

16. The average replacement dose of synthetic levothyroxine is 1.6–1.8 mcg/kg/day, which generally results in a dose of 75–125 mcg/day for women and 125–200 mcg/day for men. This dose may be appropriate as the starting dose in healthy patients with no significant co-morbidities and mild to moderate hypothyroidism (TSH concentrations of 10–50 mU/L). However, in elderly patients or those with co-morbidities (e.g., cardiovascular disease), a suitable starting dose may range from 25 to 50 mcg/day.

Pregnancy: Unique Management Issues

30. For hypothyroidism diagnosed before pregnancy:

(a) The levothyroxine dose should be adjusted to attain a TSH no higher than 2.5 mU/L prior to conception [Grade of Recommendation Inconclusive, poor quality evidence].

(b) A TSH test is indicated as soon as pregnancy is confirmed.

(c) Levothyroxine dosage may need to be increased as much as 30–50% by 4–6 weeks gestation [Level I Evidence]. 'Some authorities have suggested immediate increases in dose upon diagnosing pregnancy to avoid sequelae of hypothyroidism.' However, there is some evidence that supra-optimal levothyroxine therapy may have adverse effects, so other authorities have expressed caution against routinely increasing the dose of the levothyroxine until results of thyroid function testing are available. Further data is needed to confirm which is the safest and the most effective approach.

The facilitator will guide the discussion to ensure it is practice focused and will use a number of facilitative techniques throughout the discussion to enhance the practice integration including questioning, summarising, identification of different viewpoints, stimulating discussion of areas unexplored by the group and challenging the integration of evidence-based content into day-to-day uncertain and undifferentiated practice.

An example of connections from the presented cases to a 'real' case from their practice from a group member's feedback on the 'Hypothyroidism in Adults' module included the following comment:

> One member described a case of delayed diagnosis [of hypothyroidism] in early pregnancy and potential sequelae in terms of foetal health. He is going to write this up as a significant event and share with group members.

This excerpt captures not only the connection to a case that meant something to the group member but also a commitment to change practice and generalise the learning through a significant event auditing process.

Once a case has been thoroughly discussed, the group may review the case commentary to identify any further issues that may be important to the discussion that have not been explored. As an example, the commentary related to Mary K (see Box 6.4) from the 'Hypothyroidism in Adults' module is presented in Box 6.5.

Box 6.5 Case Commentary from the 'Hypothyroidism in Adults' Module

Case 1: Mary K, female, 61 years old

Part 1 *What would be your approach to assessment?*
A detailed history and physical examination would identify symptoms and signs to help clarify the diagnosis or to provide additional symptoms or signs of hypothyroidism. Maintaining a low threshold for considering hypothyroidism in patients of Mary's age group is recommended, as prevalence of hypothyroidism increases in women at this age. TSH would be the recommended screening test.

Part 2 *Would you consider additional investigations? And if so why?*
Her symptoms suggest hypothyroidism. Based on her history, it is possible that she is suffering from chronic lymphocytic thyroiditis (Hashimoto's thyroiditis), despite her normal neck examination. Testing her thyroid antibodies would help to clarify her diagnosis. Since her TSH is only mildly elevated, a determination of free T4 would help to rule out central hypothyroidism.

Part 3 *What would be your approach now?*
A starting dose of 50 mcg of thyroxine would be appropriate for a patient with overt primary hypothyroidism. If she was younger with no underlying disease, a starting dose of 1.6–1.8 mcg/kg would be reasonable. In the hypothyroid phase of thyroiditis, a recommended starting dose is low (25–50 mcg/day) with gradual titration based on TSH to an average daily dosage of 75–150 mcg/day.

(continued)

> **Box 6.5** (continued)
>
> She would be monitored every 6–8 weeks, with an increase in dose if her TSH were not within target range. A target of 3.0 may be appropriate for Mary. Once Mary's TSH is stable, annual monitoring would be appropriate. Ideally, she would remain on the same formulation of thyroxine. It would be important not to over treat as this *may* increase her risk for bone loss.

The discussion then moves on the next case. Most modules have three and occasionally four cases. If time is limited, the group may choose to skip a particular case if it does not reflect issues that are important to the group.

Approximately 15 minutes prior to the end of the session, the facilitator will shift the discussion to the completion of the PR-CTC tool (see Fig. 6.2). The tool is typically completed within the group setting with all members contributing. The members are asked to consider the questions listed in the PR-CTC tool. Individual members may choose one or more of the categories to complete. Often in groups that are formed within a practice setting, this will be the time when a consensus about changes within the practice setting will be established. Examples of individual and group change statements from groups' feedback on the 'Hypothyroidism in Adults' module include:

I will check TFTs [thyroid function tests] on day of consultation for patients who are pregnant that are attending to announce their pregnant state.

I will discuss hypothyroid pregnant patients with the midwife.

We will check TFTs in postpartum depressed patients.

We will be more aware of how other medication and food influences thyroxine absorption and advise patients accordingly about taking thyroxine on an empty stomach.

The meeting concludes by clarifying questions that were generated during the session and determining if the questions will be explored by group members prior to the next meeting as well as the planning for subsequent meetings. Examples of unanswered questions from groups' feedback on the 'Hypothyroidism in Adults' module include:

Does TSH rise in a normal pregnancy?

How frequently should TFTs [thyroid function tests] be monitored in pregnancy?

Does thyroxine dose requirement decrease with increasing age?

It was clear from the PR-CTC tool that a named group member had been tasked with researching the answer to each question and within a specified time frame.

At future group meetings, the facilitator will start the PBSGL meeting by clarifying issues remaining from previous sessions including questions raised for follow-up and review of previous PR-CTC statements.

History

Beginnings in Canada

In 1986, a group of eight family physicians met every 2 weeks with a peer tutor to discuss challenging clinical cases from their practices as a stimulus for discussion and as substrate for learning. This study was developed after several years of experimentation with a weekly rounds format that explored strategies to enhance the relevance of educational programmes to the unique family medicine context. A number of important issues were identified in the process of this evolving educational programme which focused on weekly case presentations by family physicians. The educational issues identified included the importance of recognising the family medicine context, the need for evidence-based information, the importance of a forum to exchange ideas with others in similar practices and the development, over time, of comfort in discussing difficult cases with peers (Premi 1974). The continual refinement of this programme culminated in the development of this research study.

This group of family physicians were drawn from 11 responses to 250 invitations to participate in a feasibility study at McMaster University in Hamilton, Ontario. The study aimed to assess the effectiveness and feasibility of a problem-based, self-directed approach to continuing medical education (CME) for family physicians. The meetings had an explicit focus on adult learning principles with participants using current knowledge and previous experience to integrate new knowledge into practice through facilitated discussion with peers.

Clinical cases were discussed to identify problems, which in turn were explored to distil a number of specific questions. These questions were then resolved with a literature search focussed on new, critically appraised review articles, and a summary was presented at a subsequent meeting or, alternatively a specialist was asked to attend. Participants reported that the process was a useful approach to CME, and the conclusion of this feasibility study was that this form of learning would be a viable approach to CME provision. Participants highlighted in particular the benefit of sharing problems and solutions with peers and the importance of considering individual patient management within their specific clinical environment:

> The complexity of illnesses in the community, the typical failure of these illnesses to conform to traditional medical formulations, the need for frequent improvisations managing clinical problems, and the uncertainty such challenges create were frequent topics of group discussion. Aware that others in their group experienced uncertainty in similar circumstances, participants said that after the course they were less likely to investigate or prescribe without clear indications to do so. (Premi 1988)

From this small beginning, the Canadian Practice-Based Small-Group Learning (PBSGL) programme has grown to involve over 5,000 participants, mainly family physicians but including also a small number of other primary care professionals. This number does not include a further 1,200 participants in Scotland, mainly general practitioners (GPs) but again with a small number of other professionals.

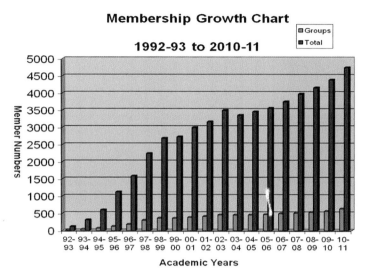

Fig. 6.3 Canadian PBSGL membership growth

Growth in Canada

Following the positive results of the feasibility study, a pilot study was developed in 1992 through the McMaster University CME programme with the endorsement of the Ontario College of Family Physicians. There was an explicit desire to build on the small-group, case-based format pioneered by McMaster's undergraduate medical programme, and the study aimed to seek effective ways of disseminating new information, while simultaneously supporting individual learning (Premi et al. 1994).

Participants organised themselves into learning groups of five to nine physicians and met in their local communities at times and places of their own choosing. The study involved 117 family physicians in 16 peer-facilitated groups with supporting 'information packages' that consisted of one or two pages of summarised practice-relevant information with one or two further pages such as patient questionnaires or treatment algorithms. The study demonstrated the readiness of participants for learner-centred and practice-based learning, in contrast to traditional information-centred approaches. The programme, which had started 8 years previously as a single-group meeting to discuss their cases, was extended across Canada and continued to evolve to meet the needs of a growing membership (Fig. 6.3).

The rapid early growth of the PBSGL programme in Canada was influenced by the implementation of new accreditation processes by the College of Family Physicians in Canada (CFPC). In 1995 a new Maintenance of Proficiency programme (MAINPRO) was introduced, requiring CFPC members to submit 250 hourly credits in a 5-year period. For members who were certificants of the college, 24 of these 250 credits had to be from the MAINPRO-C category. To be eligible for MAINPRO-C accreditation, CME programmes are required to address the key

---

Box 6.6 FMPE Mission

Our mission is to provide practising physicians with the means to maintain and enhance their professional knowledge and competence *and* to integrate that knowledge into their practices through the development, dissemination and evaluation of educational approaches and materials that are learner-centred and practice-based, using evidence-based educational principles.

---

elements of reflection and integration of newly acquired knowledge and skills into practice. The PBSGL programme provided one of the few avenues available for family physicians to gain these credits at that time.

By 1996, PBSGL had spread from its original locus as a part of McMaster University's CME programme in Southern Ontario to physicians across Canada. To reflect this national expansion, the Foundation for Medical Practice Education (FMPE) was established in Hamilton, Ontario, a not-for-profit organisation dedicated to the continuing professional development of family physicians (Box 6.6).

Collaboration with Scotland

In 2001–2002, one of the authors (RMV), a general practitioner in Scotland, spent a year on sabbatical at the Department of Family Medicine at McMaster University. One of the aims for this sabbatical period was to investigate the PBSGL programme and to assess whether it would be appropriate for GPs in the United Kingdom at a time where there was an emphasis on attendance at educational events to claim a 'postgraduate educational allowance' but without any clear or consistent focus on reflection and practice change.

The result of this analysis suggested that the programme would be equally appropriate for GPs in the UK as it is for family physicians in Canada (MacVicar 2003). NHS Education for Scotland (NES), a Special Health Board within the National Health Service (NHS) in Scotland, was sufficiently persuaded that PBSGL could have value in the Scottish system to support a pilot amongst Scottish GPs in 2003–2004. As a Special Health Board, NES is responsible for supporting health services by developing and delivering education and training for those who work in the NHS in Scotland, as captured in the NES mission statement 'to provide educational solutions that support excellence in health care for the people of Scotland'. In this Scottish pilot, 39 GPs were gathered into five groups in geographically dispersed parts of Scotland, and both a quantitative and a qualitative study of their experiences suggested that for them PBSGL was an effective and engaging learning method (MacVicar et al. 2006: Kelly et al. 2007). NES supported a roll-out of PBSGL in Scotland from 2006, and growth in membership since has followed a similar pattern to that in Canada (Fig. 6.4).

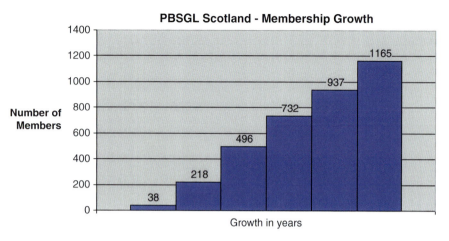

Fig. 6.4 Scottish membership growth 2006–2011

Box 6.7 PBSGL Scotland's Purpose

The aim of Practice-Based Small-Group Learning (PBSGL) is to provide health care professionals with a method of learning that improves their knowledge and skills and constructively challenges their attitudes and clinical behaviour. The method involves discussion of case-based materials in a safe and supportive environment. PBSGL is designed to integrate learning into day-to-day practice and encourages this by a seeking commitment to change within a peer-facilitated small-group setting. The methods used are learner-centred and practice-based (i.e. firmly grounded in the practice of medicine) and are firmly based upon evidence-based educational principles. We aim to continue to develop new educational approaches and materials and research these as they are developed.

The growth of PBSGL in Scotland has been nurtured by the FMPE in Canada, and this relationship has represented a mutually beneficial model of international collaboration. PBSG Learning is now an established workstream within NES and is guided by a multi-professional steering group within the organisation, the agreed purpose of which is as described in Box 6.7.

The two programmes continue to work together to develop educational materials, to share research findings and to advance strategies to enhance the implementation of new knowledge into practice.

Module Production

The FMPE currently produces 14–16 modules per year, and a robust process for module production has evolved over the years. The creation of a module involves the steps described in Box 6.8.

Box 6.8 Module Production

1. Identification of topic by members' requests, important new tests or treatments, suggestions from consultants or professional organisations or a combination of these. At this stage, an author, who is a practising family physician, is identified.
2. Needs assessment summary. An FMPE researcher identifies key articles and collates a needs assessment summary in collaboration with the author. This includes a 'gap analysis' (the gap between current practice and best practice) and a summary of barriers that are likely to impact on the implementation of best practice.
3. Development of patient cases. The author identifies appropriate cases from her/his practice that involve practice challenges and are likely to stimulate reflection on key factors and barriers identified in the 'needs assessment'.
4. Research and challenges. Researchers perform a literature search from a wide variety of sources to identify new information and guidance to bridge the gap between best available evidence and best practice and to address identified practice challenges.
5. Round-table discussion. A small group of representative family physicians, including the author and the editor, is convened with the researcher and medical writer to review and validate or revise the needs assessment summary and discuss the patient cases.
6. Drafts of module. Based on the round-table discussion the writer produces the first draft of the module which is reviewed by the author and researcher. An iterative process of further drafts follows involving the writer, author, editor and researcher.
7. Pilot test group. A 'trial run' by two volunteer groups is undertaken with specific feedback sought that is then considered and incorporated into the module.
8. Review by content experts. Two physicians with topic expertise (specialist or family physician) anonymously review the draft module to ensure accuracy and to ensure that there are no significant omissions.
9. Final draft of module. Following feedback from reviewers, the writer prepares a final revision for review by the author and editor, and a final check is undertaken prior to signing off the final copy and distributing it to members.

Evolution of the Educational Module

The modules have evolved considerably from the original feasibility study in 1988. The 'case' has always been central to PBSG Learning, and from the initial study, participants were encouraged to bring their own patient cases. Participants were encouraged to think about their previous experiences and identify cases where they struggled to address the patient's needs or where they continued to feel unclear about next steps in managing the patient's presentation. The physician presenting the case was asked to focus on those particular aspects, and the facilitator also checked to ensure the case resonated with the remaining group members.

The participants' cases at first formed the basis for the group discussion and generated a series of questions that were subsequently researched by group members and brought to the next meeting. However, the gap between meetings often meant the context of the case discussion, and the details of the issues raised were blurred and either the literature search did not get completed or the details no longer seemed relevant to the group as a whole. In addition, participants tended to bring their most complicated cases making it a challenge to identify important questions that were generalisable to the group as a whole. Despite group members being provided with a case guide, facilitators struggled with integrating these cases into the discussion. Further, the lack of resources for training facilitators at that time made handling these cases problematic.

To address this concern, starting in 1994, prepared case histories were added with the intention of stimulating discussion around all problem areas within the topic. They were not meant to replace the cases brought by group members (Premi 1994), and it is clear from an analysis of FMPE archive material that the addition of cases was undertaken after much discussion and with some trepidation. There was a concern that providing patient cases might discourage participants from discussing their own cases, but facilitators subsequently indicated that the addition of brief cases (based on real patients of the author or his/her colleagues) actually resulted in members sharing more patient challenges, as cases reminded them of similar ones of their own, stimulating a response of 'I had a patient like that....'. One year later Premi reported with some apparent relief:

> Since we added the case histories, group members report bringing more personal experiences to the discussion, not less! (Premi 1995)

The discussion within the PBSGL group has been supported in various ways from the initial expectation in 1988 that group members would research the answers to questions arising from the discussion, to information sheets presented in the 1994 pilot study that included a brief review of the literature. Modules have continued to evolve in the intervening years, and the current module including its anatomy, as well as the process for module creation, has been described above. On piloting PBSGL in Scotland, groups used the Canadian modules as produced by the FMPE, and while the modules were greatly valued, the cultural dissonance of Canadian case materials and Canadian norms and language proved an irritant for members. As a

> **Box 6.9** Examples of 'Tartanisation'
>
> **Language**
>
> - Names, e.g. 'Calum' rather than 'Chuck'
> - Working patterns, e.g. 'the surgery' rather than 'the office'
> - Medication names
>
> **Context**
>
> - Primary care management, e.g. adaptation to describe different access to investigations
> - Primary care structures, e.g. adaptation to describe different professional roles
>
> **Cultural Issues**
>
> - For example, adaptation to remove reference to aboriginal communities for Scottish modules
>
> **Epidemiology**
>
> - Adaptation to focus on UK epidemiology
>
> **Local Guidelines/Evidence Synthesis Sources**
>
> - Adaptation to provide focus on UK sources, e.g. SIGN and NICE

result, an increasingly in-depth adaptation ('tartanisation') of Canadian modules has taken place over subsequent years (see Box 6.9), and the PBSGL team in NES is now starting to produce Scottish/UK modules, de novo, adopting FMPE processes.

Communities of Practice

Over time, many PBSGL groups become communities of practice. This understanding is supported by the literature around communities of practice. Communities of practice (CoP) are defined as 'a group of people who share a concern, a set of problems or a passion about a topic, and who deepen their knowledge and expertise in this area by interacting on an ongoing basis' (Wenger et al. 2002, p. 4). Key components that underpin the development of a CoP include the development of a domain of knowledge, a community of people who care about the domain and a shared practice they are developing to be effective in their domain.

PBSGL groups form a community of family physicians within a small group that share a common practice related to the domain of family medicine. The appropriate care of the patients that makes up the practices of individual practitioners serves as the motivating force for the community. The practice is based on values, beliefs and knowledge about the role of the family physician in the diagnosis and management of individual patients and their families. Further, this common practice includes the integration of scientific evidence and community resources in the context of an ongoing relationship between the physician and the patient. The enquiries that arise while seeing patients serve as the starting point for interactions with colleagues who have similar patients, problems and goals, thus understanding not only the problem but also the context in which it developed and in which it must be solved (Saint-Onge and Wallace 2003). 'Interactions and relationships with others facing the same challenges and tasks comprise a major source of learning that enhances practice for most practitioners' (Parboosingh 2002, p. 230).

The value of the PBSGL group rests on this access to both the differing perspectives and experiences of others. The development of community is facilitated by the peer facilitators and depends on the honesty of members in discussing both successes and failures related to practice. Such an environment can only be created over time as members develop trust in and respect for the members of the group (Saint-Onge and Wallace 2003: van Winkelen and Ramsell 2003). The benefits of the transition to a community of learners include an improvement in self-assessment with opportunities to benchmark practice with others with similar practice profiles, development of practice-based learning agendas and enhanced opportunities for implementation of new knowledge into practice as participants share strategies and successes (Saint-Onge and Wallace 2003; Wenger 1998).

Pereles et al. (2002) looked at enduring small groups, including PBSGL groups, looking for evidence of CoP development. They reported that groups discussed and validated practice, learned from each other, developed a shared repertoire and shared and valued a sense of collegiality. However, they found that there was a lack of follow-up of unresolved issues and a problem with disintegration of the group if the facilitator lost interest or became fatigued. These issues have subsequently been addressed by the programme through enhanced facilitator training, opportunities for facilitators to work with a co-facilitator and the development of better tools (such as the PR-CTC tool) to enhance follow-up of identified concerns.

What Do We Know About PBSG Learning?

The PBSGL programme is grounded in the theoretical and research literature around the structure of knowledge, the role of reflection and the implementation of new knowledge into practice.

What Do We Know in Theory?

A number of authors in this book address different theoretical issues in professional learning, including concepts such as reflective practice and knowledge translation. In this section we give an account of the theoretical influences that have been most important in the origin and development of PBSGL.

Systematic reviews have suggested that a range of common educational approaches to gain new knowledge are known to have limited impact on improving professional practice (Davis et al. 1992; Oxman et al. 1995; Davis et al. 1995, 1999; Mazmanian and Davis 2002). Despite this body of evidence, current approaches to CME for general practitioners remain largely focussed on planned, formal events with tightly defined, content-orientated learning objectives. In contrast, interactive approaches to learning have been shown to be effective in changing practice, particularly when they involve small peer groups that foster trust, promote discussion of evidence focussed on real cases, provide feedback on performance and offer opportunities to practise newly learned skills (Davis et al. 1999; Marinopoulis et al. 2007).

The reason for this mismatch between current educational practice and evidence-based educational practice may relate to the growth of the evidence-based medicine movement and a perceived attendant need for the acquisition of increasing amounts of knowledge upon which to make better informed clinical decisions. The volume of output from medical research is multiplying at an unprecedented rate with over 400,000 articles added each year to the biomedical literature (Smith 1996; Davis et al. 2004). As a result of the breadth of knowledge required in their day-to-day practice, general practitioners are especially vulnerable to the impact of the ever-increasing volume of new information. The potential benefits from new knowledge have been limited by a failure to translate the new knowledge into practice including not only underuse and misuse of new knowledge but also overuse (Grol 2001; Grol and Grimshaw 2003). It has been estimated that approximately a quarter of medical care that is provided either is not beneficial or is potentially harmful (Grol and Grimshaw 2003).

The evidence-based medicine (EBM) movement began in the early 1990s, and from its earliest days, the challenges posed to the discipline of general practice have been recognised (Haynes et al. 1997). The difficulties revolve around the challenge of applying general scientific principles to individual patients in the context of routine clinical practice (Hoey 1998; Fox 2002; Gilles 2005) as well as bridging the tension between evidence-based and patient-centred practice (McColl et al. 1998). In their 1998 paper, Sweeney et al. 1998; suggest that in transposing population-derived information to the individual person, a third level of significance, 'personal significance', needs to be understood as well as statistical and clinical significance. The authors describe personal significance as the additional factors that general practitioners take into account when making decisions on implementing evidence-based decisions. These include patient-related factors such as the individual patients' health philosophy and attitudes as well as factors internal to the doctor that will include context, experience, apprehensions, failures and successes.

The historical origins of both the EBM movement and the Practice-Based Small-Group Learning programme at McMaster University and the parallel time frame over which they have developed are no coincidence. PBSGL evolved in part as a response to the need to apply the findings of EBM (which usually derived from the studies of selected populations) to individual patients. In achieving this, the various elements of the PBSGL programme (small-group process, facilitator training and support, module development and production and practice reflection) are intimately linked and interdependent. Each component is critical to the learning process and ultimately to practice change, with reflection being the key component.

As a number of chapter authors in this book have noted, Donald Schön's (1983) work highlights the centrality of reflection in how professionals learn. Schön suggested that reflection is a purposeful form of thought provoked by unease in learners when they recognise that their understanding is incomplete. He suggested that reflective practice is a spiral process that continues throughout professional life and talks particularly about working in what he calls the 'swampy lowlands' of everyday practice where the concepts learned through formal training are played out in the messy, unpredictable, undifferentiated and often emotionally charged experience of real lives. The all-encompassing nature of general practice requires an appreciation of a biopsychosocial model of illness, an understanding of the effect of the doctor-patient relationship on outcomes and the need to act as an interpreter and a witness to suffering (Heath 1995). These complex components of practice mean that complete, objective understanding of a particular patient problem will often be elusive and the unease described by Schön will be experienced on a regular basis by general practitioners. The opportunity to explore these complex issues of everyday practice with colleagues who understand the context in which patient care must occur is a major component of the PBSGL programme.

In exploring the interaction of reflection, problem-solving, physician learning and practice change, Slotnick (1999) has proposed a model based on empirical data incorporating previous work by Geertsma et al. (1982) and the foundational work of Schön (1983, 1987), Mezirow (1997) and Norman and Schmidt (1992), Schmidt, Norman, & Boshuizen (1990). These models highlighted the need for doctors to learn through 'reflecting in action' and 'reflecting on action'. The theoretical framework of learning through reflection comes from work on experiential learning and is well documented in the educational literature (Kolb 1984; Schön 1987). Slotnick proposes that the learning process begins with the identification of a specific problem the physician wishes to solve. This identification is typically triggered by three sources including 'reflection in action' while involved in practice, objective assessments of practice including audits or self-assessment programmes or through other external sources of information including clinical practice guidelines (Campbell et al. 1999). Once a problem is identified, physicians decide whether they are prepared to learn what is required to solve the problem. The physician needs to be convinced of both the relevance of the question and the potential benefit to his/her practice accrued by addressing it (Fox et al. 1989). Those questions that are not of sufficient concern are ignored at this point.

Physicians then assess the need to make the change and whether to seek new levels of competence related to the change. Part of the decision to seek new knowledge is based on an analysis of the gap between current practice and better practice. The size of the gap provokes a degree of anxiety, and the level of this anxiety influences the willingness of the physician to work at bridging the gap. If the gap is too large or too small, there may be either too much or too little anxiety and the gap is not addressed. The cost in terms of time commitment is a significant factor in deciding which problems to pursue and which resources to access. Finally, physicians determine whether resources are available to address the problem generated. One of the preferred resources for physicians includes consultation with same specialty colleagues (Haug 1997; Slotnick et al. 2001; Verhoeven et al. 1995).

As a consequence of uncertainty arising from dealing with clinical problems, Slotnick also highlighted the need for security in continuing professional development (CPD). As highlighted by Marinker and Peckham (1998), uncertainty is a defining feature of general practice, and in consequence, the need for security is of particular importance in CPD for general practitioners. In PBSGL, this security is provided within the peer-facilitated small-group format and the emergent community of learners. Facilitators, in their training, are encouraged to consider, with their group members, how the group will function and to determine 'group rules' that will include issues of confidentiality, peer support and respect.

Group discussion helps practitioners articulate and consolidate those problems that arise in everyday patient care. Further, problems that have not previously been perceived may be identified as cases are discussed. Physicians also benchmark themselves with others through the process of discussion, and this benchmarking process can be a crucial component of enhancing self-assessment thereby improving problem identification. Once aware of a gap in their practice, physicians within PBSGL are then able to draw upon the evidence-based materials as a resource for learning. Equally important, they have the opportunity not only to access the knowledge and experience of colleagues in relation to the information they need to address their gap but also to explore the integration of this knowledge into the practice environment. To address these factors fully, an important role for pattern recognition has been described. Schmidt et al. (1990) describe the ways information is organised to facilitate use in practice: disease presentations are represented as generalised experience in illness scripts, as pathophysiological descriptions and as an elaborate set of lively recollections of specific patients who suffered from that disease.

Consistent with the unique focus that general practitioners have on individual patients (McWhinney 1996), illness scripts developed by general practitioners focus on the illness experiences of individuals rather than on disease entities. Heath's description of the general practitioner's role in acknowledging and witnessing the suffering caused by illness and serving as interpreter and guardian at the interface between illness and disease intensifies this focus on illness scripts that are moulded by individual patients and the shared journey that the general practitioner experiences with the patient. In the face of such powerful illness scripts, the challenge to improve the implementation of new evidence by general practitioners could therefore be thought of as 'rescripting', involving a process of guided reflection on individual patients that GPs have seen. This focus on cases is supported by the work of Regehr and Norman (1996) who emphasise the importance of cases or problems in

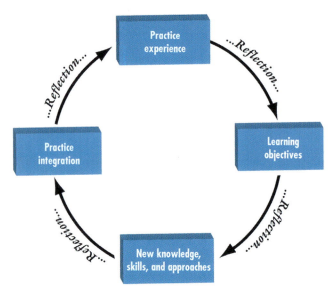

Fig. 6.5 Practice-based learning circle

concept formation and decry the tendency to consider cases as the opportunity to apply the learned rules, suggesting rather that experience with cases provides an alternative and equally useful method of reasoning. The small-group environment can facilitate the development and enhancement of these scripts through discussion of individual cases and the opportunities to explore previously unidentified gaps.

In summary, the theoretical basis for changing practice begins with the individual physician's experience of patient care (cases, problems). Through *reflection*, the physician can recognise a gap between current practice and best or better practice. Defining this gap presents an opportunity for the physician to identify learning objectives specific to their context, the family practice setting. The acquisition of new knowledge, skills and approaches to bridge this gap follows. Often, however, access to new information alone is not sufficient. The opportunity for reflection and discussion, which are necessary to help physicians identify areas where current practice requires change and to develop strategies to integrate this new approach, is provided by the peer-facilitated small-group process.

This 'practice-based learning circle' is illustrated in Fig. 6.5.

What Do We Know in Practice?

Evaluations of the Practice-Based Small-Group Learning programme have been published from the early feasibility study in the 1980s (Premi 1988) to the pilot study in the early 1990s (Premi et al. 1994) and subsequent developments on both sides of the Atlantic. Much of the work that has been carried out has focused on the experience of participants and their reports of change in practice. For example, Premi et al. (1994) reported from the PBSGL pilot that their intervention group (of 100) increased their knowledge by 12.1% compared to 50 controls taken at random from the waiting list. Further, 75 physicians reported making 127 practice changes. Similar positive evaluations on the implementation of PBSGL in Scotland suggested that practice change was likely or had happened (Overton et al. 2009). While evidence of change in knowledge and self-reported changes in practice were encouraging, they did not provide stringent evidence of a change of physician behaviour.

In contrast, Herbert et al. (2004) reported on the 'Better Prescribing Project (BPP)', a randomised control trial of case-based, learning modules (PBSGL modules) and/or individual prescribing portraits on treating hypertension in primary care in British Columbia. An analysis of the results based on almost 4,400 patients receiving treatment for hypertension did reveal modest but meaningful changes in prescribing sustained at 6 months in the group which used learning modules.

A further component of the BPP was a study by Wakefield et al. (2003) which looked at the commitment-to-change statements made by physicians in the study outlined above and compared them to the provincial pharmacy registry for 6 months before and after the educational intervention. In three out of four of the conditions studied, those physicians who expressed a commitment to change were significantly more likely to change their prescribing in the subsequent 6 months.

Linking patient outcomes to an educational intervention is fraught with difficulties with a preponderance of confounding variables. However, the ability to demonstrate an effect, albeit a modest one, is an important outcome.

PBSGL: Now and the Future

Both the Canadian and Scottish PBSGL programmes retain a significant focus on research with a shared commitment to demonstrate the effectiveness of PBSGL, to understand what it is that engages clinicians in this form of learning and to understand how it changes clinical practice.

PBSGL has been widely used in North America for a number of years as a part of family medicine residency training. The PBSGL method is used in every Canadian medical school and in some in the United States as well. PBSGL was implemented similarly as a part of GP specialty training in Scotland from 2009. A qualitative study on a group of participants in Scotland confirmed that this was a valued and effective method of learning for trainees and that it played an important role in preparing them for independent practice and independent learning (Hesselgreaves and MacVicar 2012).

The PBSGL format has been adapted by a group at McMaster University to enhance faculty development and Practice Based Small Group – Education – or PBSG ED (http://fhs.mcmaster.ca/facdev/pbsg-ed.html). This approach has been shown to be useful for a variety of health science educators including those in community practice. Teachers were able to plan changes in their teaching behaviour and subsequently reported that the majority of the planned changes were implemented (Walsh et al. 2009). This approach and these Canadian modules were used in a small study in the north of Scotland in 2011 involving groups of educational supervisors from across the primary care/secondary care and undergraduate/postgraduate interfaces to investigate whether improvements in educational practice occurred and whether there was any impact on interface issues. Interviews with participants suggested that there had been a positive impact both on their educational practice and an improved understanding of each other's roles (MacVicar et al. in press).

PBSGL in Scotland is a workstream within NHS Education for Scotland, which is a multi-professional organisation with a focus on workforce development and education across a wide variety of professions and disciplines. Following its successful implementation in Scotland for GPs and GPs in training, PBSGL is now being developed, adapted and used as a component of their CPD by other groups of professionals in Scotland. As well as nurses, many of whom have been involved in PBSGL groups, since early in their introduction to Scotland, increasing numbers of pharmacist groups with trained peer facilitators are now benefiting from this form of learning. Interest has been shown by dentists, health care chaplains and others.

As well as the maintenance and continued growth of PBSGL in Canada and in Scotland, there is growing interest in this learning method for primary care professionals from the wider international community in North America, in the United Kingdom and beyond. Both the FMPE and NES strive to support this interest and the wide implementation of this approach, adapted to local contexts through the development of local champions, and a federated approach as developed between Canada and Scotland over recent years (Boxes 6.10 and 6.11).

Box 6.10 Primary Care in Canada

Primary Care in Canada

In Canada, the publicly funded health care system, Medicare, delivers the majority of medically necessary health care services at no additional cost to the patient. Health Canada is the federal programme responsible for setting and administering national principles for the health care system. Management, organisation and delivery of health care as well as the majority of funding occur at the provincial or territorial level. Primary care is usually the first point of contact with the health care system and is accessed mainly through family/general physicians, although access through nurses or other health professionals is possible in some regions. Patients usually see a consistent family physician although patients are not limited to seeing that particular physician.

(continued)

Box 6.10 (continued)

Primary care physicians are primarily paid through fee-for-service although salaried physicians are becoming more common. Family physicians serve as the gatekeeper to the remainder of the public health system in that most referrals to specialist physicians must be made through a family physician. Many family physicians in Canada continue to provide 'cradle-to-grave' care including maternity care and delivery and in-hospital care of their acutely ill patients. However, in larger centres, many family physicians are choosing to provide office-based care only, while others are focused primarily on low-risk obstetrics, hospitalist care, palliative care and a number of other areas of focused practice.

Family physicians are trained in a 2-year residency programme after graduation from medical school. The family medicine residency programmes across Canada are in the middle of curriculum reform initiated by the accrediting body of the College of Family Physicians of Canada. The focus is on a 'Triple C curriculum': competency-based, comprehensive, focused on continuity of education and patient care and centred in family medicine. Details of the curriculum can be accessed at http://www.cfpc.ca/Triple_C/.

Box 6.11 Primary Care in the United Kingdom

Primary Care in the United Kingdom

Health care services in the United Kingdom are delivered free at the point of delivery as a part of the National Health Service, which is funded through general taxation. Private primary care practice is extremely rare as a result of the comprehensive and accessible service offered by general practitioners Each citizen is registered with a general medical practice, which generally consists of a group of general practitioners (GPs) working in partnership with either employed or closely aligned colleagues working as a primary health care team. This team includes as a core element physicians, nurses and administrative/management staff but may also include pharmacists and other allied health professionals. GPs act as primary care providers and as gatekeeper to secondary care services and are trained for the role through a 3- or 4-year training programme that includes both general practice and hospital specialty experience. GP specialty training programmes address a comprehensive curriculum that describes the competences required to practice medicine as a general practitioner in the United Kingdom (http://www.rcgp-curriculum.org.uk/).

References

Armson, H., Kinzie, S., Hawes, D., et al. (2007). Translating learning into practice: Lessons from the practice-based small group learning program. *Canadian Family Physician, 53*, 1477–1485.

Campbell, C., Parboosingh, J., Gondocz, T., et al. (1999). Study of the factors influencing the stimulus to learning recorded by physicians keeping a learning portfolio. *Journal of Continuing Education in the Health Professions, 19*, 16–24.

Davis, D., Thomson, M. A., Oxman, A. D., et al. (1992). Evidence for the effectiveness of CME: A review of 50 randomized controlled trials. *The Journal of the American Medical Association, 268*(9), 1111–1117.

Davis, D. A., Thomson, M. A., Oxman, A. D., et al. (1995). Changing physician performance. A systematic review of the effect of continuing medical education strategies [see comments]. *The Journal of the American Medical Association, 274*(9), 700–705.

Davis, D., Thomson O'Brien, M. A., Freemantle, N., et al. (1999). Impact of formal continuing medical education: Do conferences, workshops, rounds, and other traditional continuing education activities change physician behavior or health care outcomes? *The Journal of the American Medical Association, 282*(9), 867–874.

Davis, D. D., Ciurea, I., Flanagan, T. M., et al. (2004). Solving the information overload problem: A letter from Canada. *Medical Journal of Australia, 180*, S68-S71.

Fox, R. C. (2002). Medical uncertainty revisited. In G. Bendelow, M. Carpenter, C. Vautier, & S. Williams (Eds.), *Gender health and healing: The public/private divide* (pp. 236–253). London: Routledge.

Fox, R. D., Mazmanian, P. E., & Putnam, W. (1989). A theory of change and learning. In R. D. Fox, P. E. Mazmanian, & R. W. Putnam (Eds.), *Changing and learning in the lives of physicians* (pp. 161–177). New York: Praeger.

Geertsma, R. H., Parker, R. C., & Whitbourne, S. K. (1982). How physicians view the process of change in their practice behavior. *Journal of Medical Education, 57*, 752–761.

Gillies, J. C. M. (2005). *Getting it right in the consultation: Hippocrates' problem, Aristotle's answer* (Royal College of General Practitioners occasional paper, Vol. 86). London: RCGP.

Grol, R. (2001). Improving the quality of medical care: Building bridges among professional pride, payer profit, and patient satisfaction. *The Journal of the American Medical Association, 286*(20), 2578–2585.

Grol, R., & Grimshaw, J. M. (2003). From best evidence to best practice: Effective implementation or change in patients' care. *The Lancet, 362*, 1225–1230.

Haug, J. D. (1997). Physicians' preferences for information sources: A meta-analytic study. *Bulletin of the Medical Library Association, 85*, 223–232.

Haynes, B., Sackett, D. L., Guyatt, G. H., et al. (1997). Transferring evidence from research into practice: 4. Overcoming barriers to application [Editorial]. *ACP Journal Club, 126*(3), A14–A15.

Heath, I. (1995). *The mystery of general practice*. London: Nuffield Provincial Hospitals Trust.

Herbert, C. P., Wright, J. M., Maclure, M., et al. (2004). Better prescribing project: A randomized controlled trial of the impact of case-based educational modules and personal prescribing feedback on prescribing for hypertension in primary care. *Family Practice, 21*(5), 575–581.

Hesselgreaves, H., & MacVicar, R. (2012). Practice-based small group learning in GP specialty training. *Education for Primary Care, 23*(1), 27–33.

Hoey, J. (1998). The one and only Mrs. Jones. *Canadian Medical Association Journal, 159*(3), 241–242.

Kelly, D. R., Cunningham, D. E., McCalister, P., et al. (2007). Applying evidence in practice through small-group learning: A qualitative exploration of success. *Quality in Primary Care, 15*(2), 93–99.

Kolb, D. (1984). *Experiential learning: Experience as the source of learning and development*. Englewood Cliffs: Prentice Hall.

MacVicar, R. (2003). Canada's practice based small group learning programme: An innovative approach to continuing professional development. *Education for Primary Care, 14*, 431–439.

MacVicar, R., O'Rourke, J. G., Cunningham, D., et al. (2006). Applying evidence in practice through small group learning: A Scottish pilot of a Canadian programme. *Education for Primary Care, 17*(5), 465–472.

MacVicar, R., Guthrie, V., O'Rourke, J., et al. (2013). Practice-based small group learning for faculty development: An evaluation of a four month programme. *Education for Primary Care*, in press.

Marinker, M., & Peckham, M. (1998). *Clinical futures*. London: Wiley.

Marinopoulos, S. S., Dorman, T., Ratanawongsa, N., et al. (2007). *Effectiveness of continuing medical education*. Rockville: Agency for Healthcare Research and Quality. No. 07-E006.

Mazmanian, P. E., & Davis, D. A. (2002). Continuing medical education and the physician as a learner: Guide to the evidence. *The Journal of the American Medical Association, 288*(9), 1057–1060.

McColl, A., Smith, H., White, P., et al. (1998). General practitioners' perceptions of the route to evidence based medicine: A questionnaire survey. *British Medical Journal, 316*(7128), 361–365.

McWhinney, I. R. (1996). William Pickles Lecture 1996. The importance of being different. *British Journal of General Practice, 46*(408), 433–436.

Mezirow, J. (1997). Transformative learning: Theory to practice. *New Directions for Adult and Continuing Education, 74*, 5–12.

Norman, G. R., & Schmidt, H. G. (1992). The psychological basis of problem-based learning: A review of the evidence. *Academic Medicine, 67*(9), 557–565.

Overton, G. K., McCalister, P., Kelly, D., et al. (2009). Practice-based small group learning: How health professionals view their intention to change and the process of implementing change in practice. *Medical Teacher, 31*, e514–e520.

Oxman, A. D., Thomson, M. A., Davis, D. A., et al. (1995). No magic bullets: A systematic review of 102 trials of interventions to improve professional practice. *Canadian Medical Association Journal, 153*(10), 1423–1431.

Parboosingh, J. (2002). Physician communities of practice: Where learning and practice are inseparable. *Journal of Continuing Education in the Health Professions, 22*, 230–236.

Pereles, L. R., Lockyer, J., & Fidler, H. (2002). Permanent small groups: Group dynamics, learning and change. *Journal of Continuing Education in the Health Professions, 22*, 205–213.

Premi, J. (1974). Continuing medical education in family medicine: A report of eight years' experience. *Canadian Medical Association Journal, 111*(11), 1232–1233.

Premi, J. (1988). Problem-based self-directed continuing medical education in a group of practicing family physicians. *Journal of Medical Education, 63*, 484–486.

Premi, J. (1994). PBSG News. *The Foundation for Medical Practice Education*. Education. Vol. 2.

Premi, J. (1995). PBSG News. *The Foundation for Medical Practice Education*. Education. Vol. 4.

Premi, J., Shannon, S. I., Hartwick, K., et al. (1994). Practice-based small-group CME. *Academic Medicine, 69*(10), 800–802.

Regehr, G., & Norman, G. R. (1996). Issues in cognitive psychology: Implications for professional education. *Academic Medicine, 71*(9), 988–1001.

Saint-Onge, H., & Wallace, D. (2003). *Leveraging communities of practice for strategic advantage*. Burlington: Butterworth-Heinemann.

Schmidt, H. G., Norman, G. R., & Boshuizen, H. P. A. (1990). A cognitive perspective on medical expertise: Theory and implications. *Academic Medicine, 65*(10), 611–621.

Schön, D. A. (1983). *The reflective practitioner: How professionals think in action*. New York: Basic Books.

Schön, D. A. (1987). *Educating the reflective practitioner*. Retrieved June 15, 2000, from http://educ.queensu.ca/~ar/Schön87.htm

Slotnick, H. (1999). How doctors learn: Physicians' self-directed learning episodes. *Academic Medicine, 74*(10), 1106–1113.

Slotnick, H. B., Harris, T. R., & Antonenko, D. R. (2001). Changes in learning resource use across physicians' learning episodes. *Bulletin of the Medical Library Association, 89*(2), 194–203.

Smith, R. (1996). What clinical information do doctors need? *British Medical Journal, 313*(7064), 1062–1068.

Sweeney, K. G., MacAuley, D., & Pereira-Gray, D. (1998). Personal significance: The third dimension. *Lancet, 351*(9096), 134–135.

van Winkelen, C., & Ramsell, P. (2003). Why aligning value is key to designing communities. *Knowledge Management, 5*(6), 12–15.

Verhoeven, A. A., Boerma, E. J., & Meyboom-de Jong, B. (1995). Use of information sources by family physicians: A literature survey. *Bulletin of the Medical Library Association, 83*(1), 85–90.

Wakefield, J., Herbert, C., Maclure, M., et al. (2003). Commitment to change statements can predict actual change in practice. *Journal of Continuing Education in the Health Professions, 23*(2), 81–93.

Walsh, A. E., Armson, H., Wakefield, J., et al. (2009). Using a novel small-group approach to enhance feedback skills for community-based teachers. *Teaching and Learning in Medicine, 21*(1), 45–51.

Wenger, E. (1998). *Communities of practice: Learning, meaning and identity*. Cambridge: Cambridge University Press.

Wenger, E., McDermott, R., & Snyder, W. M. (2002). *Cultivating communities of practice: A guide to managing knowledge*. Boston: Harvard Business School Press.

Chapter 7
Narrative-Based Supervision

John Launer

Introduction

Narrative-based supervision is a method for discussing complex and challenging medical cases with peers and trainees. It draws on ideas from the emerging field of narrative medicine (Hunter 1991; Greenhalgh and Hurwitz 1998; Charon 2006) and is part of a comprehensive approach to family medicine developed in the United Kingdom over the last 20 years called *narrative-based primary care* (Launer 2002; Launer 2006). This approach is unusual in offering not only a method of case discussion but a set of skills for encounters with patients, a system of teaching and a theoretical base that underlies all of these. It regards all conversations with patients or between professionals as *collaborative attempts to agree on a useful and coherent story*.

In contrast to some of the other models of peer group discussion presented in this book, there is no single format for using narrative-based supervision. It can be applied in many different ways, including one-to-one conversations with peers and learners, in small groups and in large groups with or without a facilitator. Rather than prescribing any particular form of activity, our main interest is in helping people to change their way of thinking and working – with the collaborative exploration of new stories at its heart. (We use the words 'narrative' and 'story' interchangeably, and we use 'supervision' to mean any conversation between professionals aimed at improving clinical care.)

Narrative-based supervision arose initially out of a clinical training at the Tavistock Clinic in London in the mid-1990s. Participants reported that the best way to learn narrative skills for patient encounters was through *practising the same skills*

J. Launer (✉)
Tavistock Clinic, 120 Belsize Lane, London NW3 5BA, United Kingdom
e-mail: john.launer@londondeanery.ac.uk

L.S. Sommers and J. Launer (eds.), *Clinical Uncertainty in Primary Care: The Challenge of Collaborative Engagement*, DOI 10.1007/978-1-4614-6812-7_7,
© Springer Science+Business Media New York 2013

in dialogue with each other about complex clinical cases. More by accident than design, we came to place such disciplined case discussion at the heart of our training. We have continued to do so ever since, as our work has extended from the Tavistock to elsewhere in London and the UK, as well as internationally.

Narrative-based supervision promotes a view of all medical conversations, with both patients and colleagues, as intrinsically uncertain and open to multiple interpretations and outcomes. It offers precise conversational skills for engaging with colleagues' accounts of uncertainty and for helping these move towards practical and emotional resolutions. As such, it is part of a wider project to bring about cultural change in medicine, by finding opportunities for frequent, extended and focussed discussion of cases with colleagues and hence through imparting the skills for effective dialogue with patients (Launer and Halpern 2006).

This chapter describes:

- The origin and principles of narrative-based primary care
- Their application to clinical encounters
- The skills involved
- How these are used in peer supervision

The next chapter gives an account of the training methods we use to teach narrative-based supervision. A brief description of the system of general practice in the United Kingdom appears in Box 6.11 in Chapter 6.

Origin and Principles

In 1994 a group of us at the Tavistock Clinic set up a part-time course for established family physicians and their nurse colleagues (Launer and Lindsey 1997). The clinic is a postgraduate training institute for mental health professionals but also has a strong tradition of offering work discussion groups for other professions including GPs (Launer et al. 2005). The Tavistock is the place where Michael Balint worked and started the groups that bear his name (Gosling and Turquet 1964). However, our intention was to offer a skills-based training designed to address the whole range of primary care work. The members of our teaching group had a variety of backgrounds including family medicine but were all trained as family therapists as well. We believed that family medicine and family therapy could learn much from each other. We knew many people in the UK, the United States and elsewhere who shared this belief. We had no wish to turn family physicians into amateur family therapists. Rather, we aimed to help them become more therapeutic in all the work they did.

The questions we hoped to address were these:

- 'How do you practise primary care when the authority of medicine and of professionals including doctors can no longer be taken for granted?'
- 'How can you share power with patients, without letting go of evidence and science?'

- 'How do you work alongside colleagues who may have other views, other beliefs and perhaps other professions?'
- 'How can you practise humanely while following a huge agenda of preventive medicine, disease surveillance, and keeping to guidelines?'
- 'How can you hold on to optimism about the possibility of change when you see so many people who are intractably distressed?'
- 'How can you manage all of this when time and resources are so short?'
- 'How can you be a care professional and remain a caring person?'

Among the different sets of ideas that family therapists use, we hoped that a narrative approach could provide the best way of helping physicians to address such questions.

Narrative ideas have entered family therapy from the social sciences, philosophy and the humanities, where they have been deeply influential (Ricoeur 1984; Bruner 1990). Taking a narrative approach involves a move away from interpreting people's experiences ('what is really going on here?') to becoming curious about how people understand and describe their experiences ('how are people agreeing to describe what's going on?'). People taking a narrative approach are not trying to dig deep, looking for the 'underlying meaning' concealed at the bottom of everything. Instead, they see reality more like a tapestry of language that is continually being woven, with themselves as participant weavers as well as observers.

A narrative approach to medicine means seeing all medical conversations as a collaborative attempt to construct an agreed story about what is happening (Brody 1994). Patients bring initial stories that contain puzzles, questions or things that do not yet make sense. They may have a need for some practical solutions – such as a prescription, injection or operation. However, they are unlikely to accept any advice or treatment unless it also makes sense as part of their story or narrative. The same applies to conversations between colleagues.

In some clinical cases, a purely biomedical response may be the only sensible one that is worth considering. For example, if a patient asks 'is this a bunion and do I need an operation?' the best reply may sometimes simply be 'yes'. However, this is the exception rather than the rule. An opening story that seems brief and fragmentary is more likely to be the prologue to a far more elaborate one, steeped in personal meaning ('I slept really badly last night because I was so worried about my job interview, then on my way to the interview I was so distracted that I tripped over my bad toe, was in agony, made a mess of the interview, my husband is furious because we need the money…'). Exactly the same holds true when physicians engage in dialogue with each other about clinical cases.

Primary care physicians will know how it is possible only to listen to the 'thinner' version of such a story. They will also be aware of how important it is to try and engage with the 'thicker' one and how much difference it makes to the relationship with the patient, the quality of the encounter, the kind of treatment decision that is reached, and the likelihood that the physician's recommendations will be followed and the clinical outcome improved. The risks of a failure to inquire adequately into the narrative go beyond mere misdiagnosis or poor concordance with treatment: they encompass what Arthur Frank has called 'misrecognition', a fundamental failure to engage with what patients have come about and who they are (Frank 2001). They also include the risk of letting the story remain 'stuck'. Without active listening, curiosity and attentive questioning, the patient's story may remain the same as it always was, rather than evolving into something more creative and more helpful.

Narrative Medicine

When we started our course, we were virtually alone in proposing a narrative basis for understanding medical practice. Within a few years, however, narrative approaches began to have a considerable influence in medicine (Greenhalgh and Hurwitz 1998; Charon 2001). The different forms of narrative medicine that have emerged all appear to share two crucial features. One of these is the way they claim legitimacy for the individual stories of patients and doctors as a counterbalance to evidence-based medicine, while recognising that narrative is not a substitute for evidence and is not opposed to it. The other concern that unifies all the forms of narrative medicine is 'narrative competence'. This includes a number of different elements (Kalitzkus and Matthiessen 2009):

- Sensitivity to the context of the illness experience and the patient-centred perspective
- Establishing a diagnosis in an individual context instead of merely in the context of a systematic description of the disease and its aetiology
- Narrative communication skills such as exploring differences and connections, hypothesising and sharing power
- Self-reflection

We have placed an emphasis on all these aspects of narrative competence, but in one significant way our approach has differed from many other forms of narrative medicine: we also draw on the field of thought known as social constructionism.

Social constructionists point to the ways that meaning is defined by the social and cultural networks in which we find ourselves and the discourses that go on within those networks (Berger and Luckmann 1966; Gergen and Davis 1985; Harre 1986; Gergen and McNamee 1992). For doctors, social constructionism offers a way of conceptualising and addressing exactly the kinds of complex cases where not only the medical content may give rise to uncertainty ('which of two drugs should I prescribe?') but where the frames of reference are also open to question (Launer 1995; Gabbay and Le May 2010). These might include, for example:

- 'Have I been excessively influenced by drug companies?'
- 'Should I be prescribing a drug at all?'
- 'What legitimacy should I assign to the patient's view that all doctors are biased towards drug treatments?'

- 'How do I engage with colleagues who believe in promoting preventive treatment more aggressively?'
- 'How do I justify my cautious prescribing to a manager who is mainly interested in fulfilling targets for treatment?'
- 'How do I justify choosing a more expensive drug to a manager who is mainly concerned with keeping within our budget?'

Much of our teaching now addresses the dilemmas of how to remain constantly alert to the limits of absolute knowledge and certainty while remaining prepared to speak and act with conviction where it is necessary to do so. In everyday practice, this means allowing the inner voices of scepticism and of expertise to act as constant commentators on each other (Launer 1996).

A Narrative-Based Approach to a Patient Encounter

Before addressing supervision itself, the best way of demonstrating a narrative-based approach is by first describing its use in clinical practice at the simplest level. In the encounter described immediately below, the doctor is applying the rudimentary principles that provide a starting point for all narrative practice. These are:

- The doctor's precise use of questions
- The way the doctor's questions are linked closely with the patient's story exactly as it emerges
- The integration of diagnosis, reassurance, advice and treatment into the natural flow of the story rather than following any prescribed pattern

The principles being applied here are explored and developed further in the section that follows. Like other examples in these chapters, this one is partly fictionalised to protect the patient's identity. It is written in the first person, by the doctor.

'I saw a newly registered patient: an African woman in her early 40s. She came into the room with a sad and distracted expression. She told me that she had hurt her bottom the previous day. Simultaneously she took out of her handbag a number of packets of medication to show me what she was currently taking. I asked her how she had hurt her bottom and she told me that she had fallen. I enquired a bit more about how this happened, and she said that her fiancé had pushed her. When I questioned her further about this, she said they had been arguing in the car, she had got out, and he had followed her and pushed her over on the pavement. I asked if this happened a lot and she said yes it did, mainly because of her drinking. She had been an alcoholic for some time but was now trying to give up. I asked if she was getting any help for her alcohol problem and she said no, but she was a mental patient and had been getting help with her mental problems until recently when she moved away into our area.

'I asked her to tell me something about her mental problems and she said she got hallucinations, hearing and seeing things that were not there. I enquired if she had ever been admitted to hospital because of these. She said no but she had been in hospital for a few weeks during the summer for another problem. When I questioned her about this, she told me that she had a tumor. I enquired where the tumor was, and she said it was in her brain. At this point I thought that the tumor might be a delusion, so I asked her if she could show me the scar. She showed me a fresh but well healed scar behind her right ear that was entirely consistent with recent brain surgery. She then told me that it had been a 'Meningi-something', and when I suggested the word 'Meningioma', she said yes that was it. She told me the name of the consultant she was seeing for this, a neurologist I know. At the same time, I was examining the packets of medication she had laid out on my desk, and some of these were anti-epileptic pills. (The other ones were a type of sleeping tablet, and beta- blockers which might have been for anxiety, or for raised blood pressure or migraine).

'I said to her that it sounded as if her life was very difficult at the moment, and I wondered if there was anyone at home who was looking after her. She said that her fiancé did not live with her, but her children were at home. I asked her how many children she had and she started to cry, saying that she had had five children but only three were alive now. When I asked her how this came about, she told me that her first child had died soon after birth, having been born very prematurely. However, her main cause of grief was the murder of her eldest son, aged 24, which had happened 2 years ago. I expressed my sympathy, and then asked her how old her surviving children were. She explained that they were 15, 7 and 1 year old respectively.

I realised we were short of time (the encounter had taken about fifteen minutes so far), so I suggested at this point that we should attend to the problem she had originally brought to me, namely her painful bottom. I examined her briefly, reassured her that she had only been bruised, and at her request prescribed some painkillers that would not interact with her other medication. I asked her to make a follow-up appointment in a few days time. I also suggested that I should book her in to see the community mental health nurse. She agreed with both suggestions, and I gave her a written slip to hand in at the desk to fix this up. (Adapted from: 'New Stories for Old: Narrative-based primary care in the United Kingdom.' Launer 2006)

Skills for Narrative Interviewing

In both clinical work and supervision, narrative-based primary care places a great emphasis on the conversational micro-skills needed to conduct an effective narrative interview. (We use the word 'interview' as a neutral term that can apply to professional encounters either with patients or with other clinicians. It is not meant to carry the connotation of being intrusive or judgemental.) This section of the chapter identifies and explains these skills. The examples from now on all relate to professional conversations between colleagues rather than ones with patients.

The most useful set of guidelines we know for narrative interviewing comes from the Milan School – a group of family therapists working in the 1980s (Palazzoli et al. 1980; Cecchin 1987). Although their ideas predated the so-called narrative turn in the social sciences and psychology, they anticipated it in many ways and their approach is entirely consistent with it. They examined what was effective in their conversations with patients – and what was not. What they found did *not* bring about change were:

- Advice
- Looking for solutions
- Telling people what they thought was going on (interpretations)

What they found did work were conversations made up more or less entirely of questions. These were not questions for which the therapists had any answers. They were questions that, from moment to moment, invited people to look at their problems from unfamiliar and unexpected angles. Using ideas derived from Gregory Bateson, one of the pioneers of systems theory (Bateson 1972), they proposed that any change in personal understanding took place through gradual increments in a conversation and as a consequence of precise linguistic attentiveness and responsiveness on behalf of the clinician. They arrived at the notion that you could help people to change just through the process of asking them questions in a certain way. The three guidelines they offered for effective conversations were *hypothesising, circularity and neutrality.* What follows is a description of these guidelines as we have adapted them over the years for our own work.

Hypothesising

When they talked about *hypothesising*, the Milan School drew attention to the fact that it is impossible during any conversation *not* to form ideas in your mind about causes, reasons, explanations and interpretations for what the other person is describing. However there are two quite different ways of responding to this internal dialogue. On the one hand, you can assume that your own hypotheses are right and try to persuade other people of this. On the other hand, you can regard your own ideas simply as different descriptions of what is going on and use these as the basis for questions to discover if they are of any interest or use to the other person. According to the latter approach, any hypothesis is only as good as the quality and accuracy of the questions it generates.

We generally resist offering learners a list of 'good questions' since this can lead to interviews becoming studied and repetitive. Nevertheless we do on occasion suggest question stems that can encourage good technique, so long as they are applied creatively (Tomm 1988). Box 7.1 includes some of these.

Box 7.1 Examples of Useful Questions

What would you like to happen/what do you want?

What do I need to know about…?

What do you see as the main issues/your chief dilemma?

What do you think are the main contexts influencing this situation?

How do you understand…?

What explanations do you have for this?

How would you describe…?

How would x view you/what is going on?

What would x say?

Who else might have a view about this?

Has there been a situation like this before?

When x does this what does y do/how would y react?

What you have said made me curious to ask if…

How would a manager, lawyer, etc., regard this?

If you looked at this from a patient safety/ethics/consumer's/carer's perspective, what thoughts would you have?

What are the differences in beliefs/understandings/approaches between…?

What would happen if you …?

What do you think would need to happen?

Where do you think things will be in…(time)?

Supposing…?

What will happen if nothing changes?

Circularity

The second guideline offered by the Milan School – *circularity* – is the ability to create a loop of question-response-question in the interview. Whenever possible we advise people to pick up on words or phrases from the presented narrative rather than choosing these from their own vocabulary or substituting other words and phrases that may seem almost identical but may have significant differences for interviewees. Following another person's exact language is a way of showing empathy and interest through careful listening and allowing them the opportunity to imagine new ways of thinking about their dilemmas. Good interviewers can stay with the logic of the other person's narrative and follow it comfortably wherever it flows, rather than feeling that they have to follow a prescribed notion of how a professional conversation ought to go and what it must achieve. Where there are technical, medical considerations that need to be brought into the conversation, we aim to help people integrate such considerations into their questioning.

Just as good doctors can sense medical cues that are important, we have discovered that some have the ability to pick up narrative cues that carry 'life' or 'weight' and to tune out of what is superfluous. Others seem to pick cues at random from the flow of words and hence ask questions that are irrelevant or trivial. One corrective

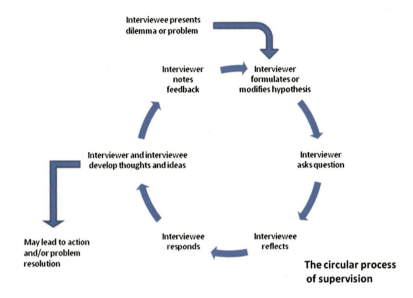

Fig. 7.1 The circular process of supervision

to this, particularly for learners, is to check constantly which among several cues it might be most helpful for them to follow and to be willing to review the conversation or wind it backwards whenever a question seems to lead down a blind alley or makes the conversation go slack (e.g. 'you mentioned earlier that there were two aspects to this problem: which of them is foremost in your mind at the moment?'). Another approach is to ask the other person how the conversation is going for them, what they are getting out of it and what is still missing for them (e.g. 'Where have we got to so far? What still remains for you to sort out in your own mind?'). Such questions, self-evidently, can be applied with equal effect in encounters with patients or in supervising colleagues.

Figure 7.1 illustrates the process of hypothesising and circularity at work. The participants here are termed 'interviewer' and 'interviewee' to indicate that the process of inquiry might apply equally to a conversation with patient and when supervising colleagues (Halpern and McKimm 2010).

Neutrality

The Milan School's third guideline of *neutrality* sometimes causes confusion because it seems to imply that interviewers are not allowed to have views or opinions of their own. This is obviously impossible. However, you can still follow the discipline of not offering your views or opinions. For most learners it can be hard to master the process of turning a hypothesis (whether conscious or intuitive) into a question and then making sure that the question doesn't give everything away by its wording or intonation. That is one of the reasons for using structured training methods. With practice the process becomes internalised and hence easier. For some people it fits so well with what they believe to be effective and ethical conversational practice that it becomes effortless. They also learn to detect when it is actually more ethical to depart from a position of neutrality when a colleague clearly indicates a need for reassurance or straightforward advice.

One way that we promote neutrality in our own training is that we discourage empathic noises (e.g. 'I hear what you're saying'), reflecting back (e.g. 'so what you're saying is…'), reformulation (e.g. 'it sounds to me as if…') and interpretation (e.g. 'I think what's really going on here is…'). We also try to avoid direct inquiry into emotions (including the ubiquitous 'how did you feel about that?'). For some clinicians this question has become an automatic response, asked without real sincerity. If someone is feeling strong emotion and chooses to express this, it is perfectly possible to allow this to happen through sensitive questioning without insisting on it. We believe a question like 'how did this affect you?' will nearly always be more helpful than a statement like 'you must have felt very angry'. Questions like these also seem to elicit richer narratives than more direct comments or interpretations. Although such comments may be said with the intention of expressing empathy, they can be experienced as clumsy and may be off the mark anyway.

We regard an important aspect of neutrality as *reflexivity*. This involves the interviewer remaining constantly alert to their own reactions – including an awareness of their feelings and prejudices as these enter their own consciousness during the interview. Interviewers may draw on this awareness in order to generate new questions. On occasion they may decide to share these sensitively with the interviewee, as a way of opening up new perspectives on the case. There is a fuller account of reflexivity by Charlotte Tulinius in Chapter 11.

From Clinical Practice to Peer Supervision

When we first started to teach narrative-based primary care in the mid-1990s, we resisted putting case discussion at the centre of our training. We wanted to distinguish ourselves from Balint groups and instead put an emphasis on skills training. As explained in the introduction to this chapter, we soon found that course participants were bringing their own stories of complex cases they wanted to discuss. In time, this activity became our main approach to teaching narrative-based practice. Although we emphasise that narrative-based primary care is at its heart a clinical approach, we also teach that peer supervision is the best medium both for learning it and for developing the skills for using it with patients.

People who attend our trainings take up narrative interviewing in a number of different ways. Some do so exclusively in their clinical work. Others use narrative-based supervision on a regular basis in one-to-one discussions, in local peer groups or in practice meetings. Box 7.2 gives a description by an experienced supervisor of how she used narrative-based supervision to help a younger colleague talk about a difficult consultation with a patient. The examples that follow, adapted from 'Narrative-Based Primary Care' (Launer 2002), show a range of different circumstances where narrative interviewing has been used to extend people's capacity to think and act in response to different difficulties in their work.

Box 7.2 A GP Supervises a Younger Colleague

In this dialogue, an experienced GP called Angela is listening to Sarah, a younger colleague. Sarah has just given an account of a consultation she had the previous day. Her patient was a large, white middle-class, middle-aged man, whose wife was a doctor. He had come requesting a referral to a hospital on the instruction of his wife. Sarah had felt frustrated that this patient's wife seemed to be suggesting a hospital referral for something that could be managed in primary care but felt that she was not able to respond to the patient in a way that would be most conducive to his health. She had written the referral for him and she did not think he had noticed her frustration but wanted to discuss what to do the next time he came. Sarah's conversation with Angela continues as follows:

Sarah: I find this man so difficult, he waltzes in and always tells me what his wife wants me to organize. I don't always think these referrals are necessary and I know I could manage him better in general practice if only he gave me the opportunity.

Angela: Is there anything else you think it would be useful for me to know about this issue?

Sarah: He works as a banker in a large successful organization and his wife is a consultant microbiologist in a local hospital and I feel intimidated by them.

Angela: Intimidated…can you tell me more about being intimidated?

Sarah: Yes I always dread it when these powerful men like him come into the surgery and make demands of me. I feel that I have to follow what they want even if I don't feel that it's the best way to manage the problem.

Angela: If he was, for instance, an unemployed small woman what difference do you think this would make to your interaction?

Sarah: Oh that would be completely different … (and Sarah went on to describe her medical management plan)

Angela: If this patient and his wife were listening to this conversation now what do you think they would say….?

Sarah: I think they would be surprised by my feeling of powerlessness and I think they would possibly accept my management. I think that they are so used to hospital medicine that they don't really know about our expertise in primary care…

Angela's comments after the conversation: Before I did narrative training I would probably have offered advice early on about how to manage the patient next time ("Yes, I find this type of patient difficult too – why don't you try this…" type of suggestion). From this conversation maybe Sarah reflected on the reasons for the consultation being difficult for her and had some space to think about the reasons she felt intimidated. It gave her an opportunity to consider how the patient and his wife view medical care from their positions, which perhaps freed her, to introduce them to the expertise she offers from a primary care point of view.

Adapted from Miller 2012: Medical conversations inviting change

Examples of Narrative-Based Supervision

One-to-One Supervision

A GP brought a case for a one-to-one discussion with a colleague trained in narrative-based supervision. The case involved a patient with a long history of pelvic pain for which no cause had ever been found, although her mother had died of uterine cancer at 42. The GP was very unsure how to go forward with this woman, who consulted often. What became clear through the colleague's questioning was that the GP felt sure the patient was depressed but over 2 or 3 years had often got into very unproductive discussions with her over this, when she vehemently denied any depression or emotional problems of any sort. He had offered her antidepressants a number of times to see if it would make a difference to her pelvic pain but she had refused. Even though he believed the mother's cause of death played a significant part in her anxiety, she repeatedly said it was irrelevant.

The supervisor widened the discussion and inquired if there were areas of her life that the GP did not know about or which he might be curious to inquire into. As a result, it became clear that the overwhelming emphasis on symptoms and diagnosis, and the GP's belief that her mother's illness weighed on the patient's mind, had prevented him from asking about a wide range of other issues including her work, her wider family and her childhood – perhaps to a surprising extent, given the nature and chronicity of the problem. With the supervisor's help, the GP chose a number of areas he might explore to find out more about her and move the consultations away from their usual 'tramlines'.

A month later, the GP reported having had a very productive consultation with the woman. He discovered she had been made redundant as a teacher at about the time the pain started and had been very disheartened at not being able to find another job. He also found out that she had actually been adopted as a child and was currently engaged in a search for her birth mother. He commented: 'I realised I'd been making the assumption that she was worried she had inherited uterine cancer from her mother. Of course she didn't know this was in my mind so she didn't even bother to explain this wasn't even her genetic mother. I think it's probably the first consultation I've ever had with her when she didn't say "Well what's causing it then?"'

A Local Peer Supervision Group

A GP brought a case to her local supervision group: this group consists of six colleagues who were all trained on the same course in narrative-based supervision and now meet monthly. She spoke about a man he looked after with severe asthma. A year before, the local chest clinic had discharged him with the instruction 'just go to your GP and ask for another course of oral steroids when you feel you need them'.

This advice was backed up with a letter from the chest clinic consultant, effectively saying the same thing. The patient was now asking for steroids with increasing frequency, sometimes on questionable grounds, but the GP felt constrained from ever saying no. One of the colleagues in the supervision group interviewed her about the case, establishing all the relevant medical information and also the history of the doctor's relationship with the patient and his family.

The supervisor then turned to the group and invited their reflections on what they had heard so far. The members of the group moved the focus from the patient onto the GP's relationship with the consultant. One of them wondered why she regarded her own authority as less than the consultant's. Others suggested some further questions the supervisor might ask her:

- 'Did she have a particularly difficult relationship with this consultant or was it a more general problem with asserting her expertise as a generalist?'
- 'Were there factors relating to her own career transition from hospital medicine to becoming a family physician?'
- 'Was the gender difference with the male consultant, or his attitude to women GPs, a factor?'

At this point the supervisor turned back to the presenting GP and asked her to comment on these questions. She said she found them really helpful: most of these factors did indeed play a part in the problem she was having. The supervisor spent the rest of the interview helping her rehearse a possible phone call to the consultant in which she could spell out why the original instruction had created a dilemma for her. The supervisor also helped her prepare some specific clinical questions for the consultant ('What spirometry results are acceptable for this patient, and what level of deterioration would indicate the need for steroids?').

The GP then found it possible to imagine ways of challenging the consultant to think about the clinical expertise of GPs – including female ones! ('What's your view of joint care plans with GPs in asthma cases, and would you be happy if we designed one together in this case?').

A Practice Meeting

A GP raised a case at a regular practice meeting facilitated by a counsellor trained in narrative-based supervision. The GP told her colleagues that she was concerned about two under-fives whose mother sometimes appeared to be drunk. The GP had made a referral to social services but then heard nothing for several weeks. Eventually she had a phone call from an administrator in social services inquiring about the 'level of surveillance' she was currently maintaining with the family. The person making the phone call seemed to imply that the GP was responsible for monitoring the risks of danger to the children and might even be blamed if something went wrong. The GP felt this was inappropriate. At the same time, she felt guilty that she had scarcely seen the family since she originally made the referral and wasn't sure if she had a duty to do so. The facilitator invited the meeting to discuss the role of GPs in child protection cases like these and the extent and limits of their colleague's responsibility in this case.

The GPs and nurses present had different views concerning how much they would want to get involved in a case like this, but all agreed that a GP could never be the 'key worker' as they had neither the training nor the time for this. One GP who had attended a child protection course the previous week said that the course leader there had given many examples of cases that had ended tragically because no one was clear who was in charge and the agencies involved all tried to pass responsibility to each other. After hearing the discussion, the presenting GP decided to contact the social worker once again and if necessary the social work manager, in order to explain that GPs do not have any formal right to carry out 'surveillance' of families and to request that the social services department should conduct a proper investigation – putting this in writing to the manager as well.

Conclusion

As these examples all show, the core of a narrative approach is the idea that almost every skill that makes for a good and effective patient encounter can also be used for talking with colleagues, either singly or in a group. Conversely, a good piece of peer supervision can model exactly how a clinician might conduct a helpful and ethical conversation with a patient or a family. Narrative-based practice and supervision are to a significant degree inseparable. They share the same philosophy and attitude and apply the same skills. They all offer the same vision of what contemporary medicine should aspire to be: a polyphonic conversation where patients, families, doctors and teams are all mutually engaged in the continual creation of new meaning. This vision also extends to narrative-based teaching, as the next chapter illustrates.

References

Bateson, G. (1972). *Steps to an ecology of mind*. New York: Ballantine.
Berger, P., & Luckmann, T. (1966). *The social construction of reality*. London: Allen Lane.
Brody, H. (1994). 'My story is broken: Can you help me fix it?' Medical ethics and the joint construction of narrative. *Literature and Medicine, 13*, 79–92.
Bruner, J. (1990). *Acts of meaning*. Cambridge: Harvard University Press.
Cecchin, G. (1987). Hypothesising, circularity and neutrality revisited: An invitation to curiosity. *Family Process, 26*, 405–413.
Charon, R. (2001) The patient–physician relationship. Narrative medicine: a model for empathy, reflection, profession and trust. *Journal of the American Medical Association, 286*, 1897–902.
Charon, R. (2006). *Narrative medicine: Honoring the stories of illness*. Oxford: Oxford University Press.
Frank, A. (2001). Experiencing illness through storytelling. In S. Tooms (Ed.), *Handbook of phenomenology and medicine*. New York: Springer.

Gabbay, J., & LeMay, A. (2010). *Practice-based evidence for healthcare: Clinical mindlines.* London: Routledge.

Gergen, K., & Davis, K. (Eds.). (1985). *The social construction of the person.* New York: Springer.

Gergen, K., & McNamee, S. (1992). *Therapy as social construction.* London: Sage.

Gosling, R., & Turquet, P. (1964). The training of general practitioners. In R. Gosling, D. Miller, et al. (Eds.), *The use of small groups in training.* London: Codicote.

Greenhalgh, T., & Hurwitz, B. (1998). *Narrative-based medicine: Dialogue and discourse in clinical practice.* London: BMJ Books.

Halpern, H., & McKimm, J. (2010). Supervision. In J. McKimm, & T. Swanwick (Eds.), Clinical teaching made easy. London: Quay Books. http://www.faculty.londondeanery.ac.uk/e-learning/supervision/the-use-of-questions. Accessed 28 Mar 2012.

Harre, R. (1986). *The social construction of emotions.* Oxford: Blackwell.

Hunter, K. M. (1991). *Doctors' stories: The narrative structure of medical knowledge.* Princeton: Princeton University Press.

Kalitzkus, V., & Matthiessen, P. (2009). Narrative-based medicine: Potential, practice and pitfalls. *The Permanente Journal 13*, 80–6. http://xnet.kp.org/permanentejournal/winter09/narrative-medicine.html. Accessed 28 Mar 2012.

Launer, J. (1995). A social constructionist approach to family medicine. *Family Systems Medicine, 13*, 379–389.

Launer, J. (1996). 'You're the doctor, doctor!' Is social constructionism a helpful stance in general practice consultations? *Journal of Family Therapy, 18*, 255–267.

Launer, J. (2002). *Narrative-based primary care: A practical guide.* Abingdon: Radcliffe.

Launer, J. (2006). New stories for old: Narrative-based primary care in the United Kingdom. *Family Systems and Health, 24*, 336–344.

Launer, J., & Halpern, H. (2006). Reflective practice and clinical supervision: An approach to promoting clinical supervision among general practitioners. *Work Based Learning in Primary Care, 4*, 171–173.

Launer, J., & Lindsey, C. (1997). Training for systemic general practice: A new approach from the Tavistock Clinic. *The British Journal of General Practice: The Journal of the Royal College of General Practitioners, 47*, 543–546.

Launer, J., Blake, S., & Daws, D. (2005). *Reflecting on reality: Psychotherapists at work in primary care.* London: Karnac.

London Deanery. *Supervision skills for clinical teachers.* http://www.faculty.londondeanery.ac.uk/supervisionskills-for-clinical-teachers. Accessed 28 Mar 2012.

Miller, L. (2012). Medical conversations inviting change. *Context, 19*, 16–19.

Palazzoli, S. M., Boscolo, L., Cecchin, G., et al. (1980). Hypothesising-circularity- neutrality: Three guidelines for the conductor of the session. *Family Process, 19*, 3–12.

Ricoeur, P. (1984). *Time and narrative* (Vol. 1). Chicago: University of Chicago Press.

Tomm, K. (1988). Interventive interviewing: Part III. Intending to ask lineal, circular, strategic or reflexive questions? *Family Process, 27*, 1–15.

Chapter 8
Training in Narrative-Based Supervision: Conversations Inviting Change

John Launer

This chapter describes training in narrative-based supervision. It covers the evolution of our training system, its structure, our approach to teaching supervision skills and what we know about outcomes. The chapter is designed to be read following the previous one, which explains the method itself.

Evolution: From Clinical Practice to Teacher Development

When we started our clinical training courses at the Tavistock Clinic, the word 'supervision' was barely used at all within medicine. Where people did use it, this was nearly always in a hierarchical or managerial way and scarcely ever in the reflective or non-judgemental way that therapists, psychologists or counsellors apply it. Partly as a result of our own work but also because of wider changes in medical culture, the idea of reflective supervision within medicine, and primary care in particular, gradually began to take root in the UK. In the late 1990s and early 2000s, we ran a series of five conferences at the Tavistock on the theme of 'supervision and support in primary care' (Burton and Launer 2003).

This converged with other changes as well. We started to get requests to run workshops for local groups of family medicine teachers, so they could apply the approach in their own teaching and clinical practice. Some of these workshops were funded by the Department of Postgraduate Medical Education at London University

J. Launer (✉)
Tavistock Clinic, 120 Belsize Lane, London NW3 5BA, United Kingdom
e-mail: john.launer@londondeanery.ac.uk

L.S. Sommers and J. Launer (eds.), *Clinical Uncertainty in Primary Care: The Challenge of Collaborative Engagement*, DOI 10.1007/978-1-4614-6812-7_8, (known as the 'London Deanery' for short). This department oversees training for around 12,000 junior doctors and dentists across London.

In 2004 the London Deanery asked us to run workshops and courses directly for them. Two or three years afterwards, they asked if we could extend these to teachers from all the other medical specialities, as well as dentistry (London Deanery 2012). This led to a major change in our profile: from a fairly esoteric approach for a self-selected group of GPs paying for a course in a specialist training centre to a mainstream supervision method taught at the biggest organisation in the UK responsible for young doctors and their clinical teachers.

Inevitably, we have had to adapt everything we teach to contexts where clinical events, and the decisions they require, can be far more technically complex and more critical than in primary care. We have had to 'get real' about the limits of narrative ideas and skills in situations where patients have more urgent needs than telling their stories and where trainees or colleagues may display problems of knowledge, attitude or performance that require their supervisors to do more than ask questions. We also try to remain as free of jargon as we possibly can. Instead of 'narrative-based supervision', we use the term *Conversations inviting change.*

In the last few years, most of our activity has moved to the London Deanery. The clientele for our trainings has changed to include clinical teachers in the medical specialties from anaesthetics and surgery to pathology and psychiatry. We have now developed a multilevel system of training from 1-day introductory workshops to extended courses where we develop the next generation of trainers to teach narrative-based supervision to others.

Our Training System

Any doctor who teaches trainees in the UK has to attend some training courses in order to obtain accreditation or reaccreditation. Some of this training is mandatory. In the case of family medicine, mandatory training for teachers (GP trainers) is extended, rigorous and demanding, but in hospital specialties, this is less so. Our own workshops and courses for clinical teachers in London are optional for everyone, although they count towards accreditation for people who do choose to come on them. We aim to attract clinical teachers from both family medicine and hospital specialities if they are interested in the same things as we are: reflective practice, dialogue, complexity, uncertainty and trainee-centredness.

Much of our teaching in narrative-based supervision now takes place in introductory 1-day workshops and 3-day courses, where clinical teachers are essentially building on supervision skills they may already possess, as well as acquiring the rudiments of a narrative-based approach. We run around twelve 1-day workshops and six 3-day courses each year. We accept up to 18 participants on each. Over the past few years, we have reached well over a thousand clinical teachers on the 1-day workshops and several hundred on the 3-day courses.

We also run a part-time certificate course at the Tavistock Clinic to produce narrative-based supervision trainers. The course lasts a year and leads to accreditation as a trainer in narrative-based supervision. Over the year we observe participants teaching in large and small groups. They also have to produce a video of themselves conducting a piece of supervision, for formal assessment. So far around 20 people have become accredited as trainers in this way, of whom around 13 have remained active trainers in narrative-based supervision.

What a Course Is Like

To give a flavour of what training in narrative-based supervision is like, here is a description of *the first day of a typical 3-day course*.

The *training team* includes five people, for around 18 participants. (We have been lucky in being able to offer this level of staffing as a result of economic expansion in the National Health Service.) The course leader is an experienced trainer who has taken responsibility for planning the course along with the other team members. Almost certainly, the course participants have never met before. Typically four or five are family physicians, two or three are psychiatrists and the rest made up from many other specialities: surgery, orthopaedics, anaesthetics, dentistry, paediatrics, sexual health, pathology and respiratory medicine – the mix is different each time. Most will have significant teaching roles in their practices or hospitals, but one or two may be coming because of a clinical rather than an educational interest in the model. All are paying a total of just over 200 GB pounds (240 US dollars) to attend all 3 days, but the course is subsidised by the London Deanery, so this represents less than half of the true cost.

Everyone has done some introductory reading: a ten-page paper outlining the principles of narrative-based supervision and containing much of the information that appears in the previous chapter of this book. They have been sent information about what to expect from the course – including the fact that they may not be admitted if they arrive late for any day. They will know that the course is going to be participatory and will be largely based on their own narratives. Box 8.1 shows the instructions they have been sent, emphasising the importance of bringing narratives with potential for further development through dialogue, rather than prepared scripts inviting mere confirmation or congratulation.

Over the years we have had to hone these instructions many times to make sure that course participants get the point. Even so, we will still get requests during the day to discuss 'why my hospital is in complete chaos', 'how guidelines for bipolar disorder need revising', 'why trainees watch the clock more than in the past' or 'how the government is destroying the NHS'. It seems that focussed, extended, case-based discussion to resolve uncertainty or anxiety is such an unfamiliar activity for some clinicians that they do not even recognise a description of it as clear and unequivocal as the one below.

Box 8.1 Preparation for Supervision Skills Training

As part of our supervision skills training we will be using real-life scenarios (not role play) for most of the day. In order to do this, we need you to provide the material. This helps to make the course relevant and also provides you with an opportunity to get help with situations that are not yet resolved in your own workplace. Please take a few minutes to think about the question below and jot down your ideas about what you might discuss. We will use the real-life scenarios in the demonstration of supervision or in the small-group work. The question we want you to answer is as follows:

What current dilemmas do I have that I would benefit from 'working through' with a supportive colleague? This can be in relation to your work as a clinician, a clinical teacher, a team member or a manager. The scenario needs to be:

Current (not already solved or in the past)
Real (not hypothetical or imaginary)
Your own (not someone else's problem)
Individual (dealing with a specific person or team, not a generic issue)
Hot (causing you concern but also suitable for sharing in confidence with the group)

Didactic Teaching

When the course starts, everyone sits in a large circle with trainers usually interspersed among participants. After the preliminaries, a reminder about confidentiality and some kind of 'bonding' exercise, a team member gives brief theoretical talk with some illustrations. The presenter will elaborate on the 'two faces' of supervision: how it sometimes involves 'looking over someone's shoulder' and sometimes 'looking after them'. She will explain how we try to use the course to help people to think about combining instructional teaching in their work with making space for reflection and helping peers and colleagues learn what they *must* do, while allowing them to discover the huge variety of what they *might* do in any complex clinical or educational situation.

Presenters talk about the principles of narrative-based supervision, but they avoid using that label or words like hypothesising. Instead, the presenter will talk about how we have distilled some thinking from many worlds – psychology, education, philosophy and elsewhere – into some basic principles that we call 'the seven Cs' (see Box 8.2). Although this mnemonic may seem simplistic, we have had consistent feedback over many years that learners find it a helpful 'aide-memoire' that allows them to hold the key principles of the approach in mind with them becoming formulaic or excessively cognitive. We have also made a point of changing the 'Cs'

Box 8.2 Conversations Inviting Change: The Seven Cs

Conversations. Effective conversations don't just describe reality, they create new understanding of it. In supervision, just as in counselling (or indeed patient consultations), conversations can be seen as interventions in their own right: the end as well as the means. Simply by taking place, they create opportunities for people to rethink and redefine their realities.

Curiosity. This is the common factor that turns conversations with colleagues from chatter into something more substantial. It should be friendly but not nosy. Curiosity invites colleagues to reframe their stories. An essential aspect of curiosity is neutrality (to people, to blame, to interpretations, to facts.) Curiosity should also extend to yourself: what are your own thoughts about the problem, and how can you prevent yourself being critical or impatient?

Contexts. This is what it is most effective to be curious about. Important contexts in consultations are families, cultures, beliefs and faith. In professional conversations, they include people's practices and professional networks, power relationships, history, geography, belief systems and values.

Complexity. Rather than looking for a 'quick fix' in every situation, it is better to consider any problem as part of an endless and infinite dance of interactions. (Think of the phosphorylation cycle – the Krebs cycle – but in three dimensions and over time and with people and conversations rather than molecules.) A sense of complexity gets away from fixed ideas of cause and effect, unchangeable problems and over-concrete solutions.

Challenge. Supervision can be seen as a form of shared activity, in which one person is challenging another to think of a different description of what is going on. What you are looking for in supervision is a better account of reality than the present one, which means a story (a narrative) that makes better sense for people of what they are going through. Sometimes this requires a bit of perturbation.

Caution. You may need to use sensitivity and monitor your own emotional responses, to make sure you are matching your questions to suit the other person and their capacity to extend their thinking at that moment. If people want straightforward advice, be prepared to give it (while being aware of its limitations).

Also, remember you're not doing therapy – on colleagues or on patients!

Care. None of the other ideas will work unless you are respectful, affectionate and attentive. Supervision, like consulting with patients, needs to be grounded in moral commitment (Launer 2010).

over the years, retaining ones with more practical resonance and discarding others that seemed too theoretical (e.g. 'circularity')

We follow this presentation almost immediately with a demonstration of supervision, where a team member asks for a participant to volunteer to be interviewed about a problem or dilemma they have brought to the course, with the rest of the course group as an audience. The demonstration is likely to address the kind of cases illustrated in the previous chapter or possibly a 'case' relating to a trainee or colleague who is causing concern.

The demonstration of narrative-based supervision generally takes about 20 minutes. We then invite discussion of what people have noticed going on in the demonstration, but we try to prevent it becoming too theoretical. We mainly want people to become attuned to the process of narrative-based interviewing. We discourage them from referring back to the actual dilemma that the volunteer brought or trying to offer them a 'solution' for it and hence dragging the whole discussion down to a conventional exercise of advice-giving, rather than keeping with the ethos of narrative empowerment that we are trying to convey. What we are trying to do is to induct the group into a form of discourse where sensitive inquiry is seen not only as a way of mapping the landscape but as the principal way of allowing colleagues to redesign that landscape as they speak.

There will be further didactic teaching on the other 2 days of the course. There will be some set reading in the weeks between each session – including a paper on questioning and a paper on systemic and narrative theory – and time for discussing these in the sessions themselves. There may be another demonstration on the last day, by which time a participant may be ready to volunteer to be the supervisor.

Small Supervision Groups

The core of our teaching and supervision practice is the *small supervision group* consisting of a supervisor, supervisee and one or more observers. It is here that supervisors learn and apply the essential guidelines of narrative-based supervision: questioning, hypothesising, circularity, neutrality and curiosity. Here a narrative-based stance starts to make sense for them and hopefully over time becomes a 'modus operandi' for addressing all the complexities and uncertainties of their everyday work. It is here too that supervisees find resolutions for their problems through being allowed enough discursive space. In the role of observers, participants see and hear the process of narrative development and change taking place in front of them.

When a small group convenes for the first time on a course, their trainer begins by reminding the group of the kinds of problems we prefer to focus on. She reassures them that by the end of the day, they will each have had a chance to take on the roles of supervisor and supervisee as well as being active observers. She explains that it is legitimate to bring any professional dilemma to the group, since we apply the same principles and skills to help with clinical cases as we do with difficulties in the workplace with trainees. The only exclusion is in relation to personal problems, which do not belong in a training of this kind or in case-based discussion.

Next, she explains that the supervisor will need to follow three simple rules as an experiment and as a way of learning the approach in its purest form. These relate to the key principles of 'hypothesising, circularity and neutrality' although we do not necessarily spell out the theoretical background at this stage:

- Only ask questions.
- Make sure that each question links directly with something the supervisee has already said.
- Withhold any suggestions, advice or interpretations until the end of the supervision, and then only offer these if the supervisor requests this.

As the course progresses, participants will have a chance to explore how to mix other forms of words or techniques into their supervision, including approaches they may have been using for years. But for now they must follow the rules. We have found consistently that this is the only way people can experience directly how hard it is to create a narrative space for someone else and how liberating it is for both parties when you succeed in doing so.

A Small Group at Work

This section gives an extended description of a typical small group at work. It conveys what actually happens in narrative-based supervision, probably more accurately than any part of these two chapters. *Although detailed, it is worth reading for anyone who wants to gain an impression of what the live work is like.* Members of our teaching group who have read it have commented that it captures the essence of our approach more than the abstract descriptions of it.

Our group on this occasion (a fictionalised one, distilled from many real ones) consists of a trainer called Salima and three group participants: Barry, Wesley and Kate. We use a minimum of three people per group so that there can be a range of different views. Generally speaking, we will mix people from different specialities on a course, but in this example, the group participants and the trainer are all GPs.

Having listened to the trainer's introduction, Kate offers to bring a clinical case that is bothering her – a young woman she has seen the previous day. Barry offers to supervise her on this. Salima as trainer helps them to rearrange the seating. Barry and Kate face each other as supervisor and supervisee. Wesley sits alongside Barry as an observer, and Salima sits a very small distance away from the group but where she can see all three of them clearly.

Barry begins his inquiry by posing some questions he has picked up from the demonstration interview:

"Is there anything I need to know about you or your team, to make sense of what you're going to tell me?"

"Are you the only professional involved or are there others?..."

[Comment: People are often struck by the emphasis we place on understanding contexts before going for content. However, we encourage carefully graded questions of the kind Barry has asked here. Such questions help to build trust, especially between colleagues who may not know each other. They establish information that may turn out to be essential later – or that emerges when the supervisor has already advanced too far on the basis of incorrect assumptions. They also encourage the supervisee to start conceptualising the problem from an interactional point of view.]

At this point, Barry asks Kate to tell him about her patient. She tells him about a 16-year-old girl called Cherie whom she has seen a number of times in her clinic. Cherie has already had multiple sexual partners, is casual about contraception and is possibly a substance abuser although she denies this. As it happens, Kate also knows and sees Cherie's mother, who attends the same clinic and is HIV positive and on a methadone programme. Cherie and her mother seem to have a lot of secrets from each other, which Kate believes is unhealthy.

Kate now elaborates on the mother's history, going into detail. Barry nods encouragingly, frequently says '*Mmm*' and looks highly engaged, but he does not pose any further questions. Salima, the trainer, requests the group's permission to 'freeze frame' the conversation and asks Barry what is going through his mind:

Barry: '*I'm feeling a bit overwhelmed. I thought my opening questions were good but now I'm not sure if I should interrupt. She said she wanted to talk about Cherie but now she's only talking about the mother*'.
Salima: '*What do you think Kate wants from this conversation?*'
Barry: '*To be honest, at this moment I haven't a clue!*'

[Comment: Barry is a good listener. However, Kate needs more than 'just listening'. If all that Barry does is to listen without asking some questions to help her focus her thoughts, he may be infected by Kate's own apparent sense of being overwhelmed, without offering her any chance of developing a clearer narrative. Salima's intervention was effectively a teaching point to draw his attention to this process.]

Barry turns back to Kate and asks her why she brought the case to supervision and what she wants to get out of it. Kate, who has heard Salima's exchange with Barry, is clearly relieved by the question. She says there are two related things that are really bothering her about the case. Firstly, Cherie is refusing to give a blood sample for HIV and drug testing, even though the results would make a big difference to the kind of help Kate could offer. Secondly, Kate would like to enlist the mother's help in persuading her to do so but she doesn't know if it's possible without the risk of breaking confidences on both sides.

The conversation progresses. Barry does well in exploring these dilemmas. Some of his questions seem to imitate types of question that were asked in the demonstration earlier but miss the mark as far as Kate is concerned. Others are spot on, including an inquiry about how she has managed in similar sets of circumstances in the past. After a while, Salima pauses the conversation again to ask Barry how he thinks he is doing. He reflects that the supervision seems to be moving forward: Salima agrees and congratulates him on some particularly telling questions. She also says she would now like to bring the observer into the conversation. She asks: Wesley: *'What are you noticing? Have you had any thoughts about other questions that Barry might ask Kate?'*

Wesley is clearly pleased to have been brought into the exercise. He was looking a bit bored (which is one of the reasons Salima intervened as she did) and now offers a list of things he thinks Kate should and should not do. He talks about informed consent in relation to the blood tests, rules of confidentiality in relation to 16-year-olds and their parents and how careful you have to be to avoid complaints these days. Salima asks him *'Could you turn any of those points into a question for Barry to ask?'* Wesley looks puzzled and says, *'No, I think Barry is doing just fine. But Kate needs to be jolly careful with these two women. I got into hot water in a case just like this'.*

[Comment: Some course participants apparently cannot observe the process of a conversation rather than the content, and they cannot stop themselves giving advice. When this happens, the trainer's main responsibility is to keep everyone focussed on the main tasks, namely, to make sure the supervisee gets some appropriate help with her dilemmas and that the supervisor learns some new skills. When this particular observer gets his chance to act as supervisor in the afternoon, the trainer may need to intervene more often and be more directive with him. If a course member is still not 'getting it' on the second day, the team may need to discuss how to address this, at a debriefing during a break.]

Salima turns back to Barry and recommends the standard tactic used at this point in narrative-based supervision. Rather than choosing the next question himself, he might just ask Kate what is going through her head at the moment or if there is anything she has heard in the group conversation that has given her some new ideas.

To the surprise of both Salima and Barry, Kate says that she has found some of Wesley's ideas helpful. They have made her realise that she had overcommitted herself in her own mind to a campaign of persuasion in relation to both Cherie and her mother: persuading Cherie to have blood tests, persuading them to talk to each other more, persuading the mother to persuade the daughter and so on. *'Maybe I should chill out and let Cherie make her own choices. I could try to build up trust with her like I did with her mum. Anyway, I need to read up more on confidentiality and when you can breach it. I take risks sometimes and I know I shouldn't'.*

Barry is curious about Kate's response. Picking up on her phrases, he asks her what *'chilling out'* with Cherie would involve and how Kate would know when she had *'built up trust'*. Following her responses to these questions, he asks her where she thinks she might find up-to-date information about confidentiality and when to breach it. *'Perhaps I can ask Wesley over lunch'*, she replies, and all four of them laugh.

Salima, sensing a good moment to finish, suggests that Barry should ask Kate to review what she has got out of the conversation. She says she feels far more relaxed about the situation and is actually now beginning to think of personal reasons why she was so exercised by it in the first place. Barry blushes and says, *'Did I miss something important?'* Kate replies, *'No, it wouldn't have been appropriate to talk about here – it's about my own daughter and a problem she's been having. I don't want to go into it, but it was really helpful to make the link. I wouldn't have thought of it without your questions'.*

Salima asks Wesley to offer his comments. He says he is pleased that his counsel was helpful and disarms everyone by apologising for getting 'carried away' earlier, because of his own previous experience of a complaint. Finally, Barry gives feedback on his own performance. In retrospect, he says he thinks the context-setting questions at the beginning were probably unnecessary. He also explains he has learned a lot from Wesley's comments: sometimes you can deprive people by not giving advice when they actually want it and that *'being carried away'* spontaneously may be more effective than sticking to the rules. He also confesses that he might have *'gone for the jugular'* with his own trainees, asking them straight away who the girl or her mother reminded them of in their own families and no doubt making it impossible for them to reflect on this as a result.

[Comment: This vignette demonstrates the potential of narrative-based supervision to generate unexpected and even paradoxical learning. It also shows how hard it is to pin down what is 'right' and 'wrong' in supervision, from the issue of giving advice to the dilemma about whether to inquire about personal experience in the context of professional work. There are no simple rules about how to integrate the 'pure' model with the other kinds of conversations that physicians use and may feel more comfortable about. The crucial question is what this small group might have learned, or not learned, if Salima had not insisted on such strict rules to start with, but had given them licence to supervise in any way they pleased.]

Large Supervision Groups

The reasons for including large-group work in our courses are:

- They can be even more effective than small groups in illustrating the power of multiple perspectives and ideas.
- They demonstrate that case discussion in large groups, if conducted with a consistent and disciplined approach, can be a useful way of helping a colleague address a clinical dilemma.

We use a variety of structured methods for large groups, all employing Tom Andersen's concept of the 'reflecting team' (Andersen 1987, see also Chapter 11). Our commonest approach is as follows. The supervisor and supervisee sit at the front of the room, facing each other. The task of the supervisor is to conduct the supervision in exactly the same way as in a small group, mainly through the use of questions. A trainer sits alongside the supervisor, available in case the supervisor wants to take a break to discuss how the interview is going or explore possible ways forward. We encourage supervisors to take breaks like this regularly during interviews in front of a large group, just as we do in small-group work. Sometimes the trainer will initiate these if the supervisor does not.

As well as these three core individuals, five or six other people sit a small distance away, where they can observe the interview and act as a reflecting team. When breaks take place in the interview, the supervisor then has the option not only of talking to the trainer but also asking for the views of the reflecting team. (Alternatively the trainer may make a proposal that they should do so.) The members of reflecting team then hold a separate conversation among themselves. They might comment on the progress of the interview, offer hypotheses about the supervisee's story or suggest further questions the supervisor might ask. Sometimes the supervisor or trainer will join in this discussion, but generally the team just talk among themselves for a few minutes.

The supervisee can listen to all of this but without taking part. This gives supervisees a rest but also allows the team discussion to remain focussed and not to turn into a chat where lots of people are throwing random ideas at the supervisee without this being channelled through the supervisor. On occasion a supervisee will say that they really want the team to come up with suggestions about what do in the particular case. Our general rule as in small group work is: '*withhold any advice to the end, and only if the person bringing the case explicitly asks for this*'. This is because we believe that actions that emerge through dialogue and are self-determined are preferable to other people's ideas.

When the interview resumes, we ask that supervisors always say, '*Is there anything you've heard from the reflecting team that you'd like to respond to, of have you had any other new thoughts of your own?*' The reason for insisting on this kind of formulation is to ensure that supervisors do not colonise the narrative by choosing a hypothesis, question or piece of advice that caught their own fancy but instead allow the supervisee to keep control of the emerging narrative and its direction.

At the conclusion of a large-group discussion of this kind, supervisors will generally ask supervisees to review what they have learned from the conversation, what questions or contributions from the reflecting team have been most helpful, whether any significant unresolved issues remain and where they might take such issues for further discussion. The trainer might then hold a discussion with the supervisor and reflecting team about the process of the interview, in order to bring out teaching points, but will ask them not to comment further on the content of the case itself.

The purpose of this, once again, is to leave supervisees in full charge of their story and where they want to take it now that the supervision is over. We ask both in small-group and large-group work that no one should talk further about their cases during the breaks or over lunch. What we hope to promote by these kinds of discipline is that peer supervision – or supervision as part of training – is a conversation that should be as focussed and as professionally disciplined as any encounter with a patient.

If the overall course group has more than the nine or ten people involved in this process, we ask everyone else to sit silently in a circle around the room, so the three core participants and reflecting team are in a 'virtual fishbowl'. At the end, we invite these passive observers to comment on the entire process including the effectiveness of the reflecting team.

Outcomes

How does one judge the effectiveness of a complex, multifaceted approach to medical practice that includes a philosophical take on medicine, a repertoire of techniques to enact that philosophy in medical conversations and a range of training activities delivered within specific institutions? In one respect at least, narrative-based supervision has been a striking success. It has introduced a radically challenging view of what medical conversations might be into the heart of the postgraduate medical training establishment in London, including the social constructionist ideas that underlie them. It has made this view accessible to a range of specialists who would in normal circumstances have had no exposure to ideas or training methods beyond conventional ones and has imparted skills consistent with that view.

As well as influencing training, we have had some modest success in promoting the model in or near UK workplaces. Some of our trainers have managed to set up peer supervision groups in their own localities. Currently there are four of five of these across London, usually meeting for one evening a month. In addition, a number of our trainers offer regular case discussion sessions within their own practices or neighbouring ones, broadly applying the principles and methods used on our courses. A number of GP speciality programmes have also adopted our model of case-based discussion in place of more traditional Balint-style discussions.

Beyond that, the model has acquired enough of a national and international reputation for us to receive regular invitations from around the UK and more widely to deliver 'one-off' presentations workshops or courses. So far we have done this in Finland, Denmark, Norway, Turkey, Israel, Japan, the United States, Canada and Australia. Sometimes we find that ideas and techniques from our teaching have been absorbed into local postgraduate trainings or continuing professional development, particularly in family medicine. However, the only place where a parallel movement to the one in London is clearly taking off is in Israel, where there is a cohort of family medicine teachers who are enthusiastic about the approach. At the time of writing, a similar movement is also starting up in Norway.

In one country where our approach has been taught – and where narrative ideas have had influence from other sources – there is evidence that narrative skills have a specific effect on the capacity of doctors to engage empathically with their patients. In interviews with Danish GPs about their encounters with patients who had psychological problems, Davidsen and Reventlow found that doctors had a 'global and consistent style' in the way that they gave accounts of their work. This style ranged from the purely biomedical to a focus on the doctor's view or the doctor-patient relationship to a narrative approach. They report: 'Doctors who took a narrative approach became more deeply involved with the patient and exhibited a greater engagement, than did the rest of the participants. They stressed that the narrative was the pathway to emotional engagement and empathy with the patient, and participation in co-construction of the story was considered an empathic approach' (Davidsen and Reventlow 2011).

The most robust evidence we have for the effects of our courses comes from an independent evaluation that the London Deanery commissioned in 2010 from a team of researchers from Cardiff University (Bullock et al. 2011). They carried out an intensive study of a 3-day course, using audio and video recordings. They also asked a number of participants to keep audio diaries describing their use of learned skills between course sessions. They looked in depth at all the data and examined three levels of learning according to a standard model of educational research (Kirkpatrick and Kirkpatrick 2006):

1. Reaction or satisfaction with the programme
2. Demonstration of learning
3. Extent to which new learning is applied to practice

The full report extends to 124 pages, but the most salient findings included the following:

- Participants gave a clear endorsement of the core activity of the course: the opportunity to practise supervision in small groups. Although they found practising the new questioning techniques in these groups challenging, they valued the high-quality feedback that was generally provided by the trainers.
- Modelling of the 'seven Cs' by trainers was the most effective way of conveying a narrative stance. Course participants were able to apply this model even when their questioning did not necessarily 'fit the rules'. As a result, both trainers and participants were sometimes able to produce positive outcomes in supervision even when being didactic, so long as their overall stance was facilitative. Conversely, it was possible for some people at some times to 'talk the talk' but with negative outcomes because significant elements of the 'seven Cs' were lacking.
- There was variability among trainers, in participants' views of 'noncore' activities like role play and in how well strong emotion was handled in the groups.
- Out of six participants studied in depth, five considered they had made progress in their own development, although analysis of their supervision performance showed this was not all equal. For example, one participant 'seemed to have embodied this way of being, demonstrating an impact on himself as a person', while another 'appeared to employ the techniques as a way of bringing the interactant around to a prescribed conclusion rather than enabling them to explore fully the situation for themselves'.

These findings are congruent with our experience as trainers. They fit well with the vignette of small-group work described above, where the carefully crafted open questions at the beginning of the supervision seem in retrospect to have been redundant, while the apparently blustering interventions of a tyro achieved an unexpectedly positive outcome.

As the report points out, it is the overall tolerance of the narrative stance that allows even *discordant* contributions from trainers or participants to have a positive effect, when a fundamentalist application of narrative techniques alone would be purely negative. We have responded to the report by making changes in our courses and by constantly reminding ourselves that the techniques are a route to a vision, and not vice versa. Whenever a dialogue indicates that you should move a different direction, that is exactly what should happen. In the last resort, narrative-based supervision and practice are about the centrality of effective dialogue in medicine and in the way that all human beings create meaning.

References

Andersen, T. (1987). The reflecting team: dialogue and meta-dialogue in clinical work. *Family Process, 26*, 415–28.

Bullock, A., Monrouxe, L., & Atwell, C. (2011). Evaluation of the London deanery training course 'Supervision skills for clinical teachers' (working paper 141). Cardiff: University of Cardiff School of Social Sciences. http://www.cardiff.ac.uk/socsi/resources/wp141.pdf. Accessed 28 Mar 2012.

Burton, J., & Launer, J. (Eds.). (2003). *Supervision and support in primary care*. Oxford: Radcliffe.

Davidsen, A. S., & Reventlow, S. (2011). Narratives about patients with psychological problems illustrate different professional roles among general practitioners. *Journal of Health Psychology, 16*, 959–968.

Kirkpatrick, D. L., & Kirkpatrick, J. D. (2006). *Evaluating training programs* (3rd ed.). San Francisco, CA: Berett-Koehler.

Launer, J. (2010). Supervision, mentoring and coaching. In T. Swanwick (Ed.), *Understanding medical education: Evidence, theory and practice*. Edinburgh: Association for the Study of Medical Education.

London Deanery. (2012). Supervision skills for clinical teachers. http://www.faculty.londondeanery.ac.uk/supervision-skills-for-clinical-teachers. Accessed 28 Mar 2012.

Chapter 9
Practice Inquiry: Uncertainty Learning in Primary Care Practice

Lucia Siegel Sommers

Most primary care clinicians in nonacademic settings lack a practice-based collegial forum for addressing the clinical uncertainty inherent in their work. Practice Inquiry comprises a set of small group methods designed explicitly for engaging case-based clinical uncertainty. Clinical uncertainty is defined as confusion and puzzlement around the diagnostic, management, relationship, prognostic, and/or ethical issues raised by an individual patient case. For the clinician small group that meets over time, these collaborative learning methods offer in-depth facilitated case discussion for addressing real-time patient uncertainties with empathic support, intellectual curiosity, and attention to process.

Practice Inquiry targets clinicians at three levels: practicing primary care clinicians, postgraduate trainees, and medical students. This chapter describes Practice Inquiry for practicing primary clinicians and includes:

- *Beginnings*. This section describes the need for a workplace learning setting where clinician colleagues collaborate to address individual patients' clinical uncertainties (Sommers et al. 2007).
- *Practice Inquiry in the colleague group*. This section illustrates how colleagues collaborate on an uncertainty case. ("Colleagues" refers to physicians, nurse practitioners, and physician assistants in primary care settings who attend Practice Inquiry colleague group meetings and present patients from their own patient panels.)

Electronic supplementary material: The online version of this chapter (doi:10.1007/978-1-4614-6812-7_9) contains supplementary material, which is available to authorized users.

L. Siegel Sommers (✉)
Department of Family and Community Medicine, University of California, San Francisco, 2393 Filbert Street, San Francisco 94123, CA, USA (Residence)
e-mail: Lucia.Sommers@ucsf.edu

L.S. Sommers and J. Launer (eds.), *Clinical Uncertainty in Primary Care: The Challenge of Collaborative Engagement*, DOI 10.1007/978-1-4614-6812-7_9,
© Springer Science+Business Media New York 2013

- *Conceptual framework.* This section reviews the rationales underlying Practice Inquiry's focus on the colleague group, case-based clinical uncertainty, inputs to clinical judgment, follow-up, and group facilitation.
- An *"inquiry practice."* This section conceptualizes the larger primary care setting within which Practice Inquiry would ideally dwell along with two other forms of collaborative learning under development: *Practice Epidemiology*, a set of strategies for describing patient panels to improve care, and *Practice Mining*, a framework for initiating potentially useful investigations into unexpected and perplexing patient care phenomena observed by clinicians in the course of caring for their patients.

Practice Inquiry as an integral curriculum focus in three US Family Medicine residency programs is described in Chapter 10. A description of Practice Inquiry as a curriculum focus within a longitudinal medical school clerkship is found in On-line Resource #1.

Beginnings

Three events converged in the mid- to late 1990s in San Francisco, California, to provide impetus for Practice Inquiry: the creation of the "Curriculum Template," (Sommers and Marton 2000) a document outlining a novel approach for continuing medical education (CME) in managed care settings; the launch of an office-practice rotation for third year residents at an internal medicine postgraduate training program; and, in the same training program, the initiation of a primary care case conference where residents presented their case-based dilemmas. All three initiatives dealt with preparing clinicians for the twenty-first-century world of primary care medicine in the United States (see Box 9.1).

First, in 1994, a group of California health care policy makers and clinical educators were tasked to assess the CME needs of clinicians in managed care organizations and recommend a comprehensive curricular approach to addressing those needs. The resulting "Curriculum Template" provided a blueprint for a CME curriculum that integrated four core content areas – relationship-centered care, evidence-based practice, team functioning, and reflective practice – and postulated that collegial learning should happen as part of daily practice, "not something occurring outside the routine activities of the physician" (Confessore 1997). The Template outlined a small group learning approach with clinicians meeting in "colleague groups" during set-aside time and using the clinicians' own cases as the substrate for learning. The template writers had been inspired by the Balint group model, a time-honored method for individual case discussion with emphasis on the clinician–patient relationship (see Chapters 4 and 5) and a more recent Canadian

Box 9.1 Primary Care in the United States

Governance of the US Health care System: The US has a market-based health care system largely dependent on the private ownership of health care resources and the purchase of private health insurance. The federal government, through the Department of Health and Human Services and state and local governments, provides public health insurance coverage for the elderly, the disabled, and low income individuals; operates or funds care delivery programs for low-income medically underserved populations, military personnel and veterans, and Native Americans; and monitors, regulates, and evaluates the delivery of health care services. There is no central governing body that manages or otherwise exerts global control of the health care delivery system.

Breakdown of Health Insurance Coverage: In 2010, 64% of individuals reported having coverage through a private health insurance plan, predominantly employer-based; 31% reported having coverage through a government health insurance plan; and 16% reported having no health insurance (*estimates by type of coverage are not mutually exclusive as individuals can be covered by more than one type of health insurance plan during the year*) (DeNavas-Walt et al. 2010).

Primary Care Clinicians: Primary care is provided by physicians, nurse practitioners, and physician assistants. Primary care physicians (PCPs) are doctors of medicine (M.D.) and osteopathy (D.O.) who have completed a 3-year accredited residency program in family medicine, general internal medicine, or general pediatrics. Approximately 30% of US physicians are primary care physicians (COGME 2010), with an estimated 90 PCPs per 100,000 people (GAO 2008).

Nurse practitioners (NPs) are registered nurses who have completed an accredited masters or doctoral level educational program in advanced practice nursing. NPs are certified by an individual state's nurse practice act to either practice independently or through a required collaborative agreement with a physician. Approximately 52% of NPs practice primary care (AHRQ 2011), with an estimated 28 primary care NPs per 100,000 people (GAO 2008).

Physician assistants (PAs) are individuals who have completed a 24–30 month accredited physician assistant education program, generally receiving a master of science degree, and are licensed by states to practice medicine with the supervision of a physician. Approximately 43% of PAs practice primary care, (AHRQ 2011) with an estimated eight primary care PAs per 100,000 people (GAO 2008).

(continued)

Box 9.1 (continued)

Organizational Contexts in Which Primary Care Services Are Provided:
Over 80% of patient visits to primary care delivery sites occur in physician
offices (Hing and Uddin 2010). These sites are predominantly independent
and physician-owned, small- to medium-sized group practices. Most of these
"private practice" PCPs affiliate with networks of independent physicians
that contract with managed care health insurance plans offered by
employers, unions, and state governments; participating PCPs provide care
to individuals and families enrolled in a given health plan, in accordance
with a plan's scope of services and the network's performance parameters.

Office-based physicians are reimbursed largely through a fee-for-service
payment mechanism based on a national fee schedule that reimburses physicians for specific services provided at each office visit; between visit coordination of care functions are not reimbursed. The current fee schedule is
weighted disproportionately toward in-hospital and procedural services,
resulting in significantly lower overall income levels for PCPs relative to specialist physicians (Berenson and Rich 2010).

Increasingly, PCPs are assuming positions as salaried employees in private
and public health care organizations, including group-model health maintenance organizations, hospital system-owned practices, community health
center networks, and local government-run integrated delivery systems. In
some organizations, salaries are based on incentive-driven compensation
formulas.

Health care Reform and the Patient-Centered Medical Home: Recently
enacted health care reform legislation is prioritizing the development of large,
"accountable," and integrated health care delivery systems that coordinate
health services across the care continuum (Kocher et al. 2010). A new primary
care delivery model, the Patient Centered Medical Home (PCMH), is envisioned to serve as a core infrastructure of these systems (Davis et al. 2011).
Implementation and evaluation of the PCMH model are currently underway
(Grumbach and Grundy 2010).

small group approach to CME incorporating evidence-based medicine (EBM) concepts to address case dilemmas (see Chapter 6).

Second, in 1998, at the internal medicine residency program of St. Mary's
Medical Center in San Francisco, California, my faculty colleagues and I piloted an
office-practice rotation that placed residents with general internists who were program graduates practicing in the community. Despite having had initial concerns
about seeing fewer patients, these new teachers uniformly gave the pilot rotation
high grades. The residents, we learned, provided relief from "hamster care" – each

clinician, following their assigned patients, straightforward and complex, one by one, day after day at a 15-minute clip (Morrison and Smith 2000). When the residents saw patients with them, the clinicians found themselves getting "off the wheel." They took time to step back, listen and reflect on the resident's presentation of the clinician's own patients. In this teaching context, the clinicians reported becoming more deliberate in their assessment of their patients' problems and relying less on automatic, reflexive habits such as referral to specialists (Barnett et al. 2012). Seeing patients together opened up occasions for sharing how clinicians use a most precious commodity – clinical judgment, what Montgomery defines as "the practical reasoning or phronesis that enables physicians to fit their knowledge and experience to the circumstance of each patient." (2006). Klass talks about students learning medicine from their teachers and peers, highlighting a critical dimension of this fitting process:

> Call it what you will - detailing, apprenticeship, peer mentorship or discussion groups are all different responses to the necessity for judgment to be 'come upon' in practice…unlike information and knowledge, the transfer of judgment demands a working collaboration. (2004)

With the license to practice medicine comes the independence from supervision and the opportunity to exercise one's unique clinical judgment. Is the consequence of this independence the clinician's virtual isolation from mentors and colleagues whose "working collaboration," as Klass points out, is critical for honing clinical judgment? The office-practice rotation embedded learning directly into practice, allowing for the kind of informal learning that Coles talks about in Chapter 3. Unfortunately, with more emphasis on productivity coming from integrated health systems that own or contract with primary care practices (Kocher and Sahni 2011), as of 2012, only one of the original seven community-based teachers still welcomes residents in their practice.

Third, in 1998, a "working collaboration" also characterized the focus of a new, one-hour primary care teaching conference held weekly for residents prior to seeing their scheduled continuity patients in the medical clinic. Over the years, the clinic had increasingly enrolled patients presenting with complex medical and psychosocial problems. Struggling to sort out their patients' diagnostic and management dilemmas and under time constraints to see more patients, the residents had limited opportunity during clinic to "present" their patients for one-on-one teaching. The new teaching conference created a learning space similar to that of traditional bedside rounds where residents could share and discuss specific patients scheduled for that day's clinic session and put to use their newly-acquired EBM skills. With facilitation by a physician teacher and a behavioral scientist, the residents collaborated in a form of peer mentorship to think through and plan strategies for addressing their patients' multifaceted dilemmas and acknowledge the clinical uncertainty that Atkinson (1984) and Ludmerer (1999) maintain had been overlooked if not denied during their earlier medical training.

Envisioning life after residency, graduating residents wondered how they would manage in their new practice positions when confronted with case-based uncertainties and 15-minute appointment slots. Would such conferences devoted to actual case dilemmas be available? We reminded them how they had been trained for "graded and progressive responsibility" with the ultimate goal of becoming independent physicians and "self-directed learners" (ACGME 2009; Slotnick 1999). Once in practice, we assured them they would find resources for coping with and even *tolerating* clinical uncertainty, a well-noted capability of generalist physicians (Thomson 1978; Epstein and Hundert 2002; Ghosh 2004; Mamede et al. 2007a).

Practice Inquiry (PI) in the Colleague Group

The office-practice rotation and the new clinic conference taught us valuable lessons about how clinicians learn together. Keeping in mind the Curriculum Template's original CME mandate, we decided to ask our community-based teachers and other clinician colleagues in the San Francisco Bay Area to join us in exploring the question that we were now prompted to ask: *What would happen if, once out of training, in their workplace settings, primary care clinicians had set-aside time to meet with their peers in facilitated small groups and discuss patients that stumped them, caused them worry, or for whom what they were doing was not working?*

We wondered whether community-based practitioners, such as our office-practice teachers, would make time for such collegial work given that their practice lives were becoming increasingly constricted due to larger patient loads, proliferating practice guidelines, and administrative hassles (Sommers et al. 2001). In proposing that set-aside time to address uncertainties would benefit primary care clinicians, we were emboldened by Trisha Greenhalgh's advocacy for an "evidence-based, Balint group" (2002) where clinicians would not have to choose "between evidence-based medicine and old-fashioned clinical intuition," a setting where uncertainty could be actively *engaged* and not merely *tolerated*.

Box 9.2 The CME Programs

Practice Inquiry: Improving Clinical Judgment and Clinical Practice at the Department of Family and Community Medicine at University of California, San Francisco (UCSF), and at Kaiser Permanente Medical Center Oakland, California

The Practice Inquiry CME Program at UCSF based in the Department of Family and Community Medicine began in 2005 preceded by 2½ years of pilot work. As of Spring 2013, seven PI groups are part of the program. Two PI groups have been meeting in Kaiser Permanente Medical Centers based in the Department of Medicine; one group has been CME-certified since 2005, and the other group is currently applying for accredited CME status. In the US, most states require physicians and mid-level practitioners to obtain "CME credits" in order for licensure renewal.

(continued)

Box 9.2 (continued)

Practice Inquiry Groups

Group site (in Northern California)	Affiliation	First meet-ing	Current members	Meeting frequency/ time	Facilitation
1. Maxine Hall Health Center (San Francisco)	CHC (publicly funded)	2002	6 PCPs 1 NP	Every other month	LS
2. Asian Health Services (Oakland)	CHC (publicly funded)	2004	22 PCPs 1 PA	Weekly	MD member
3. Kaiser Permanente (Oakland)	Private nonprofit HMO	2004	4–7 PCPs 2–3 special-ists	Twice monthly	MD member
4. Lakeshore UCSF FM Faculty Practice (San Francisco)	Private, nonprofit, and university sponsored	2005	6 PCPs 2 NPs	Monthly	LS MD members
5. Potrero Hill Health Center (San Francisco)	CHC (publicly funded)	2006	5 PCPs 1 NP 1 Specialist	Every other month	LS
6. Baywest (San Francisco)	Private practice	2006	3 PCPs 1 NP	Monthly, on hold recruiting members	LS
7. Axis Health Center (Pleasanton)	CHC (publicly funded)	2009	6–8 PCPs 1 NP	Monthly	LS MD member
8. Sutter East Bay Foundation (Albany)	Hospital system-owned PCP group practice	2010	6 PCPs 2 NPs	Monthly	LS
9. Kaiser Permanente (Richmond)	Private nonprofit HMO	2010	5–7 PCPs 2–3 special-ists	Weekly	MD member

PCP primary care physician, *NP* nurse practitioner, *PA* physician assistant, *LS* Lucia Sommers, *CHC* community health center

Practice Inquiry colleague group pilot work began in 2001 in several small group private practices, one large group private practice, three community health centers, and one Kaiser Permanente ambulatory care practice. In 2005, the CME Office of the School of Medicine, University of California, San Francisco (UCSF), accredited PI colleague groups for AMA PRA Category 1 Credit™ for physicians and mid-level practitioners. A similar program was accredited at Kaiser Permanente, Oakland, California. (See Box 9.2 for PI colleague group sites and On-line Resource #2 for CME program details: funding, objectives, participation requirements, key statistics, program evaluation, and the PI Questionnaire, "Your Feedback about Practice Inquiry").

A Scenario

The colleague group scenario described below uses the *single-case* Practice Inquiry discussion format. (See On-line Resource #4 for multiple-case discussion formats.) The scenario is based on an actual patient case presented in a well-established San Francisco colleague group of seven clinicians (Case details have been modified to safeguard patient confidentiality.). The clinicians work together in the same clinic and meet monthly at noon around a table in the lunchroom. A group member serves as facilitator.

The single case format includes eight phases that, given a moderately complex case, is completed in 50–60 minutes. Experienced colleague groups move more quickly and may discuss two or three cases during one meeting. In this scenario, each group phase begins with a request or question from the group facilitator which starts discussion and guides inquiry, followed by initial responses from the case presenter or colleague group members. Following this initial dialogue, the purpose

The Eight Phases of a Practice Inquiry Colleague Group

1. The Uncertainty Statement

2. The Uncertainty Narrative

3. Additional Information

4. Presenter's Question(s)

5. Inputs to Judgment

6. *the blend*

7. Implications for Practice

8. Conclusion

Fig. 9.1

of each group phase is described and relevant theoretical perspectives regarding clinical judgment, decision-making, clinician behavior and small group process are highlighted, sometimes referencing conversation that occurred later in the group. The eight PI colleague group phases are displayed in Fig. 9.1.

Phase I: The Uncertainty Statement

> **Facilitator (to the presenter):** "Please start our session by telling us about your dilemma."
>
> **Presenter:** "I don't know whether this patient has CHF, may be developing a pulmonary problem, or both. I've done what I think is a good initial work-up but maybe I'm forgetting something."

The colleague presenting the case (case presenter) describes a real-time uncertainty involving the care of a patient. Starting the discussion with an "I don't know" statement is a bold move and one with which new groups rightfully struggle. The task requires removing one's "mask of infallibility" and "cloak of competence" (Gorovitz and MacIntyre 1976; Haas and Shaffir 1977). It requires setting aside one's role as an authoritarian figure that can "mitigate ambiguity and uncertainty" (Rodning 1992) and making a statement about confusion, surprise, or dismay about the care of an individual patient. The task also necessitates that presenters not deny or disregard uncertainties nor should they simply accept and normalize them (Atkinson 1984; Light 1979; Katz 1984).

In making the uncertainty statement, the case presenter foregoes the mantra of the classic patient presentation (e.g., "This is a 60-year-old diabetic female with sudden onset of…."). This formulaic ritual prompts clinicians to present an ordered array of facts about the patient that often delays the unspoken punch line of "I don't know what is going on here!" Foregoing this ritual allows the case presenter to focus instead on what is important to learn now. This need to learn and to do better for the patient trumps the fear of revealing inadequacy as a clinician, the emotion that Gerrity and colleagues suggest motivates clinicians' underlying reactions to uncertainty. These reactions express themselves as anxiety, concern about bad outcomes, and reluctance to disclose uncertainty to patients and mistakes to other clinicians (1992; 1995).

For the presenter's colleagues, seeing one of their own come forward with an uncertainty statement is both disarming (How can I ignore this colleague's request?) and validating (I'm not the only one who sometimes doesn't know). Logistically, it announces the topic of initial focus and activates colleagues' recall of their own experiences with similar patients.

The early research of Renee Fox on medical students offers guidance on how clinicians appreciate the uncertainty statement within the context of a colleague group:

> There are three basic types of uncertainty around which the process of 'training for uncertainty' in medical school centers is based. There are the uncertainties that originate in the impossibility of commanding all the vast knowledge and complex skills of continually

advancing modern medicine, the uncertainties that stem from the many gaps in medical knowledge and limitations in medical understanding and effectiveness that nonetheless exist, and *the uncertainties connected with distinguishing between personal ignorance and ineptitude and the lacunae and incapacities of the field of medicine itself.* (Fox 1957, italics added)

In the colleague group, the third type of uncertainty expresses itself when the case presenter tells colleagues "I've done what I think is a good initial work-up but maybe I'm forgetting something." They hear their colleague ask, "Is it me? Is it because I don't have the knowledge to deal with this problem? Then again, maybe I've done what I'm supposed to do and should rest easy." Hearing these concerns, colleagues cannot help but reflect, "If this were my patient, what would I do?"

Phase 2: The Uncertainty Narrative

Facilitator (to the presenter): "Now, tell us what you want us to know about your patient and the uncertainty so that we're in the best position to help."

Presenter: "Mr. D is an 87-year-old Latino male, long-time patient who I've always enjoyed seeing since he and I love soccer. He is widowed and now lives alone in a studio apartment on a small pension. He has managed to care for himself, takes long walks, and is on meds for hypertension and diabetes. Our clinical pharmacist has been working with him for the past year or so and his diabetes has been in somewhat better control. He also reports that after seeing the nutritionist, he eats less of his beloved chicharrones and pan dulce. Despite all this, he was hospitalized 6 weeks ago for a heart attack. Somehow I hadn't checked his cholesterol for a while and it was through the roof. I feel really awful about this. In the last month, he has developed wheezing; he is a former smoker and says he quit when he was about 60. I gave him salbuterol and beclomethasone inhalers but I'm not sure it's helping. Maybe we have to give it more time.... I am wondering if this could be cardiac. I know this sounds strange to say but despite his years and his conditions...oh yes, did I mention, that he also has rheumatoid arthritis? Despite all of this, I really see him as quite vital. But now, I'm worried .... he seems quite out of it - he's just not himself. I'm playing telephone tag with the cardiologist and his daughter. His chest x-ray is ambiguous - a slightly enlarged heart, hyperinflation of lungs, and blunting of costophrenic angles bilaterally; the echo is pending."

To describe the uncertainty, in contrast to how trainees "present" patients to their physician teachers, the clinician tells a story. Past medical history items (e.g., rheumatoid arthritis), for example, are referenced throughout the narrative; other items are left out (e.g., hospitalization details). If the chart is brought to the meeting, it is not passed around. The presenter controls the storytelling.

Recalling what they know about the presenter as a person and clinician, the colleague group's first task is to listen attentively to the uncertainty narrative. The colleagues listen for how the presenter thinks and feels. They recognize the heuristics based in the intuitive, 'System 1' mode of reasoning where easily-accessed, automatic knowledge is revealed with ease (e.g., "Despite all of this, I really see him as quite vital. But now, I'm worried…..he seems quite out of it – he's just not himself.") At the same time they are comfortable with their colleague's use of the more analytic formulations found in 'System 2' thinking (e.g., "His chest x-ray is ambiguous…. a slightly enlarged heart, hyperinflation of lungs….") (Croskerry 2009). As the colleagues listen to the patient story, they, too, could react intuitively (e.g., "Early dementia?") Then, more thoughtfully, they might ask themselves, "What are other causes of confusion?". Dhaliwal describes such back and forth reasoning, stating, "Expert clinical judgment is characterized by an adroit self-regulatory sense of when intuition is insufficient and analysis is necessary" (2011). Alternatively, in mentioning only a small number of potentially correlated cues (e.g., cough, chest x-ray findings), the presenter could be using "fast and frugal heuristics" that adjust reasoning to the specific setting and patient context (Gigerenzer and Gaissmaier 2011).

Phase 3: Additional Information

> **Facilitator (to colleagues):** "What additional information would help you to better understand the uncertainty for this patient? Let's limit this to 3-4 simple questions."

> **Colleagues:**
> - "What medications is he on?"
> - "Does he have clinical signs of CHF, neck veins, or edema?"
> - "How functional is he now?"
> - "When did his wife die? How is he managing?"

The colleagues actively elicit additional data important to their understanding of the case. To avoid overwhelming the presenter, the facilitator limits the number of questions. Each question posed becomes a window that opens up a potential topic of interest. While listening and responding to these questions, the presenter's memory of illness scripts/trajectories become activated and updated for "connecting the dots" (Lloyd and Reyna 2009; Hertwig et al. 2013). Could Mr. D's cardiac status be more compromised than originally thought? Is he still taking long walks with his dog? Feeling more at ease, the presenter mentions, "As I think about it, I'm realizing that possibly Mr. D was more short of breath, maybe even confused, at our last visit." Colleagues' simple questions spark new insights that the presenter then articulates. From these insights, colleagues gain better awareness of the presenter's automatic, tacit knowledge–working knowledge about Mr. D that the presenter has gained over the years but cannot easily put into words. As discussion continues, colleagues give "language to practice" since tacit knowledge is best passed on through social interaction (Mattingly and Fleming 1994; Fenton et al. 2001).

Phase 4: Presenter's Initial Question

> **Facilitator (to the presenter):** "Now that we have additional information about Mr. D, provide us with a question to start discussion."

> **Presenter:** "I know that other things could be going on here, but I don't want Mr. D to suffer an acute event at home. How to prevent this?"

The original uncertainty takes on new dimensions as the presenter hears colleagues' questions, recalls more of Mr. D's symptoms, and worries how the patient might die alone, suddenly, at home. This is where discussion needs to start. To show respect and offer validation, colleagues exhibit patience. They might want to begin somewhere else (e.g., Mr. D's cognitive functioning), but they appreciate the value of beginning "where the presenter is." Increasingly, primary care clinicians are said to be suffering from "information chaos" (Beasley et al. 2011). Smith suggests that just as commonly clinicians' questions reveal their need for psychological support, affirmation, commiseration, and feedback. He adds, "such 'information needs' are never likely to be met by computer or by books or journals and may be one explanation why doctors tend to turn first to colleagues for information." 1996)

Phase 5: Inputs to Judgment

> **Facilitator:** "We all now know what's on our presenter's mind. Rather than answer the question directly, consider asking another question, one that might open a new direction previously not considered. You can also make an observation or request more information."

Colleagues:

- "I can see why this patient is worrying you…. sorting out the cardiac from the pulmonary issues can be tricky. In residency we ordered a BNP (Brain Naturetic Peptide) to sort it out."
- "I've had a couple of patients where the cardiologist has ordered that test. Since I went to medical school awhile back, I'm not clear how it helps. We should look it up."
- "Your relationship with him seems really solid. What would it be like to talk with him about missing that cholesterol panel?"
- "You've known this patient for a long time. Tell us more about what you mean when you say, 'He's not himself.'"
- "I'm curious about his mood. Does he still light up when you talk soccer?"

The facilitator assists the presenter to consider colleagues' questions and observations at a pace allowing for careful listening and reflection. Colleagues commonly make "inputs to judgment" in five arenas:

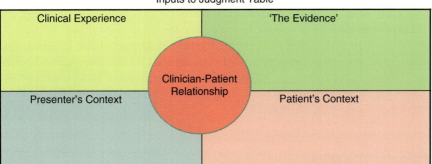

Fig. 9.2

- Clinical experience (e.g., how does heart failure typically present following a heart attack?)
- "The evidence" (e.g., what test characteristics for the BNP test are important to consider in a patient like Mr. D?)
- Clinician context (e.g., what is the impact of the presenter's regret in making decisions for Mr. D?)
- Patient context (e.g., what is important to know about Mr. D and his worldview?)
- Patient–clinician relationship (e.g., how can "soccer talk" be diagnostic?)

The five arenas are graphically displayed on the "Inputs to Judgment" table that the facilitator draws on a whiteboard and uses to document colleagues' inputs in the five arenas. (See Fig. 9.2 and On-line Resource #5 for guidance on using the table.)

One or more of these arenas fit prominently in several well-known approaches to clinical thinking. These include patient-centered care (Levenstein et al. 1986), relationship-centered care (Tresolini 1994), evidence-based medicine (Sackett et al. 1991), Balint Groups (see Chapters 4 and 5), and cognitive and affective de-biasing (Croskerry and Norman 2008). In Practice Inquiry, each input arena bears equal scrutiny for its contribution to engaging the case-based uncertainty. The deliberate consideration of these arenas encourages colleagues to access special expertise and offer novel opinion early in the discussion before conclusions are drawn (Christensen et al. 2000).

Covering the above input arenas in this phase is important, but just as valuable is *how* colleagues ask questions and make observations that encourage presenters to think out loud, reveal assumptions, and voice expectations. For this to happen, colleagues refrain from giving straight advice (e.g., If this were my patient, I would....), hidden advice (e.g., How do you think he would do on the Clock Drawing Test?), or offering interpretation (e.g., It seems to me that what is going on here is…).

Useful inquiry modes include reflecting back what the presenter said, being respectfully curious about something the presenter mentions but does not elaborate, and using the presenter's own words to craft hypotheses about what could be going on. (See Chapter 7, section "Skills for Narrative Interviewing.") In responding, the presenter makes connections across input to judgment categories (e.g., the presenter's sense of *this* patient in contrast to colleagues' experiences with older cardiac patients). Colleagues listen for their colleague's assumptions and expectations (e.g., "I was really hoping that the inhalers would fix the cough.") and encourage speculative thinking that gently challenges them. Evidence that colleagues have struck the right tenor in question-asking becomes apparent when the presenter, feeling at ease, offers additional information: "Did I mention? My older brother recently died at home after a heart attack. Maybe this figured more into Mr. D's case than I realized."

Phase 6: The Blend

> **Facilitator (to the presenter and colleagues):** "We've now heard several questions and observations that might be useful to our presenter in thinking about the dilemma."
>
> **(And then to the presenter):** "How is this sounding to you?"
>
> **Presenter:** "You're right, my own sense of Mr. D as 'vital' and able to withstand this illness has so clouded my thinking that depression and medication effects didn't cross my mind, or…I hate to think about it, early dementia. I'm now realizing that I haven't had any sort of advanced directives discussion with him."

In this phase the facilitator guides the group in refocusing on the new inputs to judgment that have emerged through discussion. The work from this point on is one of synthesis and integration, a Practice Inquiry process called "the blend." *The blend* involves a synthesis of the inputs, now reconstituted through the group's collaborative reasoning, to form new perspectives on the original uncertainty. Although synthesis work can begin earlier, the group members' reasoning together now focuses explicitly on:

- Reappraising earlier thinking *and* feelings (e.g., the gut reaction of Mr. D. being 'vital') (Stolper et al. 2011)
- Revisiting assumptions (e.g., advocating dietary restrictions to optimize the cardiac status of an 87-year-old who loves his chicharrones and pan dulce)
- Recognizing the impact of affective and cognitive biases on perceptions and actions (e.g., the case presenter's positive feelings toward Mr. D which made the lipid panel oversight that much worse) (Croskerry and Norman 2008)
- Rehearsing how to clarify patient preferences through consulting Mr. D as if he were at the table (e.g., a colleague role-plays Mr. D. complaining about his dietary restrictions)

Seen in this regenerative way, *the blend* presents a significant challenge. For this patient, it constitutes the particular "know-how" to sort out cardiac and pulmonary causes and balance diagnostic and therapeutic strategies with concerns for quality-of-life. *The blend* involves the colleagues in implicitly referencing what Gabbay and May (2010) describe as "mindlines," flexible and internalized concepts about

certain practices or types of patients that have evolved over time within the colleague group (e.g., caring for the older patient with cardiac or pulmonary problems
or both). The task becomes one of updating the group's explicit knowledge base
(e.g., engage in literature review, "curbside" local experts) and of helping the
presenter create an expanded narrative upon which practice is reconstructed (Coles
2002; Carr 1995). Doing *the blend* is also enhanced by the group's "heedful inter-
relating," a learned behavior that relies upon "knowledge generated by the richness
of the connections between the individuals" and illustrated when one colleague
says to the presenter, "Tell us more about what you mean when you say, 'He's not
himself.'" (Boreham 2000)

Phase 7: Implications for Practice

Facilitator (to the presenter): "We're almost out of time. Where would you say
you are now with Mr. D?"

Presenter: "I'll be thinking a lot about how to sort out Mr. D's cognitive and
emotional status. Getting him to talk soccer could help. If he doesn't light up,
there's a problem…. I'll be getting in touch with the cardiologist about the echo
and find out about a BNP…what else? Oh yes, a review article for us on BNP."

Reflecting upon *the blend* and its implications for practice reconstruction, the
presenter considers how to proceed. As colleagues listen to these reflections, they
may feel compelled to add something left out. They must do this with great care.
The presenter needs time to assess what has been said and consider how the new
directions envisioned may prove useful or become blind alleys. Much as in Balint
groups, these directions are not directives or action plans to which the presenter
must commit. Rather they are options for next steps designed to learn more about
the uncertainty by acting on it and seeing what happens next (Rudolph et al. 2009;
McKenna et al. 2013). Unlike the solitary deliberations of individual clinicians, this
reconstructive work occurs among colleagues who practice their craft in similar
workshops using comparable materials.

As a group, the colleagues gain wisdom through wrestling with reducible and
irreducible uncertainty and in the process build a collective case repertoire. They
become increasingly knowledgeable about each other's strengths and challenges
(e.g. who knows about cardiac drugs, who struggles with limit-setting) and become
better coaches for each other (Gawande 2011). Together they learn "good- enough
holding of anxiety," a valuable skill for engaging clinical uncertainty (Innes et al.
2005). When practiced consistently in the colleague group, the 'good-enough
holding' skill can transfer to one-on-one clinician-patient interactions and support
the shared decision-making that is particularly useful "when clinical evidence is
low" (Han 2013, Politi et al. 2013).

The ultimate value of the group's work on *the blend* becomes clearer when the case
presenter returns with follow-up. Was Mr. D depressed or showing early-onset dementia? Was there evidence of heart failure? How is Mr. D doing now? Case follow-up not

only feeds colleagues' curiosity, but the case's denouement or continuing drama adds to its luster as the colleagues' newest 'virtual' patient. Could Mr. D enter their memory banks as a classic cardiac patient at the beginning of a downhill spiral? Then again, 2 months later, the group could learn that he is back taking daily walks.

Phase 8: Conclusion

> **Facilitator (to the presenter and colleagues):** "So, in summary, what have we done together…and where are we now?"

> **Presenter:** "Thank you all for helping me look at Mr. D more realistically. "Heartwarming" patients can be just as tough as the "heartsinks!"

> **Colleagues:**
> - "This discussion helps me rethink my assessment of a dear older woman patient who had benefitted from anti-depressants but recently has become a bit befuddled."
> - "Talking soccer! Now that's really powerful. Let's make use of these special connections we have with patients when we're stuck."
> - "Wouldn't it be great to get an 'App' for our smart phones to alert us to over-due screening tests? But then again…"
> - "Our way of working on cases reminds me of the 5 blind men and the ele-phant; we need each other to put these beasts together!"

Appreciating one's "knowns and unknowns" (Fenton et al. 2009) occurs as colleagues are prompted to reflect on their patient panels in light of Mr. D (e.g., Which of my patients are labeled as depressed who might have early dementia?). How flexible am I as a communicator? (e.g., Do I use patients' hobbies as functional markers?) What knowledge gaps and knowledge stores are realized? (e.g., After some thought, I actually remember how BNP works). Such opportunities for unstructured, shared reflection encourage "reflexivity," the self-conscious account of knowledge production as it is produced (Baarts et al. 2000). Engaging in this collaborative work as the patient case unfolds in real time provides a tangible immediacy to reflexivity and places it in the service of perfecting judgment (Weiner 2004; Epstein et al. 2008).

Equally important in this group phase is the opportunity to reflect upon the group's capacity to formulate and use *meta-level* strategies to engage uncertainty. An example of a meta-level strategy comes from the colleague who refers to making use of "these special connections we have with patients when we're stuck" (e.g., talking soccer). This form of double-loop learning (Rushmer and Davies 2004) involves the group in explicitly keeping track of meta-level strategies that generalize across cases and can be called up for use in future cases. (See On-line Resource # 6 for examples of meta-level uncertainty engagement strategies.)

A related task is the group's careful noticing of how it learns. This triple-loop learning (Rushmer and Davies 2004; Regehr 2010) occurs through paying attention to the way the group engages in uncertainty work – how, meeting after meeting, as one colleague comments, "We need each other to put these beasts together."

Conceptual Framework

The scholarship of Renee Fox, Donald Schön, and Karl Weick has been pivotal to the conceptual development of Practice Inquiry. Renee Fox's understanding of how clinical uncertainty is perceived by clinicians has influenced the expression of uncertainty in the PI colleague group setting. Similarly, the writings of Karl Weick and Donald Schön on the relationship of cognition and action in organizational actors have informed the "uncertainty engagement" aspects of colleague groups, the process by which clinical professionals working in organizations collaborate in addressing and inquiring case-based uncertainty. Both Weick and Schön drew upon a social constructionist tradition that helped them appreciate the problem-setting and sensemaking capacities of individuals and groups (Magala 2002; Kinsella 2006).

We have been drawn to Schön for his celebration of professional practice and see it as the requisite substrate for colleague group work:

> Perhaps there is an epistemology of practice that takes fuller account of the competence practitioners sometimes display in situations of uncertainty, complexity, uniqueness, and conflict. Perhaps there is a way of looking at problem-setting and *intuitive artistry* that presents these activities as describable and as susceptible to a kind of rigor that falls outside the boundaries of technical rationality. (1995)

This "way of looking at problem-setting and intuitive artistry" becomes fully manifested in the PI colleague group as clinicians deliberate on case-based uncertainty.

Weick describes key organizational functions in human as opposed to mechanistic terms. His emphasis on the collective aspects of "sensemaking," "mindfulness," "improvisation," and "galumphing" (i.e., purposeful playfulness,) has informed our understanding of how clinicians in a group come together for validation, tangible support, and professional growth (Weick 2001; Coutu 2003). In describing "enactment," Weick could be referencing the talk – reflection cycles of a colleague group:

> At the heart of enactment is the idea that cognition lies in the path of the action. Action precedes cognition and focuses cognition. The sensemaking sequence implied in the phrase, 'How can I know what I think until I see what I say?' involves the action of talking which lays down the traces that are examined so that cognitions can be inferred. These inferred cognitions then become preconceptions which partially affect the next episode of talk… (2001)

Colleague group discourse allows for the "seeing of what's said" by understanding eyes and ears. The group's sensemaking support becomes relied upon as colleagues collaboratively engage uncertainty cases meeting after meeting.

While Weick and Schön have impacted PI's development directly, their work has also influenced educators and researchers in medical education, cognitive and social psychology, and organizational development whose scholarship, in turn, is referenced throughout this chapter. Schön's concept of reflection in and on action has been adapted for clinical contexts by Epstein(1999), Coles (2002), Moulton and colleagues (2007), and Mamede and colleagues (2007b). These educators and researchers explore how the individual clinician, contending with uncertainty, engages in reflective work. Frankford and colleagues (2000), Bleakley (2006), and Mann (2011) have expanded this focus beyond the individual to envision reflection processes in small group settings and organization-wide for both improving patient care and sustaining professional work.

Weick's concepts of collective sensemaking and improvisation become relevant to clinicians in patient care settings through the work of Miller and colleagues (2001), Wears and Nemeth (2007), and Rudolph and colleagues (2009). These educators and researchers explore how interaction through talk and improvisation provide an antidote to practicing medicine by algorithm. Weick and Schön have also provided a substantial platform for Stacey (1995) and Lave and Wenger (1991). Their concepts pertaining to professionals working in "complex adaptive systems" and "communities of practice" have, in turn, enriched PI development through interpretation by Parboosignh (2002), Innes and colleagues (2005), and Greenhalgh and Wieringa (2011). These scholars underscore the knowledge creating capacities (in contrast to knowledge translating ones) unleashed when clinicians interact with patients as well as each other.

To develop the small group as the setting for collaborative engagement of uncertainty, we have been influenced by the focused learning approaches embodied in three, clinician-oriented, approaches to small group work: Balint groups, problem-based small group learning (PBSGL) groups (as described by John Premi in 1988), and narrative-based supervision (NBS) groups. Each approach in its current form is presented in one or more chapters of this book.

Below we describe concepts integral to Practice Inquiry's five core components: the colleague group, case-based clinical uncertainty, inputs to clinical judgment, follow-up, and group facilitation. Each component supports both uniformity of process across groups and individual group uniqueness.

The Colleague Group

Sharing individual uncertainty cases on an on-going, scheduled basis is the essence of Practice Inquiry colleague group work. Despite learning medicine in hospital-based ward teams, US physicians have few formal opportunities after postgraduate training to learn in small group settings. Not so in Western Europe. Michael Balint first introduced Balint Groups in the 1950s in the UK (see Chapters 4 and 5) and Launer and Burton began working with narrative-based supervision groups in the 1990s (see Chapters 7 and 8). Continuing professional development for physicians in Sweden, Denmark, Scotland, and Canada – as well as Ireland (O'Riordan 2000) – has relied heavily on small group learning using a variety of approaches (See Chapters 6, 11, and 12).

In PI, clinicians attend colleague groups voluntarily and consider each other as professional equals. Offering advice and feedback for care improvement, they interact on a routine basis with the express purpose of engaging case-based uncertainty. Colleague groups offer a stark contrast to a health care organization's QI/QA management program that oversees clinician performance by monitoring adherence to screening criteria (Landon 2012; Kizer and Kirsh 2012). While performance monitoring is important for assuring compliance to population-based quality indicators, Parboosingh and colleagues have noted, "Failure to take advantage of practitioner interactivity may explain in part the disappointingly low mean rate of practice improvement reported in studies on the effectiveness of practice improvement projects" (2011).

PI group size is ideally 7–8 members. Age, gender, and physician/mid-level practitioner mix should reflect the clinicians with patients at the practice site. Unlike a health care team where some members have non-fiduciary relationships with patients, colleague group membership is limited to clinicians with full accountability for the consequences of medical error, an attribute that Lester suggests, allows clinicians to identify strongly with one another in the sense of "there but for the grace of God go I" (Lester and Twitter 2001). The "psychological safety" thus created paves the way for collaborative learning (Marold et al. 2012).

Compared with other learning formats such as lecture or performance feedback, small group interaction in some studies has been shown to facilitate practice change (Davis 2011; Forsetlund et al. 2009). This may occur because in these gatherings the stage is set for creating "connexional experiences," interactions that allow participants to go beyond the boundaries of self and feel part of a larger whole. When connexional experiences occur between doctor and patient, as described by Suchman and Mathews, they can "reframe the doctor's task to make clinical uncertainty more tolerable" (1988). Colleague groups, as settings for clinicians to 'bear witness' to each other's worries, misgivings or mistakes (Carmack 2010), hark back to hospital attending rounds and conferences that Bosk detailed as "occupational rituals" for managing uncertainty (1980). More recently, Prasad described the fundamental purpose of mortality and morbidity conferences as ritually anchoring medical professionals through "defining their sense of what is means to be a doctor;" quality improvement, patient outcomes, and systems improvement, he suggests, are secondary issues (2010). When clinicians, thus, share their clinical uncertainties in colleague group settings, could such collaborative engagement lead to effective uncertainty engagement that over time translates into practice change?

Case-Based Clinical Uncertainty

In Practice Inquiry, the combined focus on the *individual patient* and *clinical uncertainty* is unusual given the current structure and focus of both quality assurance/quality improvement (QA/QI) and CME programs in the US. From the 1970s onward starting in hospital settings, QA/QI and CME programs defined their unit of analysis as the patient group as opposed to the individual patient. The medical audit has been the methodology of choice for connecting knowledge deficiencies to CME solutions and also, along with other tools, for connecting system problems to QI/QA solution processes (Brown and Uhl 1970; Kibbe et al. 1993; Shojania et al. 2012). Although audits with feedback have been a CME mainstay and Continuous Quality Improvement methods have dominated hospital as well as ambulatory care quality initiatives, evidence of clinician behavior change resulting from either modality or in combination with other strategies has often been lacking (Sommers et al. 1984; Bowie et al. 2012; Ivers et al. 2012).

PI, in contrast to a medical audit, or the average QI project or CME program, focuses first on the individual case and second on the implications of the patient case for improving care for other patients. PI functions in ways similar to Tumor Boards in hospital settings where there is high potential to directly impact the care of a specific patient (Gagliardi et al. 2007). In PI, a presenter can put new learning into action almost immediately following a meeting. Furthermore, through virtual contact with colleagues' dilemma patients, clinicians can reflect on their own patient panels with new appreciations that come from incorporating the new case-based learning into their experience base. Most QI/QA programs lack these direct effects, as their objective is to reduce "unwarranted" practice variation through monitoring patient care more globally using evidence-based criteria that vary in relevance to individual patients (Miller et al. 2001; Mercuri and Gafni 2011). As Blumenthal notes,

> One reason why some physicians are frustrated with current quality measurement efforts is that they seem not to assess what physicians feel they were trained to do and take the most pride in: to make countless daily decisions about diagnosis and treatment using copious, incomplete, confusing, and changing information, under time pressure and in the face of an ambiguous medical literature. (2004)

To become a PI case, a patient must attract attention as a quandary or a puzzle which resides in the caregiving. It is just such instances of 'not knowing' that all variety of experiential learning theorists – Weick (1969), Schön (1983), Kolb (1984), Mezirow (1990), Eraut (1994) – and the clinical educators influenced by their work – Miller (1967), Knowles (1996), Slotnick (1999), Fish and Coles (1998), Crabtree (2003) – believe are critical for high quality adult learning. The messy indeterminacy of the unscripted, that which is 'not in the book,' is the stock-in-trade for professionals whatever their expertise. As Light points out, "Regardless how technically developed a professional field is, it will define the treatment of problematic cases as its true work" (Light 1979) (See On-Line Resource #3 for representative uncertainty cases and the Practice Inquiry Clinical Uncertainty Taxonomy).

Inputs to Judgment and "the Blend"

According to EBM advocates, good clinicians integrate or blend their clinical expertise with "the conscientious, explicit, and judicious use of current best evidence" in the service of making decisions for the individual patient (Sackett et al. 1991).

While challenging what EBM advocates exclude from this integration (e.g., non-experimental evidence), EBM critics also point out how little guidance is offered for doing this critical synthesis work particularly when faced with clinical uncertainty (Feinstein and Horwitz 1997, Wears and Nemeth 2007, Tonelli 2001). Yet regardless of differences, EBM fans as well as critics do share one belief: the task of integration – that is, *the blend* of clinical experience, evidence, and the unique patient, clinician, and relationship contexts necessary for puzzling through a case-based uncertainty – belongs exclusively to the individual clinician working independently.

First, the clinician must find relevant evidence-based guidelines and decide how to apply them to the individual patient. Second, she should recognize the cognitive and emotional biases that surface when applying evidence to a patient and employ an array of cognitive tools to prevent error caused by these biases (e.g., increase knowledge through simulation exercises, improve intuitive and deliberate decision-making by 'slowing down,' selectively get help from others and from decision support tools; Moulton et al. 2007; Graber et al. 2012). Lastly, to prepare oneself for the difficult work of *the blend* and guard against error, the clinician is advised to use mindfulness techniques to develop "resilience," an antidote to compassion fatigue and burnout (Beckman et al. 2012; Zwack and Schweitzer 2013).

The blend, thus, is viewed as a process that is quintessentially what doctors do alone in their heads (Berg 1995). To suggest otherwise is antithetical to medical education's training for progressive independence, freedom from supervision, and self-direction in lifelong learning (Kennedy et al. 2009; Bleakley 2010).

How problematic is this notion of the clinician, reasoning alone, for the daily work of primary care? For the majority of patients in a clinician's patient panel, doing *the blend* by themselves presents few problems. But for 5% or 10% of patients – no one knows for sure – the slowing down and being mindful is not working. Markers such as repeat hospitalizations or frequent emergency room visits indicate problems with *the blend* and signal diagnostic error.

In Practice Inquiry, *the blend* evolves from conversations in which colleagues ask questions that are curious and imaginative while showing concern and empathy (see Chapters 7 and 8). Beyond providing validation and new ideas, colleagues also convey a strong interest in doing something very special – accompanying case presenters to a familiar learning place, a place reminiscent of the best of their training years where they first experienced peers and mentors learning together at the bedside. Premi underscores this value when he notes, "Each individual must make personal contributions to the learning activities of the group" (1988).

The quality of *the blend* may well depend on the group's ability to use its collective "adaptive expertise" (Mylopoulos and Woods 2009). In meeting over time, colleagues collaborate in engaging uncertainty to both manage the case at hand and make the knowledge created available to other patients. Strategies for managing a chronic pain patient, for example, discussed at one meeting are refined using a second pain case presented at a subsequent meeting. Over the months, a clinic-wide policy for managing chronic pain patients could materialize through what Mylopoulos and Scardamalia would call "collaborative, iterative idea improvement" (2008).

In jointly constructing frameworks for engaging uncertainty as "shared mental models" (Custer et al. 2012), colleagues participate in *knowledge creation* oriented to the patient under discussion but potentially benefiting other patients as well.

Follow-Up

Colleagues in Practice Inquiry do three types of follow-up: follow-up on *patients* discussed (once presented, colleagues want updates on outcomes); follow-up on recurring *topics* that colleagues identify through case discussion via review of case logs; and follow-up on colleagues' *capabilities* as collaborative learners.

In primary care, systematic, post-visit follow-up of individual patient outcomes is largely non-existent, making it difficult for clinicians to prevent cognitive skill decay and overconfidence (Croskerry and Norman 2008; Weaver et al. 2012). To calibrate decision-making and "educate intuition" (Hogarth 2001), clinicians not only require information on how their patients are doing but how *they* themselves are doing (Schiff 2008). Balla and colleagues' findings from their qualitative study of GP's after-hours care decision-making for high-risk patients corroborate the need for case review and feedback. In their interviews of GPs, a key request was for "formal opportunities for reflection in a safe and supportive environment" (2012). In such settings, following up on patient cases reminds clinicians that even the best plans can fail because of what Innes and colleagues call "the unpredictable nature" of consultation outcomes (2005).

Follow-up on recurring topics occurs most typically when, on hearing the uncertainty statement for a new case, the facilitator or a colleague makes a mental note, saying to themselves, "Oh, boy… Another one of these!" Consulting the case log shows that indeed, one of "these" has been presented two or three times previously. (See example of case log in On-line Resource #2.) Attention to the recurring topic (e.g., "incidentalomas" in asymptomatic patients) could result in inviting an expert (e.g., endocrinologist) to attend an upcoming colleague group meeting. meeting; instead of showing slides, the invited guest listens to case summaries, provides advice on specifics, and offers general guidance.

Follow-up on the colleague group's collaborative learning involves turning its "gaze" upon itself (Iedema et al. 2006). It must make time periodically to (1) explicitly discuss group process (e.g., conversation stoppers and starters); (2) assess relevancy of uncertainty cases presented to health care needs of the community; and (3) review the group's impact on its practice setting (e.g., value of new clinic policies resulting from presentations of uncertainty cases.)

Colleague Group Facilitation

When facilitating a Practice Inquiry colleague group, it helps to appreciate the group as a "complex adaptive system" (CAS), a dynamic network of relationships which change and adapt with information flow (Miller et al. 1998; Plsek and

Greenhalgh 2001). Guided by CAS-oriented concepts, Kimball and colleagues offer three, general facilitation strategies to assure transparency in facilitation methods, a valuable attribute in adult learning (2005):

- "Engage the whole system first." (In PI, this translates into focusing on the *whole* patient whose uncertainty could have implications for the *whole* organization.)
- "Use simple rules." (In PI this translates into gentle reminders such as "listen carefully," "be curious," and "reflect first.")
- "Create an edge." (In PI this translates into conversation tactics that shift direction, air alternatives and expose dichotomies.)

Colleague groups are encouraged to *deliberately* collaborate in uncertainty engagement, that is, to value the conscious, explicit process of *together* tackling a case. Simultaneously, to prevent an overly rigid practice, groups can learn "improvisation" skills – ways to be imaginative and creative in conversation. Engstrom's concept of "deliberate practice" (as interpreted in clinical setting by Balla et al. 2009 and Van de Wiel et al. 2011) and Weick's concept of "improvisation" (as interpreted in clinical setting by McKenna et al. 2013) provide complementary, facilitative guidance when they are combined in the colleague group:

Deliberate practice		Improvisation
Stay focused	< >	Appreciate tangents
Maintain motivation	< >	Engage in play
Practice routines	< >	Value serendipity
Correct via feedback	< >	Explore error

Specific facilitation methods for each colleague group phase are found in On-line Resource #6. These methods can be helpful to deal with group process problems such as 'group think' (a result of groups reducing internal conflict through reaching consensus without sufficient analysis of alternatives), and 'group polarization' (the tendency for groups, influenced by a subset of members, to make decisions that are more extreme than ones they would make as individuals; Marold et al. 2012; Redelmeier & Dickenson 2012). Most importantly, learning colleague group facilitation skills is best done through observing groups; participating in groups; facilitating groups followed by focused feedback; and attending Balint, PBSGL, or NBS program facilitator trainings (See Chapters 4, 6, and 8.).

Building an *Inquiry Practice*

In this section, Practice Inquiry is placed within an *inquiry practice* – a hypothetical organizational setting that could foster the formal integration and continuing development of collaborative learning and practice improvement in US health care delivery systems.

Inspired by Frankford and colleagues' concept of a "reflective practice organization," an *inquiry practice* is a primary care entity (e.g., a large group practice, a health center) in which education and service are explicitly combined to allow clinicians to learn together from their patient panels and invest that learning directly into improving care for patients (2000). In combining education and practice explicitly, these practices would develop strong links to their individual communities for assuring "responsive medical professionalism" (Frankford et al. 2000; Poses 2003; Elwyn et al. 2010). This concerted commitment to learning would require ongoing vigilance since *inquiry practices* would dwell within quasi-governmental/private entities such as "patient-centered medical homes" (PCMH) and accountable care organizations and operate under payment systems such as the "Physician Quality Reporting System" that reimburses clinicians based on performance measures (Cassell and Jain 2012).

Practice Inquiry, as described above, along with two other collaborative learning methods under development – "Practice Epidemiology" and "Practice Mining" (see below) – are examples of structured opportunities for learning from practice in colleague group settings. All three methods are meant to encourage new approaches to collaborative learning inspired by the innovative, inquiry-oriented concepts of the many educators and researchers cited in this chapter.

Why would a PCMH want an *inquiry practice* within its walls? First, in offering supportive climates for collaborative learning in practice, an *inquiry practice* would attract high-quality primary care clinicians, a treasured commodity in these times of low medical student interest in primary care specialties (Council on Graduate Medical Education 2010). Second, it could help position the larger organization to become a responsive "learning culture." This entails the development of the survival-enhancing quality of "adaptive reserve"– the capacity to learn from error, reorganize, and keep moving (Miller et al. 2010; Bohmer 2011). Last, an *inquiry practice's* collaborative learning capacities could provide the missing link between the health care organization's one-size-fits-all performance monitoring systems (Kizer and Kirsh 2012) and the individual clinician's discretionary, person-centered practice. (Clinicians may better appreciate these systems if they were charged with studying their patients' illnesses and care patterns to better inform monitoring criteria).

Specifications for an *Inquiry Practice*

The major reorganizational efforts occurring in US primary care today provide ample opportunities for *inquiry practice* development. PCMH infrastructures under construction could include specifications calling for primary care clinicians to drive the learning culture inherent in an *inquiry practice*. By expanding upon PCMH mission statements, specifications could include:

- *Reaffirming primary care principles as central to health care systems.* Following Loxtercamp's observation (2001) that professionals publically "profess" their beliefs, an *inquiry practice* would advertise to its patients and community that primary care is essential to a community's well-being and that the primary care clinician's task is to provide "person-focused care" using a "generalist approach" (Starfield 2011; Stange 2009). Such care is grounded in the clinician's and patient's long-term relationship through which patient and clinician *together* build knowledge and skills to address new health problems as they arise. Given the challenges of maintaining these relationships over time, an *inquiry practice* sustains its clinicians by nurturing qualities of compassionate witnessing and reflection (Sturmberg and Cilliers 2009).

- *Envisioning health care organizations as complex adaptive systems.* In understanding itself as a dynamic, relationship-oriented entity, an *inquiry practice* would devote significant effort to boundary-spanning through sharing results of case-based work. The patients that come to PI colleague groups often fly under the QA/QI radar and prompt potentially disruptive questions (e.g., What constitutes health maintenance for obese patients? Do higher doses of chronic pain medications show commensurate gains in functionning?) In bringing these cases to other groups within the organization for commentary and exploration, the boundaries of an *inquiry practice* would be expanded to include all clinic staff. Additionally, as Frankford and colleagues propose (2000), in a "reflective practice organization," a variety of heterogeneous small groups would cut across hierarchies and disciplines to engage in collaborative learning. (See Chapter 10, for the New Hampshire Dartmouth Family Medicine Residency's *interdisciplinary* PI groups.) Similar to clinician colleague groups, these interdisciplinary groups would encourage discussion of problematic one-on-one patient interactions, identify types of patients whose behaviors increase health risks, and examine care-related phenomena that surprise or cause concern. Case-based discussion of individual patients and caregiving relationships could help balance the preoccupation many health organizations have with re-engineering care processes.

- *Evolving as a learning community where clinicians have protected time to become students of their patients.* A colleague group's identity in an *inquiry practice* is forged by a dedication to enhance clinical judgment in the service of patient care improvement. Since primary care clinicians' clinical judgment is the foundation upon which the whole primary care enterprise rests, organizations that rely upon primary care clinicians would appreciate this judgment function as integral to the organization's overall success. It would be, thus, in the organization's best interests to create protective time for collaborative learning aimed at enhancing judgment. Although CME educators have advocated "practice-based learning and improvement" (PBLI) as essential for continuing professional development (Moore and Pennington 2003), most PBLI initiatives privilege neither *collegial* learning nor set-aside time for small group work despite evidence of potential value (Owen et al. 1989; Siriwardena et al. 2008; Safran et al. 2006; Davis 2011). Frankford and colleagues' hypothetical collaborative learning groups (2000) and Soubhi and colleagues' proposed learning communities (2010) designed for primary care settings call for organizations to support this collegial work through set-aside time.

- *Facilitating clinician collaboration in the care of complex patients.* The critical
  need for clinician resource redistribution due to increasing demands for primary
  care services and the increasing number of complex patients cared for in primary
  care settings call for clinicians in an *inquiry practice* to collaborate in two additional challenges (Katerndahl et al., 2011; Blumenthal 2012):

  – Devising schemas for differentiating complex patients from the larger patient
    pool and transitioning them between care-intensity levels (See "Practice
    Epidemiology" below)
  – Organizing support functions housed in colleague groups for formulating and
    updating clinical rationales for the care of complex patients

As important as nonclinician care management is for care coordination
(Altschuler et al. 2012; Doty et al. 2012), in colleague group settings, colleagues
would present individual complex patients for guidance on *clinical* coordination
and decision-making that would reflect what Hewson and colleagues described as
"strategic medical management" – "a way to deal with uncertainty through deliberate actions that protect against premature closure, misdiagnosis, unnecessary
tests, and unnecessary expenses" (1996).

In carrying out a collaborative form of "strategic medical management" review,
colleague groups would focus on "high leverage" patient care tasks - ones that Eidus
and colleagues (2012) suggest influence short-term and long-term clinical and
economic patient outcomes. These tasks could include assessing benefits versus
harms of additional diagnostic testing suggested by specialists, considering the
significance of clinically occult disease found through preventive testing, and
deliberating on quality-of-life considerations for different therapeutic options. This
review function would also build in supports such as point-of-care, live consultation
with specialists (Lister 2012) and the colleague group, itself, serving as an internal
consultant prior to specialist referral (Kinnersley et al. 1999). "Comprehensivist" is
the term Tinetti and colleagues use to describe primary care clinicians with skills
and expertise required "to supervise care that requires integration across all the
patient's conditions within the context of the patient's health goals and priorities"
(2012). Ideally, in an *inquiry practice*, clinicians would be supported by a
payment system conducive to such comprehensivist-directed care (Merrell and
Berenson 2010).

Practice Epidemiology

Unlike Practice Inquiry that focuses on the individual dilemma patient, Practice
Epidemiology (PE), a second form of learning unique to an *inquiry practice*, directs
attention to the patient panels of colleague group members. Provided with reports
from automated databases. the colleague group uses PE methods to define across-
panel quality of care gaps and oversee *clinically–relevant* panel management.

First, to use PE for addressing quality of care gaps, colleague groups would navigate user-friendly automated databases ideally designed with their input. Having access to patient demographic, clinical, and utilization data, they would review their panels and categorize patients into risk groups. Risk group formation and categorization would entail applying *clinical judgment* designations to define constructs such as "symptom status" (stable/unstable) or "functional capacity" (good/poor). (These are designations that only primary care clinicians can make resulting from long-term, close relationships with patients.) For example, in the colleague group setting, each clinician would reflect on a list of 30 of their patients aged 75 and older and categorize them by both symptom status and functional capacity. Colleagues could focus discussion on patients in the combined "unstable symptoms/poor functional capacity category" and ask questions such as "How well do we understand these patients' preferences for end-of-life care?"

When PE is carried out over time with different patient groups, the results could provide windows into clinicians' panels to address important questions and illuminate unrecognized needs. Could clinician-directed PE exercises potentially yield as many if not more actionable quality problems than strategies that rely upon administrative databases with externally derived monitoring criteria? Additionally, compared to reliance on externally designed, performance measurement systems to encourage evidence-based practices, would there be fewer adverse consequences through using PE methods to design clinically relevant, *internal* monitoring processes? (e.g., over-testing coming from "obedience to measures"; Lee and Walter 2011; Powell et al. 2012; Kizer and Kirsh 2012). "*Quality-improving*" work, thus, becomes grounded in colleagues' clinical observations informed by data from systems they help design.

Second, in the setting of an *inquiry practice*, PE could provide a clinician-centric form of panel management whereby colleagues collaborate in using tools for population-based care (Ibrahim et al. 2001; Neuwirth et al. 2007) at the level of their own patient panels and thus decide how their time should be apportioned based on patient and service complexity. In colleague groups, clinicians would work with similar databases used for identifying quality gaps, but now in the service of guiding resource allocation decisions. In the US, most patients currently receive 15-minutes appointments regardless of number and complexity of problems, levels of disability, and utilization patterns. Potentially better ways to spend clinician time could include:

- Participating with a health educator and eight patients who take medication for diabetes and hypertension in a 60-minute group visit
- Telephoning a health aide visiting a homebound patient for medication reconciliation for 15 minutes
- Weekly emailing to patients with asthma in response to symptom diaries

The average primary care setting is not currently financially or administratively capable of supporting an infrastructure to negotiate clinically defined visit needs (Casalino 2010). This should not deter clinicians from trying out PE approaches for defining "share the care" arrangements and determining which types of patients and services they need to manage versus those nonphysicians could support (Ghorob and Bodenheimer 2012).

Plans are already in place at sites undergoing PCMH transformation efforts, using administrative databases, to "complexity-score" patients and "load-balance" clinician panels accordingly (Santa Clara Valley Medical Center 2011). A study by Grant and colleagues showed how physicians differed from automated algorithms in the way they defined 'complexity' in their patients (2011). Freund and colleagues (2012) used both a risk model derived from a database *and* clinician judgment to select patients for case management. Like Grant, they also found little overlap in cases selected by each method. In Coleman and colleagues' study where physicians were asked to select patients they wanted to retain for continued management in the face of "balancing" their patient panels, those retained were older, sicker, long-time patients (2010).

In contrast to a computerized algorithm for identifying complex patients, a PE process done in a colleague group setting could encourage clinicians to assess patient need for non-clinician case or disease management through using their continuity relationship-derived knowledge of patients, their families and communities. Clinicians would not only select the appropriate case or disease management intervention, but also define their own relationship with the patient in the short term. PE processes could help colleague groups define and work through such clinical management decisions as: Which kinds of patients need a twice-a month, half-hour visit with a physician to closely follow several unstable chronic conditions? Which patients need monthly visits with a non-clinician health coach for monitoring a single stable chronic disease and semi-annual visits with a nurse practitioner?

Practice Mining

Practice Inquiry colleague group discussion over the years has revealed that clinicians provided with set-aside time could use their practices to "pan for gold," that is, spot phenomena that they alone know to look for and when burnished through study, could inform practice improvement. In these sightings, they recognize events, interactions, and the unfolding of stories potentially important to their patient's health. Over the years, individual clinician members of SF Bay Area colleague groups have noted several such phenomena:

- Patients spontaneously stop taking antidepressants. What happens to their functioning and quality of life?
- Increasingly more elderly and demented patients have pacemakers. How to manage this given a family's desire for comfort care?
- Many morbidly obese patients may never lose weight but nonetheless need routine health maintenance. What does "health maintenance" entail for these patients?

"Practice Mining" is a form of collaborative learning that would prepare colleagues to attend critically to what they are experiencing daily: noticing unique or recurring phenomena of potential importance; naming phenomena; using multiple methods (e.g., quantification, description through story or visual arts) to characterize their evolution; and sharing observations within the colleague group to gauge interest, input, and collaboration (White 2000). Phenomena would include patient behaviors (e.g., response to treatment), clinician–patient relationship dynamics (e.g., impact of culture), and clinician behavior (e.g., abilities to vary clinician-patient communication style). The phenomena clinicians choose to observe would determine investigation method; simple investigational methods would be recommended given limited time and resources. To inspire but not intimidate, colleagues would read examples of Feinstein's "clinimetric" approaches (Sledge and Feinstein 1997), Berger's portrait of a country doctor (1967), or Hames' (1971) efforts to describe his practice. Based on colleague group member participation and support, particular questions of interest such as those cited above would be explored by the group for a 6–8-month time period or long enough to see if collaboration with university-based researchers and community organizations could lead to fruitful projects.

Why should an *inquiry practice* engage in Practice Mining? At a time when primary care clinicians risk becoming clinically "deskilled" through increasing use of electronic medical records, clinical guidelines, and decreased contact with hospitalized patients (Hoff 2011), PM would encourage clinicians to refocus on generalists' traditional expertise – to observe, assess, and exercise judgment in the best interests of individual patients for whom the convergence of lifestyle, pathogens, heredity, and modes of coping result in suffering (Feinstein 1994; Reeve et al. 2011).

Secondly, PM would call on clinicians to pay attention to how medicine's advances meet the human condition. From their unique vantage point in the life of their patients, primary care clinicians can note symptom expression in medically unexplained, "contested" conditions such as fibromyalgia (Swoboda 2008); gauge usefulness of clinical guidelines in caring for patients, both simple and complex (Lipman and Price 2000; Fried et al. 2011); and catalogue circumstances where "overdiagnosis" could potentiate risk of iatrogenesis (Hoffman and Cooper 2012).

Thirdly, PM could do what Kienle and Kiene describe as "skimming off the knowledge pool that is built up through clinicians' daily experience" (2011). With a similar goal in mind, it could organize "evidence farming," Hay and colleagues' term for gathering results of local communities' efforts to apply evidence-based guidelines to their own patient populations (2008). Lastly, to counter images of primary care as "boring paperwork and just coordinating care" (Chen 2009), incorporating PM in an *inquiry practice* could help attract intellectually curious, creative young clinicians essential to meeting the twenty-first-century care needs of patients and their communities.

Conclusion

Han and colleagues suggest that "the ultimate challenge for clinical practice and research is to understand more precisely what coping with uncertainty entails and how it can be promoted" (2011). Practice Inquiry is a set of methods that supports primary care clinicians in the collaborative engagement of case-based clinical uncertainty. In the "medical homes" of tomorrow, as described in this chapter, simple architecture could create space for clinician small groups to do this explicit, structured work.

In the San Francisco Bay Area between 2002 and 2012, 220 primary care clinicians have had sustained participation (three or more meetings for at least 1 year) in PI colleague groups. These groups have been based in group practices linked with a nonprofit hospital system, three public-funded community health center networks, a state-run university medical center, and a staff model health maintenance organization. These clinicians' ongoing commitment to PI work has been supported by the CME program of the Department of Family and Community Medicine at the University of California, San Francisco, and by a similar program at the Kaiser Permanente Medical Center in Oakland, California. Practice Inquiry has been sustained through medical director leadership of these group practices and community health centers and through the volunteer support of physician and non-physician educators who have served as group facilitators. This book has been inspired, in large part, by the dedication of the individual groups in continuing to meet regularly, of the facilitators in continuing to work with their groups and refine their skills, and of the sponsoring organizations in believing in the value of PI.

Renee Fox in her 2000 essay, "Medical Uncertainty, Revisited," categorizes the 21st century clinical uncertainties primary care clinicians face today and includes, among others, genomic medicine, population-based care models supported by evidence-based guidelines, iatrogenic effects of rapidly expanding technology, and bioethical questions about the definition of life and of death. In completing the annual PI Questionnaire with the question, "What have you liked best about PI colleague group meetings?", a group member responded by underscoring the reality of today's uncertainties: "I value the opportunity to critically evaluate cases in the context of the complex primary care environment of NOW" (See PI Questionnaire, On-line Resource #2). Reengineering primary care practice settings to become more efficient at care delivery and information management is expected to yield clinicians more time to spend with patients in the "primary care environment of NOW." The PI experience, however, suggests that no amount of individual knowledge management and communications skills training can substitute for collegial collaboration in actively engaging these new (as well as old) uncertainties.

What Practice Inquiry, Practice Epidemiology and Practice Mining have in common is a focus on supporting primary care clinicians in becoming better at what they were trained to do and what they value most – using clinical judgment in the service of addressing individual patient problems. The creation of primary care settings where this can happen ideally would embody *inquiry practice*-like principles.

These include the centrality of primary care in large-scale health care systems; involvement of all providers across disciplines and organization levels in small group learning around the patients they care for; and, very importantly, close primary care clinician collaboration in the care of complex patients. Creating settings where lofty goals such as these are transformed into straightforward, clear realities is the hope and challenge for collaborative engagement of uncertainty.

In responding to the "what-do-you-like-best" item on the PI Questionnaire, another colleague framed this hope and challenge with quiet simplicity: "We have become better colleagues to each other." Provided with this support, engaging clinical uncertainty could become an "intrinsic motivator" (Cassel and Jain 2012) for clinicians that would strengthen professional responsibility and commitment to patients during these times when accountable care organizations and Physician Quality Reporting are changing the caregiving landscape.

Acknowledgements Drs. Peter Sommers, Rodger Shepherd, Keith Marton, Kim Duir, Amiesha Panchal, and John Rapp were instrumental in the development of Practice Inquiry, *inquiry practice* concepts, and the review of chapter drafts.

References

Accreditation Council for Graduate Medical Education. (2009). *Internal medicine 1*.

Altschuler, J., Margolius, D., Bodenheimer, T., et al. (2012). Estimating a reasonable patient panel size for primary care physicians with team-based task delegation. *Annals of Family Medicine, 10*(5), 396–400.

Atkinson, P. (1984). Training for certainty. *Social Science and Medicine, 19*(9), 949–956.

Baarts, C., Tulinius, C., & Reventlow, S. (2000). Reflexivity – A strategy for a patient-centred approach in general practice. *Family Practice, 17*, 430–434.

Balla, J. I., Heneghan, C., Glasziou, P., et al. (2009). A model for reflection for good clinical practice. *Journal of Evaluation in Clinical Practice, 15*(6), 964–969.

Balla, J., Heneghan, C., Thompson, M., et al. (2012). Clinical decision making in a high-risk primary care environment: A qualitative study in the UK. *BMJ Open, 2*, e000414. Print 2012.

Balsa, A. I., Seiler, N., McGuire, T. G., et al. (2003). Clinical uncertainty and healthcare disparities. *American Journal of Law and Medicine, 29*(2–3), 203–219.

Barnett, M. L., Song, Z., & Landon, B. E. (2012). Trends in physician referrals in the United States, 1999–2009. *Archives of Internal Medicine, 172*(2), 163–170.

Beasley, J. W., Wetterneck, T. B., Temte, J., et al. (2011). Information chaos in primary care: Implications for physician performance and patient safety. *Journal of the American Board of Family Medicine, 24*(6), 745–751.

Beckman, H. B., Wendland, M., Mooney, C., et al. (2012). The impact of a program in mindful communication on primary care physicians. *Academic Medicine: Journal of the Association of American Medical Colleges, 87*(6), 815–819.

Berenson, R. A., & Rich, E. C. (2010). *US Approaches to Physician Payment: The Deconstruction of Primary Care. Journal of General Internal Medicine, 25*(6), 613–8.

Berger, J., & Mohn, J. (1967). *A fortunate man: The story of a country doctor*. New York: Pantheon Books.

Berg, M. (1995) Turning a practice into a science: reconceptualizing postwar medical practice. *Social Studies of Science, 25*(3), 437–76.

Bleakley, A. (2006). Broadening conceptions of learning in medical education: The message from teamworking. *Medical Education, 40*, 150–157.

Bleakley, A. (2010). Blunting Occam's razor: Aligning medical education with studies of complexity. *Journal of Evaluation in Clinical Practice, 16*, 849–855.

Blumenthal, D. (2004). Decisions, decisions: Why the quality of medical decisions matters. *Health Affairs (Millwood)*, (Suppl Variation), VAR124–VAR127.

Blumenthal, D. (2012). Performance improvement in health care – Seizing the moment. *The New England Journal of Medicine, 366*, 1953–1955.

Bohmer, R. M. J. (2011). The four habits of high-value health care organizations. *The New England Journal of Medicine, 365*(22), 2045–2047.

Boreham, N. C. (2000). Collective professional knowledge. *Medical Education, 34*, 505–506.

Bosk, C. L. (1980). Occupational rituals in patient management. *The New England Journal of Medicine, 303*(2), 71–76.

Bowie, P., Bradley, N. A., & Rushmer, R. (2012). Clinical audit and quality improvement – Time for a rethink? *Journal of Evaluation in Clinical Practice, 18*, 42–48.

Brown, C. R., Jr., & Uhl, H. S. (1970). Mandatory continuing education. Sense or nonsense? *The Journal of the American Medical Association, 213*(10), 1660–1668.

Carmack, H. J. (2010). Bearing witness to the ethics of practice: Storying physicians' medical mistake narratives. *Health Communication, 25*(5), 449–458.

Carr, W. (1995). *For education: Towards critical educational inquiry*. Buckingham: Open University Press.

Casalino, L. P. (2010). Analysis & commentary. A Martian's prescription for primary care: Overhaul the physician's workday. *Health Affairs (Millwood), 29*(5), 785–790.

Cassel, C. K., & Jain, S. H. (2012). Assessing individual physician performance: Does measurement suppress motivation? *The Journal of the American Medical Association, 307*(24), 2595–2596.

Chen, P. (2009). Primary care's image problem. *New York Times,* 12 Nov 2009.

Christensen, C., Larson, J. R., Jr., Abbott, A., et al. (2000). Decision making of clinical teams: Communication patterns and diagnostic error. *Medical Decision Making, 20*(1), 45–50.

Coleman, K., Reid, R. J., Johnson, E., et al. (2010). Implications of reassigning patients for the medical home: A case study. *Annals of Family Medicine, 8*(6), 493–498.

Coles, C. (2002). Developing professional judgment. *The Journal of Continuing Education in the Health Professions, 22*(1), 3–10.

Confessore, S. J. (1997). Building a learning organization: Communities of practice, self-directed learning, and continuing medical education. *The Journal of Continuing Education in the Health Professions, 17*(1), 5–11.

Council of Graduate Medical Education. (2010). *Council of Graduate Medical Education (COGME) Twentieth Report: Advancing Primary Care*. Rockville: Council of Graduate Medical Education. http://www.hrsa.gov/advisorycommittees/bhpradvisory/cogme/Reports/twentiethreport.pdf. Accessed on 1 May 2012.

Council on Graduate Medical Education. (2010). *Advancing care needs* (Twentieth Report). Dec 2010, (pp. 1–53).

Coutu, D. L. (2003). Sense and reliability: A conversation with celebrated psychologist Karl E. Weick. *Harvard Business Review, 81*(4), 84–93.

Crabtree, B. F. (2003). Primary care practices are full of surprises! *Health Care Management Review, 28*(3), 279–283.

Croskerry, P. (2003). Cognitive forcing strategies in clinical decisionmaking. *Annals of Emergency Medicine, 41*(1), 110–120.

Croskerry, P. (2009). A universal model of diagnostic reasoning. *Academic Medicine, 84*(8), 1022–1028.

Croskerry, P., & Norman, G. (2008). Overconfidence in clinical decision making. *The American Journal of Medicine, 121*(5 Suppl), S24–S29.

Custer, J. W., White, E., Fackler, J. C., et al. (2012). A qualitative study of expert and team cognition on complex patients in the pediatric intensive care unit. *Pediatric Critical Care Medicine, 13*(3), 278–284.

Davis, D. (2011). Can CME, save lives? The results of a Swedish, evidence-based continuing education intervention. *Annals of Family Medicine, 9*(3), 198–200.

Davis, K., Abrams, M., & Stremikis, K. (2011). How the affordable care act will strengthen the nation's primary care foundation. *Journal of General Internal Medicine, 26*(10), 1201–1203.

DeNavas-Walt, C., Proctor, B. D., & Smith, J. C., (2010) U.S. Census Bureau Current Population Reports. *Income, poverty, and health insurance coverage in the United States: 2009* (pp. 60–238). Washington, DC: U.S. Government Printing Office.

Dhaliwal, G. (2011). Going with your gut. *Journal of General Internal Medicine, 26*(2), 107–109.

Doty, M. M., Fryer, A. K., & Audet, A. M. (2012). The role of care coordinators in improving care coordination: The patient's perspective. *Archives of Internal Medicine, 172*(7), 587–588.

Eidus, R., Pace, W. D., & Staton, E. W. (2012). Managing patient populations in primary care: points of leverage. *J Am Board Fam Med, 25*(2), 238–244.

Elwyn, G., Crowe, S., Fenton, M., et al. (2010). Identifying and prioritizing uncertainties: Patient and clinician engagement in the identification of research questions. *Journal of Evaluation in Clinical Practice, 16*(3), 627–631.

Epstein, R. M. (1999). Mindful practice. *The Journal of the American Medical Association, 282*(9), 833–856.

Epstein, R. M., & Hundert, E. M. (2002). Defining and assessing professional competence. *The Journal of the American Medical Association, 28*(2), 226–234.

Epstein, R. M., Siegel, D. J., & Silberman, J. (2008). Self-monitoring in clinical practice: A challenge for medical educators. *The Journal of Continuing Education in the Health Professions, 28*(1), 5–13.

Eraut, M. (1994). *Developing professional knowledge and competence*. London: Falmer.

Feinstein, A. R. (1994). "Clinical judgment" revisited: The distraction of quantitative models. *Annals of Internal Medicine, 120*(9), 799–805.

Feinstein, A. R., & Horwitz, R. I. (1997). Problems in the "evidence" of "evidence-based medicine". *The American Journal of Medicine, 103*, 529–535.

Fenton, E., Harvey, J., Griffiths, F., et al. (2001). Reflections from organization science on the development of primary health care research networks. *Family Practice, 18*(5), 540–544.

Fenton, M., Brice, A., & Chalmers, I. (2009). Harvesting and publishing patients' unanswered questions about the effects of treatments. In P. Littlejohns & M. Rawlins (Eds.), *Patients, the public and priorities in healthcare* (pp. 165–80). Abington: Radcliffe.

Fish, D., & Coles, C. (1998). *Developing professional judgment in health care: Learning through the critical appreciation of practice*. Oxford: Butterworth-Heinemann.

Forsetlund, L., Bjørndal, A., Rashidian, A., et al. (2009). Continuing education meetings and workshops: Effects on professional practice and health care outcomes. *Cochrane Database of Systematic Reviews, 15*(2), CD003030.

Fox, R. C. (1957). Training for uncertainty. In R. K. Merton, G. G. Reader, & P. Kendall (Eds.), *The student-physician: Introductory studies in the sociology of medical education*. Cambridge: Harvard University Press.

Fox, R. C. (2000). Medical uncertainty revisited. In G. Albrecht, R. Fitzpatrick, & S. Scrimshaw (Eds.), *Handbook of social studies in health and medicine* (pp. 409–25). London: Sage.

Frankford, D. M., Patterson, M. A., & Konrad, T. R. (2000). Transforming practice organizations to foster lifelong learning and commitment to medical professionalism. *Academic Medicine, 75*(7), 708–717.

Freund, T., Wensing, M., Geissler, S., et al. (2012). Primary care physicians' experiences with case finding for practice-based care management. *The American Journal of Managed Care, 18*(4), e155–e161.

Fried, T. R., Tinetti, M. E., & Iannone, L. (2011). Primary care clinicians' experiences with treatment decision making for older persons with multiple conditions. *Archives of Internal Medicine, 171*(1), 75–80.

Gabbay, J., & LeMay, A. (2010). *Practice-based evidence for healthcare: Clinical mindlines*. London: Routledge.

Gagliardi, A. R., Wright, F. C., Anderson, M. A. B., et al. (2007). The role of collegial interaction in continuing professional development. *The Journal of Continuing Education in the Health Professions, 27*(4), 214–219.

Gawande, A. (2011). Top athletes and singers have coaches. Should you? *The New Yorker* (pp. 44–53) 3 Oct 2011.

Gerrity, M. S., Earp, J. A. L., DeVellis, R. F., et al. (1992). Uncertainty and professional work: Perceptions of physicians in clinical practice. *American Journal of Sociology, 97*(4), 1022–1051.

Gerrity, M. S., White, K. P., DeVellis, R. F., et al. (1995). Physicians' reactions to uncertainty: Refining the constructs and scales. *Motivation and Emotion, 19*(3), 175–191.

Ghorob, A., & Bodenheimer, T. (2012). Sharing the care to improve access to primary care. *The New England Journal of Medicine, 366*(21), 1955–1957.

Ghosh, A. K. (2004). On the challenges of using evidence-based information: The role of clinical uncertainty. *The Journal of Laboratory and Clinical Medicine, 144*(2), 60–64.

Gigerenzer, G., & Gaissmaier, W. (2011). Heuristic decision making. *Annual Review of Psychology, 62*, 451–482.

Gorovitz, S., & MacIntyre, A. (1976). Toward a theory of medical fallibility. *The Journal of Medicine and Philosophy, 1*(1), 51–71.

Graber, M. L., Kissam, S., Payne, V. L., et al. (2012). Cognitive interventions to reduce diagnostic error: a narrative review. *BMJ Quality and Safety 21*(7), 535–557.

Grant, R. W., Ashburner, J. M., Hong, C. C., et al. (2011). Defining patient complexity from the primary care physician's perspective. *Annals of Internal Medicine, 155*(12), 797–804. W251-255.

Greenhaigh, T. (2002). Intuition and evidence – Uneasy bedfellows? *The British Journal of General Practice, 52*(478), 395–400.

Greenhalgh, T., & Wieringa, S. (2011). Is it time to drop the "knowledge translation" metaphor? A critical literature review. *Journal of the Royal Society of Medicine, 104*(12), 501–509.

Grumbach, K., & Grundy, P. (2010). *Outcomes of Implementing Patient-Centered Medical Home Interventions: A Review of the Evidence from Prospective Evaluation Studies in the United States*. Retrieved from Patient-Centered Primary Care Collaborative July 10, 2012: http:/www.pcpcc.net/files/ evidence_outcomes_in_pcmh.pdf.

Haas, J., & Shaffir, W. (1977). The professionalization of medical students: Developing competence and a cloak of competence. *Symbolic Interaction, 1*(1), 71–88.

Hames, C. G. (1971). Evans County cardiovascular and cerebrovascular epidemiologic study. *Archives of Internal Medicine, 128*, 883–886.

Han, P. K., Klein, W. M., & Arora, N. K. (2011). Varieties of uncertainty in health care: A conceptual taxonomy. *Medical Decision Making, 31*(6), 828–838.

Han, P. K. (2013). Conceptual, methodological, and ethical problems in communicating uncertainty in clinical evidence. *Medical Care Research and Review, 70*(1 Suppl), 14S–36S.

Hay, M. C., Weisner, T. S., Subramanian, S., et al. (2008). Harnessing experience: Exploring the gap between evidence-based medicine and clinical practice. *Journal of Evaluation in Clinical Practice, 14*, 707–713.

Hertwig, R., Meier, N., Nickel, C., et al. (2013). Correlates of Diagnostic Accuracy in Patients with Nonspecific Complaints. *Medical Decision Making, Jan 7*. [Epub ahead of print].

Hewson, M. G., Kindy, P. J., Van Kirk, J., et al. (1996). Strategies for managing uncertainty and complexity. *Journal of General Internal Management, 11*, 481–485.

Hing, E., & Uddin, S. (2010). *Visits to primary care delivery sites: United States, 2008* (NCHS data brief, Vol. 47). Hyattsville: National Center for Health Statistics.

Hoff, T. (2011). Deskilling and adaptation among primary care physicians using two work innovations. *Health Care Management Review, 36*(4), 338–348.

Hoffman, J. R., & Cooper, R. J. (2012). Overdiagnosis of disease: A modern epidemic overdiagnosis of disease. *Archives of Internal Medicine, 172*(15), 1123–1124. doi:10.1001/archinternmed.2012.3319.

Hogarth, R. M. (2001). *Educating Intuition. Chicago*: University of Chicago Press.

Ibrahim, M. A., Savitz, L. A., Carey, T. S., et al. (2001). Population-based health principles in medical and public health practice. *Journal of Public Health Management and Practice, 7*(3), 75–81.

Iedema, R. A., Jorm, C., Long, D., et al. (2006). Turning the medical gaze in upon itself: Root cause analysis and the investigation of clinical error. *Social Science and Medicine, 62*(7), 1605–1615.

Innes, A. D., Campion, P. D., & Griffiths, F. E. (2005). Complex consultations and the 'edge of chaos. *The British Journal of General Practice, 55*, 47–52.

Ivers, N., Jamtvedt, G., Flottorp, S., et al. (2012). Audit and feedback: Effects on professional practice and healthcare outcomes. *Cochrane Database of Systematic Reviews, 6*, CD000259.

Katerndahl, D., Wood, R., & Jaén, C. R. (2011). Family medicine outpatient encounters are more complex than those of cardiology and psychiatry. *Journal of the American Board of Family Medicine, 24*(1), 6–15.

Katz, J. (1984). *The silent world of doctor and patient.* Baltimore: Johns Hopkins University Press.

Kennedy, T. J. T., Regehr, G., Baker, G. R., et al. (2009). "It's a cultural expectation …" the pressure on medical trainees to work independently in clinical practice. *Medical Education, 43*, 645–653.

Kibbe, D. C., Bentz, E., & McLaughlin, C. P. (1993). Continuous quality improvement for continuity of care. *The Journal of Family Practice, 36*(3), 304–308.

Kienle, G. S., & Kiene, H. (2011). Clinical judgement and the medical profession. *Journal of Evaluation in Clinical Practice, 17*(4), 621–627.

Kimball, L., Silber, T., & Weinstein, N. (2005). Dynamic facilitation: Emerging design principles from the new science of complexity. In S. Schulman (Ed.), *The IAF group facilitation handbook* (pp. 225–240). San Francisco: Jossey-Bass.

Kinnersley, P., Rapport, F. M., Owen, P., et al. (1999). In-house referral: A primary care alternative to immediate secondary care referral? *Family Practice, 16*(6), 558–561.

Kinsella, E. A. (2006). Constructivist underpinnings in Donald Schön's theory of reflective practice: Echoes of Nelson Goodman. *Reflective Practice, 7*(3), 277–286.

Kizer, K. W., & Kirsh, S. R. (2012). The doubled edged sword of performance measurement. *Journal of General Internal Medicine, 27*(4), 395–397.

Klass, D. J. (2004). Will e-learning improve clinical judgment? *British Medical Journal, 328*(7449), 1147–1148.

Knowles, M. (1996). Andragogy: An emerging technology for adult learning. In R. Edwards, A. Hanson, & P. Raggatt (Eds.), *Boundaries of adult learning.* New York: Routledge.

Kocher, R., & Sahni, N. R. (2011). Hospitals' race to employ physicians – The logic behind a money-losing proposition. *The New England Journal of Medicine, 364*(19), 1790–1793.

Kocher, R., Emanuel, E. J., & DeParle, N. A. (2010). The affordable care act and the future of clinical medicine: The opportunities and challenges. *Annals of Internal Medicine, 153*(8), 536–539.

Kolb, D. A. (1984). *Experiential learning.* Englewood Cliffs: Prentice-Hall.

Landon, B. E. (2012). Use of quality indicators in patient care: A senior primary care physician trying to take good care of his patients. *The Journal of the American Medical Association, 307*(9), 956–964.

Lave, J., & Wenger, E. (1991). *Legitimate peripheral participation in communities of practice situated learning: Legitimate peripheral participation.* Cambridge: Cambridge University Press.

Lee, S. J., & Walter, L. C. (2011). Quality indicators for older adults: Preventing unintended harms. *The Journal of the American Medical Association, 306*(13), 1481–1482.

Lester, H., & Tritter, J. Q. (2001). Medical error: A discussion of the medical construction of error and suggestions for reforms of medical education to decrease error. *Medical Education, 35*(9), 855–861.

Levenstein, J. H., McCracken, E. C., McWhinney, I. R., et al. (1986). The patient-centred clinical method. 1. A model for the doctor-patient interaction in family medicine. *Family Practice, 3*(1), 24–30.

Light, D., Jr. (1979). Uncertainty and control in professional training. *Journal of Health and Social Behavior, 20*(4), 310–322.

Lipman, T., & Price, D. (2000). Decision making, evidence, audit, and education: Case study of antibiotic prescribing in general practice. *British Medical Journal, 320*(7242), 1114–1118.

Lister, G. (2012). 2011 Joseph W. St Geme Jr lecture: Five things I'd like to see changed in American pediatrics, five lessons I've learned. *Pediatrics, 129*(5), 961–967.

Lloyd, F. J., & Reyna, V. F. (2009). Clinical gist and medical education: Connecting the dots. *The Journal of the American Medical Association, 302*(12), 1332–1333.

Loxterkamp, D. (2001). A vow of connectedness: Views from the road to Beaver's farm. *Family Medicine, 33*(4), 244–247.

Ludmerer K. M. (1999). *Time to Heal: American medical education from the turn of the century to the era of managed care*. New York: Oxford University Press.

Magala, S. (2002). *Organizing as improvisations (methodological temptations of social constructivism)* (ERIM report series research in management #2002-76-ORG). Rotterdam: Erasmus Research Institute of Management.

Mamede, S., Schmidt, H. G., & Rikers, R. (2007a). Diagnostic errors and reflective practice in medicine. *Journal of Evaluation in Clinical Practice, 13*(1), 138–145.

Mamede, S., Schmidt, H. G., Rikers, R. M., et al. (2007b). Breaking down automaticity: Case ambiguity and the shift to reflective approaches in clinical reasoning. *Medical Education, 41*(12), 1185–1192.

Mann, K. V. (2011). Theoretical perspectives in medical education: Past experience and future possibilities. *Medical Education, 45*, 60–68.

Mattingly, C., & Fleming, M. H. (1994). *Clinical reasoning: Forms of inquiry in a therapeutic practice*. Philadelphia: F. A. Davis Company.

McKenna, K., Leykum, L. K., & McDaniel, R. R., Jr. (2013). The role of improvising in patient care. *Health Care Management Review, 38*38(1), 1–8.

Mercuri, M., & Gafni, A. (2011). Medical practice variations: What the literature tells us (or does not) about what are warranted and unwarranted variations. *Journal of Evaluation in Clinical Practice, 17*(4), 671–677.

Merrell, K., & Berenson, R. A. (2010). Structuring payment for medical homes. *Health Affairs (Millwood), 29*(5), 852–858.

Meyers, D., Peikes, D., Dale, S., et al. (2011). *Improving evaluations of the medical home* (AHRQ publication No. 11–0091). Rockville: Agency for Healthcare Research and Quality.

Mezirow, J. (1990). *Fostering critical reflection in adulthood: A guide to transformative and emancipatory learning*. San Francisco: Jossey-Bass.

Miller, G. E. (1967). Continuing education for what? *Journal of Medical Education, 42*, 320–326.

Miller, W. L., Crabtree, B. F., McDaniel, R., et al. (1998). Understanding change in primary care practice using complexity theory. *The Journal of Family Practice, 46*(5), 369–376.

Miller, W. L., McDaniel, R. R., Crabtree, B. F., et al. (2001). Practice jazz: Understanding variation in family practices using complexity science. *The Journal of Family Practice, 50*(10), 872–878.

Miller, W. L., Crabtree, B. F., Nutting, P. A., et al. (2010). Primary care practice development: A relationship-centered approach. *Annals of Family Medicine, 8*(S1), S68–S77.

Montgomery, K. (2006). *How doctors think: Clinical judgment and the practice of medicine*. New York: Oxford University Press.

Moore, D. E., Jr., & Pennington, F. C. (2003). Practice-based learning and improvement. *The Journal of Continuing Education in the Health Professions, 23*(Suppl 1), S73–S80.

Morrison, I., & Smith, R. (2000). Hamster health care. *British Medical Journal, 321*(7276), 1541–1542.

Moulton, C. A., Regehr, G., Mylopoulos, M., et al. (2007). Slowing down when you should: A new model of expert judgment. *Academic Medicine, 82*(10 Suppl), S109–S116.

Mylopoulos, M., & Scardamalia, M. (2008). Doctors' perspectives on their innovations in daily practice: Implications for knowledge building in health care. *Medical Education, 42*, 975–981.

Mylopoulos, M., & Woods, N. N. (2009). Having our cake and eating it too: Seeking the best of both worlds in expertise research. *Medical Education, 43*, 406–413.

Neuwirth, E. B., Schmittdiel, J. A., Tallman, K., et al. (2007). Understanding panel management: A comparative study of an emerging approach to population care. *The Permanente Journal, 11*(3), 12–20.

O'Riordan, M. (2000). Continuing medical education in Irish general practice. *Scandinavian Journal of Primary Health Care, 18*(3), 137–138.

Owen, P. A., Allery, L. A., Harding, K. G., et al. (1989). General practitioner's continuing medical education within and outside their practice. *British Medical Journal, 299*(6993), 238–240.

Parboosingh, J. T. (2002). Physician communities of practice: Where learning and practice are inseparable. *The Journal of Continuing Education in the Health Professions, 22*(4), 230–236.

Parboosingh, I. J., Reed, V. A., Caldwell Palmer, J., et al. (2011). Enhancing practice improvement by facilitating practitioner interactivity: New roles for providers of continuing medical education. *The Journal of Continuing Education in the Health Professions, 31*(2), 122–127.

Plsek, P. E., & Greenhalgh, T. (2001). Complexity science: The challenge of complexity in health care. *British Medical Journal, 323*(7313), 625–628.

Politi, M. C., Lewis, C. L., & Frosch, D. L. (2013). Supporting shared decisions when clinical evidence is low. *Medical Care Research and Review, 70(1 Suppl),* 113S–128S.

Poses, R. M. (2003). A cautionary tale: The dysfunction of American health care. *European Journal of Internal Medicine, 14*(2), 123–130.

Powell, A. A., White, K. M., Partin, M. R., et al. (2012). Unintended consequences of implementing a national performance measurement system into local practice. *Journal of General Internal Medicine, 27*(4), 405–412.

Prasad, V. (2010). Reclaiming the morbidity and mortality conference: Between Codman and Kundera. *Medical Humanities, 36*(2), 108–111.

Premi, J. (1988). Problem based, self directed continuing medical education in a group of practicing family physicians. *Journal of Medical Education, 63*, 484–486.

Primary Care Professionals. (2008). *Recent supply trends, projections, and valuation of services* (GAO-08-472 T). Washington, DC: U.S. Govt. Accountability Office.

Primary Care Workforce Facts and Stats No. 2. *The number of nurse practitioners and physician assistants practicing primary care in the United States.* AHRQ Publication No. 12-P001-3-EF; Oct 2011.

Redelmeier, D. A., & Dickinson, V. M. (2012). Judging whether a patient is actually improving: More pitfalls from the science of human perception. *Journal of General Internal Medicine, 27*(9), 1195–1199.

Reeve, J., Irving, G., & Dowriek, C. F. (2011). Can generalism help revive the primary healthcare vision? *Journal of the Royal Society of Medicine, 104*, 395–400.

Regehr, G. (2010). It's not rocket science: Rethinking our metaphors for research in health professions education. *Medical Education, 2010*(44), 31–39.

Rodning, C. B. (1992). Coping with ambiguity and uncertainty in patient-physician relationships: I. Leadership of a physician. *The Journal of Medical Humanities, 13*(2), 91–101.

Rudolph, J. W., & Morrison, J. B. (2008). Sidestepping superstitious learning, ambiguity, and other roadblocks: A feedback model of diagnostic problem solving. *The American Journal of Medicine, 121*(5 Suppl), S34–S37.

Rudolph, J. W., Morrison, J. B., & Carroll, J. S. (2009). The dynamics of action-oriented problem solving: Linking interpretation and choice. *Academy of Management Review, 34*(4), 733–756.

Rushmer, R., & Davies, H. T. O. (2004). Unlearning in health care. *Qual Saf Health Care, 13*(Suppl II), ii10–ii15.

Sackett, D. L., Haynes, R. B., Guyatt, G. H., et al. (1991). *Clinical epidemiology: A basic science for clinical medicine* (2nd ed.). Boston: Little Brown.

Safran, D. G., Miller, W., & Beckman, H. (2006). Organizational dimensions of relationship-centered care: Theory, evidence, and practice. *Journal of General Internal Medicine, 21*(S1), S9–S15.

Santa Clara Valley Medical Center. Delivery System Reform Incentive Pool Plan. Feb 2011, 1–61.

Schiff, G. D. (2008). Minimizing diagnostic error: The importance of follow-up and feedback. *The American Journal of Medicine, 121*(5A), S38–S42.

Schön, D. A. (1983). *The reflective practitioner*. New York: Basic Books.

Schon, D. A. (1995). The new scholarship requires a new epistemology. *Change, 37*(6), 26–35.

Shojania, K., Silver, I., & Levinson, W. (2012). Continuing medical education and quality improvement: A match made in heaven? *Annals of Internal Medicine, 156*, 305–308.

Singh, H., Giardina, T. D., Meyer, A. N., et al. (2013). Types and origins of diagnostic errors in primary care settings. *JAMA Internal Medicine, 173*(6), 418–425.

Siriwardena, A. N., Middlemass, J. B., Ward, K., et al. (2008). Drivers for change in primary care of diabetes following a protected learning time educational event: Interview study of practitioners. *BMC Medical Education, 8*, 4.

Sledge, W. H., & Feinstein, A. R. (1997). A clinimetric approach to the components of the patient-physician relationship. *The Journal of the American Medical Association, 278*(23), 2043–2048.

Slotnick, H. B. (1999). How doctors learn: Physicians' self-directed learning episodes. *Academic Medicine, 74*(10), 1106–1117.

Smith, R. (1996). What clinical information do doctors need? *British Medical Journal, 313*(7064), 1062–1068.

Sommers, L. S., & Marton, K. (2000). The curriculum template: Creating continuing medical education curricula for physicians in practice in managed care settings. *The Western Journal of Medicine, 173*(5), 337–340.

Sommers, L. S., Sholtz, R., Shepherd, R. M., et al. (1984). Physician involvement in quality assurance. *Medical Care, 22*(12), 1115–1138.

Sommers, L. S., Hacker, T. W., Schneider, D. M., et al. (2001). A descriptive study of managed-care hassles in 26 practices. *The Western Journal of Medicine, 174*(3), 175–179.

Sommers, L. S., Morgan, L., Johnson, L., et al. (2007). Practice inquiry: Clinical uncertainty as a focus for small-group learning and practice improvement. *Journal of General Internal Medicine, 22*(2), 246–252.

Soubhi, H., Bayliss, E. A., Fortin, M., et al. (2010). Learning and caring in communities of practice: Using relationships and collective learning to improve primary care for patients with multimorbidity. *Annals of Family Medicine, 8*(2), 170–177.

Stacey, R. D. (1995). The science of complexity: An alternative perspective for strategic change processes. *Strategic Management Journal, 16*(6), 477–495.

Stange, K. C. (2009). The generalist approach. *Annals of Family Medicine, 7*(3), 198–203.

Starfield, B. (2011). Is patient-centered care the same as person-focused care? *The Permanente Journal, 15*(2), 63–69.

Stolper, E., Van de Wiel, M., Van Royen, P., et al. (2011). Gut feelings as a third track in general practitioners' diagnostic reasoning. *Journal of General Internal Medicine, 26*(2), 197–203.

Sturmberg, J. P., & Cilliers, P. (2009). Time and the consultation–an argument for a 'certain slowness'. *Journal of Evaluation in Clinical Practice, 15*(5), 881–885.

Suchman, A. L., & Matthews, D. A. (1988). What makes the patient-doctor relationship therapeutic? Exploring the connexional dimension of medical care. *Annals of Internal Medicine, 108*(1), 125–130.

Swoboda, D. A. (2008). Negotiating the diagnostic uncertainty of contested illnesses: Physician practices and paradigms. *Health, 12*(4), 453–478.

Thomson, G. H. (1978). Tolerating uncertainty in family medicine. *The Journal of the Royal College of General Practitioners, 28*(191), 343–346.

Tinetti, M. E., Fried, T. R., & Boyd, C. M. (2012). Designing health care for the most common chronic condition – Multimorbidity. *The Journal of the American Medical Association, 307*(23), 2493–2494.

Tonelli, M. R. (2001). The limits of evidence-based medicine. *Respiratory Care, 46*(12), 1435–1440.

Tresolini C. Health Professions Education and Relationship-centered Care: Report of the Pew-Fetzer Task Force on Advancing Psychosocial Education. San Francisco, Calif: Pew Health Commission; 1994. The Pew-Fetzer Task Force.

Van de Wiel, M. W., Van den Bossche, P., Janssen, S., et al. (2011). Exploring deliberate practice in medicine: How do physicians learn in the workplace? *Advances in Health Sciences Education: Theory and Practice, 16*(1), 81–95.

Wears, R. L., & Nemeth, C. P. (2007). Replacing hindsight with insight: Toward better understanding of diagnostic failures. *Annals of Emergency Medicine, 49*(2), 206–209.

Weaver, S. J., Newman-Toker, D. E., & Rosen, M. A. (2012). Reducing cognitive skill decay and diagnostic error: theory-based practices for continuing education in health care. *Journal of Continuing Education in the Health Professions, 32*(4), 269–278.

Weick, K. E. (1969). *The social psychology of organizing.* New York: Random House.

Weick, K. E. (2001). *Making sense of the organization.* Oxford: Blackwell.

Weiner, S. J. (2004). Contextualizing medical decisions to individualize care: Lessons from the qualitative sciences. *Journal of General Internal Medicine, 19*(3), 281–285.

White, K. L. (2000). Fundamental research at primary care level. *The Lancet, 355,* 1904–1906.

Zwack, J., & Schweitzer, J. (2013). If every fifth physician is affected by burnout, what about the other four? Resilience strategies of experienced physicians. *Academic Medicine, 88*(3), 382–389.

Chapter 10
Using Practice Inquiry to Engage Uncertainty in Residency Education

Tina Kenyon, Claudia W. Allen, and Alan Siegel

In primary care specialties, coping with uncertainty is accepted as part of the territory. In discussing stress from uncertainty throughout a physician's career, Bovier and Perneger state: "Uncertainty shapes many decisions made by clinicians every day and is so ubiquitous that physicians must learn to tolerate ambiguity if they are to provide quality care to patients who suffer from complex conditions"(Bovier and Perneger 2007; Rizzo 1993; Hewson et al. 1996; Griffiths et al. 2005; Geller et al. 1990). This complexity attracts many physicians to primary care, but the challenge of *learning* uncertainty cannot be addressed through "experience" alone. Using experiential learning methods, it requires support and reinforcement during postgraduate training.

Practice Inquiry (PI), a set of methods for clinicians to engage case-based clinical uncertainty in small group settings, has been used by practicing clinicians in the San Francisco Bay Area since 2002 (Sommers et al. 2007, also see Chapter 9). These methods are aimed at enhancing clinical judgment through collegial collaboration. During prescheduled, dedicated time, primary care providers with patient panels meet in facilitated small groups to discuss individual patients for whom they

Electronic supplementary material: The online version of this chapter (doi:10.1007/978-1-4614-6812-7_10) contains supplementary material, which is available to authorized users.

T. Kenyon, ACSW (✉)
NHDFMR, 250 Pleasant Street, Concord, NH 03301, USA
e-mail: tkenyon@crhc.org

C.W. Allen, Ph.D.
Department of Family Medicine, University of Virginia Health System, PO Box 800729, Charlottesville, VA 22908-0729, USA
e-mail: claudiaallen@virginia.edu

A. Siegel, M.D.
Contra Costa Family Medicine Residency Program, 2500 Alhambra Avenue, Martinez, CA 94553, USA
e-mail: alan.siegel@hsd.cccounty.us

L.S. Sommers and J. Launer (eds.), *Clinical Uncertainty in Primary Care: The Challenge of Collaborative Engagement*, DOI 10.1007/978-1-4614-6812-7_10,
© Springer Science+Business Media New York 2013

are experiencing clinical uncertainty, that is, diagnostic, therapeutic, prognostic, ethical, and/or clinician-patient relationship dilemmas.

As a framework for helping socialize learners to engage clinical uncertainty, PI lends itself well to the breadth and depth of family medicine education and explicitly showcases uncertainty as a phenomenon worthy of exploration and strategic management in its own right. This chapter describes the Practice Inquiry experience in three family medicine residency programs: New Hampshire Dartmouth Family Medicine Residency in Concord, New Hampshire (NHDFMR), The University of Virginia Family Medicine Residency in Charlottesville (UVAFMR), and the Contra Costa Family Medicine Residency in Martinez, California (CCFMR). The first section of the chapter provides background on the need for work focused on clinical uncertainty in postgraduate medical education. In Boxes 10.1, 10.2, and 10.3, specific approaches to using PI methods in each of the three residency programs are outlined. The second section gives an assessment of PI's value from the perspective of the faculty who facilitate the resident PI groups at each of the respective programs (authors TK, CA, and AS; "faculty" refer to individuals who hold university academic appointments in the residency program). In the third section, plans for continued implementation and expansion of PI in each program are discussed. Recommendations for introducing PI in residency programs are provided in the chapter's final section.

Impact of Uncertainty on Clinicians and Students

How does omnipresent uncertainty impact students and physicians in the early stages of their professional socialization? How does the educational process prepare physicians to successfully manage uncertainty and address complexity in primary care? Experiences with residents in three training programs as well as observations in the literature suggest three reasons why clinical uncertainty requires explicit attention within the residency program curriculum.

First, complexity in primary care and the frequency with which it defies algorithmic solution take an emotional toll on young physicians, negatively affecting their personal wellness and professional performance. Several researchers have documented that physicians feel stressed by uncertainty (An et al. 2009; Ghosh 2004), and their reaction to stress can be associated with higher medical costs and negative effects on patient care (Evans and Trotter 2009). Awareness of medicine as an uncertain science typically begins in medical school (Light 1979). The nature of uncertainty and the confusion inherent in it have been described by Renee Fox: "There are three basic types of uncertainty around which the process of 'training for uncertainty' in medical school centers is based: (a) uncertainties that originate in the impossibility of commanding all the vast knowledge and complex skills of continually advancing modern medicine; (b) uncertainties that stem from the many gaps in medical knowledge and limitations in medical understanding and effectiveness that nonetheless exist; and (c) uncertainties connected with distinguishing between personal ignorance and ineptitude and the lacunae and incapacities of the field of medicine itself"(Fox 1957). As difficult as it is for experienced physicians, uncertainty presents an added challenge for young physicians, who, often unsure about their knowledge and skills or whether the relevant knowledge exists to begin with, struggle with distinguishing between these two possibilities (Atkinson 1984; Schor et al. 2000).

Second, clinical uncertainty is exacerbated in underserved and vulnerable patient populations with high prevalence of chronic medical problems, complicated by cultural differences and psychological challenges. Left unaddressed, this complexity can deter young physicians from caring for vulnerable populations. Wayne and colleagues found an association between intolerance of ambiguity and decline in medical students' attitudes toward the underserved (Wayne et al. 2011). Students who perceived novel or complex situations as threatening developed more negative attitudes to treating underserved populations. The authors suggest that these attitudes result from the high level of complexity presented by underserved patients and propose that "attention to, and practice with, ambiguous situations (in medical school) may help moderate decreases in attitudes toward underserved populations." To the extent that residency programs strive to graduate capable and committed physicians who care for the most vulnerable patients, Wayne and colleagues argue, medical education must offer students tools to respond to these challenges.

Third, if properly engaged, uncertainty and complexity can be the fulcrum around which physicians' capabilities as clinicians can be expanded. Engaging uncertainty allows residents to move beyond algorithmic competence to begin a conscious process of using clinical judgment (Fraser and Greenhalgh 2001). Other professional disciplines (e.g., business, law) recognize that expanding capacity to navigate difficulty and complexity is key to excellent performance. Giving people permission to acknowledge complexity and uncertainty without fear of reprisal is a fundamental step (Pink 2009; LaBarre 2011). The "hidden" curriculum in medical school discourages students from tackling uncertainty. When a student is publicly embarrassed for not having "the answer," the lesson learned is to hide uncertainty (Kelly 2004). The medical student brings these powerful, negative experiences with them to residency training. Building a culture of encouragement for trainees to ask questions and learn through revealing uncertainty is, however, a challenging process. Being open about knowledge and skill deficits requires positive reinforcement through faculty and peer role modeling of uncertainty engagement through such methods as literature searching and consultation with team members as well as specialists.

In postgraduate training, the many competing demands on trainees' time necessitate a variety of fine-tuned educational methods to support residents in "finding answers" to questions: perfecting skills in taking a history and performing physical exams, diagnostic decision-making, and identifying treatment plans with their teachers. Woven through this learning process is the realization that answers may not always be forthcoming. While uncertainty in patient care is apparent to trainees, it is not always highlighted as its own unique challenge.

With the wide range of content and complexities in family medicine, uncertainty is the only certainty. In many residency programs, the process of engaging uncertainty within the physician-patient relationship is addressed through resident participation in Balint groups (see Chapters 4 and 5). In PI, as in Balint (Dornfest and Ransom 2012; Launer 2007), the power of the group supports the uncertainty learning process. Unlike Balint, PI provides the group an opportunity to explore any type of clinical conundrum involving a clinician and a patient. PI uniquely expands the conversation to include medical literature, other group members' experience, and the patient/practitioner/team/health system interface. It fosters conversation on potential action steps to improve patient care. Having a broader perspective of the patient care context opens up previously overlooked options and positions learners to see beyond their own perspectives.

In Boxes 10.1, 10.2, and 10.3, each residency program's specific curricular approaches to using PI group methods are outlined within the following sections: small group discussion formats, group composition, facilitation, meetings, and evaluation.

Practice Inquiry's Value to the FM Residency Curriculum: An Assessment by Three Faculty Small Group Facilitators

This section explores how Practice Inquiry (PI) contributes overall value to postgraduate training in family medicine in three family medicine residency programs and why the authors believe PI should be integrated into program curricula despite the many competing educational demands. The overall objective of PI in the residency setting is to provide a successful experience in uncertainty engagement. Two overarching themes around residents' development of competency in uncertainty engagement have emerged: through reflecting "out loud," residents learn to share perspectives and gain insights relevant to their professional development, bringing reflection from an *internal* to an *external* process; and, in contrast to reasoning alone through uncertainty, residents learn how to involve *their peers* in contributing reflections and expertise to inform the reasoning process. Six important components of these themes and how they are addressed through PI are discussed below.

The Developmental Task of Becoming Comfortable with Disclosing Uncertainty to Peers

The "hidden curriculum" in medical training places a premium on rapidly knowing the right answer and overlooking knowledge gaps (Kelly 2004). For uncertainty to become a learning opportunity, medical education must encourage learners to openly wrestle with complexity and identify problems that defy algorithms. The ability to "watch and wait," for example, involves comfort with the unknowable.

Part of professional development is crafting a lifelong learning style, cultivating curiosity, learning how to identify one's knowledge limits, and appreciating the value of relying on one's team and colleagues to support these tasks. Although medical education teaches learners to seek explicit answers to patients' problems, answers based on evidence or expert opinion may not always be available. In this "gray zone" of uncertainty, PI provides a framework for uncertainty engagement that is reflected in the "Inputs to Judgment Table" (see Chapter 9): What does the literature say? What do my colleagues think? What is the patient telling me and not telling me, verbally, behaviorally, as well as through the physical examination? How does what I don't know impact my management of this patient? Perhaps there is "an answer," but the resident has yet to find it. When an acceptable answer is not apparent, despite multiple investigations, learning how to be "comfortable with being uncomfortable" is the strategy of choice.

In addition to becoming comfortable with the challenges of finding answers, residents gain comfort in disclosing uncertainty in the PI group. As a group of peers, they systematically drill down to find unexplored clues. This may include technical knowledge, approaches to decision-making, or a hidden bias about patients. In this safe group, residents are able to ask: "I am not supposed to be judgmental toward my patients, but maybe I am, and how is that affecting my care?" By sharing and listening, they gain trust in each other and become more comfortable being who they are and voicing thoughts without fear that teachers and peers will lose confidence in them or evaluate them negatively. In the course of sharing cases, the trainees experience how it *feels,* in a protected setting, to disclose uncertainty to peers as well as to teachers and the sense of relief it offers. Positive experiences with uncertainty engagement in residency could lead to continuing PI-like activity after graduation.

Using PI to Reframe "The Problem Patient" into "A Patient with a Problem"

Physicians attracted to primary care specialties are interested in establishing longitudinal relationships with patients. Physician-patient dynamics are multifaceted and complex since physicians and patients bring their mental frames, beliefs, emotions, and personalities to the relationship. After a resident has "tried everything" with a patient without success, the PI group provides a setting for learners to expand their problem-solving lens. By examining the situation with input from peers, residents can practice reframing. One useful reframing technique is for the group to generate a list of questions to ask the patient. In one PI group session, residents discussed a recent immigrant patient who was severely debilitated by panic attacks which he attributed to heart "crises." Peers encouraged the resident to pose questions to the patient that explored the man's earlier life in his village back home, the meaning of health problems in his culture, and his relationship with his wife and in his job. In case follow-up, the resident reported uncovering "missing pieces" in the man's story. These "pieces" provided important clues about how the patient was framing his symptoms and why reassurance alone was not working. The patient welcomed the resident's new questions, focusing on him as a person as well as on his illness. The caregiving process became more satisfying for both patient and resident.

When residents are "stuck," PI can help expand the frame and allow the doctor to understand the patient on many levels, for example, as a person in the broader context of their world, how the patient interacts with various team members, and what the medical literature may provide about the patient's problems. Specific patient cases discussed in the PI group can generalize and offer a broader context for reframing the difficult doctor-patient relationships that other residents may also be experiencing. Residents have offered feedback such as, "I tried this (i.e., a strategy discussed in a recent PI session) with a couple of my other challenging patients, and I can't believe how well it worked." Small successes encourage curiosity about the challenges of working with difficult patients. Sharing what works and creating strategies together help redefine these cases from "problem patients" to being "patients with problems."

"By the Book": Incorporating the Complementary Skills of Information Mastery into Practice Inquiry

Information mastery skills enhance the effectiveness of Practice Inquiry. Merely locating articles in the medical literature pertinent to an uncertainty case under discussion does not ensure the articles' applicability to the case. Additional uncertainty can arise about the value of "the evidence" they contain. Did a pharmaceutical company sponsor the drug trial? Are sound reasons given for excluding certain patient groups? Locating resources and scrutinizing the context and quality of the evidence behind the recommendations are the skills practiced in the small group setting. Another dimension of information mastery includes selecting and managing diagnostic resources. What testing makes sense in this patient's situation? How will it provide useful diagnostic data? What about cost considerations? Case-based PI group discussion enables sharing opinions about the often difficult process of exploring available resources, assessing the evidence quality, and integrating what is learned into care planning options for the individual patient. Practicing these skills in the group is also valued by the residents who are increasingly using them at the point of care.

Changing Patterns of Uncertainty

A principle goal of medical training is to show steady increase in competence and capability. When asked what most concerns new first-year residents, many will identify the fear of contributing to patient morbidity and mortality. In the second year, this changes as residents become concerned about their effectiveness as a team leader and teacher for junior residents and medical students. In the third year, the resident's focus shifts to preparing for postresidency practice and the impending lack of a supervising physician. As competence grows in treating common conditions such as hypertension, for example, uncertainty shifts to more complex presentations, for example, how to treat hypertension in a refugee population with culturally specific health practices. In the PI group, residents collaborate in tackling these more advanced presentations and use each other's growing experience to prepare for their next developmental milestone – independent practice.

Seeing the "Aha" Moment: Incorporating a Strengths Perspective and Recognizing Growth

Practice Inquiry fosters a "strengths-based" approach to both patients and learners through the use of the "Inputs to Judgment Table" (Weick et al. 1989). The table prompts residents to consider the various inputs to judgment available to them when discussing an uncertainty case: relevant "evidence" from the medical literature, colleagues' experience pertinent to the patient, strengths that reside in both the patient and resident, and the positive aspects present in the clinician-patient relationship. When these attributes are discussed in the PI group, the resident can practice *inquiring* into the patient's explanatory models for understanding what goals are the most salient and how best to fashion effective interventions. Discussion of these inputs helps the resident recognize the "person-in-situation" and translate that broader vision to the health care team (Richmond 1922). The new perspective can sometimes change the team's reaction to the patient from frustration to empathy and from resignation to renewed commitment to devise new strategies. After a PI discussion about a needed diagnostic study, a resident concluded, "It's now clearer to me that the patient's reluctance to get this test could be coming from her poor tolerance of a previous test. Perhaps I can work with the specialist to figure out another test for this condition which may make her more comfortable."

Using the "Inputs to Judgment Table" also allows the group to identify biases and see barriers arising from their behavior and attitudes toward patients. While residents may not recognize how they are gaining in self-awareness skills, PI facilitators are in a unique position to reference this learning at appropriate times in the group session. These discussions become particularly useful in capturing "aha" moments, those moments in the group when insights that have accrued over time become clarified and allow for transformational learning.

Transferable Skills

Practice Inquiry fosters and reinforces transferable patient care, self-reflection, and collaborative practice skills. Several of these skills and how they transfer include:

- Reimagining patients and caregiving situations with "new eyes" transfers to modeling a biopsychosocial worldview that interfaces with the clinical literature, the experiences of one's peers, and the involvement of the health care team.

- Accentuating a "strengths-based" perspective transfers to modeling clinician-patient communication for care planning and education that emphasizes positives in the patient's life and in the clinician-patient relationship (Weick et al. 1989).

- Encouraging an attitude of curiosity, inquiry, and reflection transfers into mindful practice in all arenas of patient care, resulting in the ability to encourage collaborative "wondering aloud" and disclosing uncertainty (e.g., slowing down to call attention to what is happening during a patient encounter is equivalent to the practice of "time-outs" in the operating room).

- Enhancing respect across disciplines transfers into more frequent consultation and collaborative problem-solving within the health care team, a "we're all in this together" ethic that research suggests translates into greater work satisfaction (Bovier and Perneger 2007).

What's Ahead for Practice Inquiry in the Programs at New Hampshire Dartmouth, Virginia, and Contra Costa

New Hampshire Dartmouth

The PI model will continue in several different group settings. In addition to the third-year PI resident group that began in 2007 (meeting monthly throughout the academic year), a PI group for faculty and four, interdisciplinary team PI groups in the outpatient clinic help inculcate the value of uncertainty engagement.

The PI faculty group has been meeting for 2 years and, in addition to using individual patient case formats, has experimented with two other formats: a "special topic" format and "Educational Inquiry." In the "special topic" format, a focused question is discussed such as "What happens when the consultant and the primary care physician disagree on the patient's treatment plan?" Patient cases are used to illustrate the dilemma. In "Education Inquiry" (EI), using resident-faculty situations as context, faculty bring uncertainty related to learning situations or individual learners. For example, a faculty member wanted to explore possible approaches to a medical student who received extensive improvement feedback for poor performance but responded to that feedback with minimal change; the student then requested a letter of recommendation. In cases involving individual learners, the EI group helps the faculty member consider questions such as: What are contributing factors? When is the concern most evident? How does the learner view the problem? In providing a structured forum to discuss challenging teacher-learner interactions, faculty members receive support and expertise from colleagues, leading to new insights and possible interventions. While informal "curbside" conversation is the usual approach (as with patient care problems), using an "inquiry" format with educational uncertainty provides time for focused discussion. The faculty group uses Practice Inquiry or Educational Inquiry as needs dictate; meetings take place monthly, are well attended, and receive positive evaluations. (See On-line Resource #7 for description of Educational Inquiry.)

Last year, PI groups began in the four interdisciplinary teams. A PI interdisciplinary group includes nurses, medical assistants, integrated care managers, and faculty and resident physicians in the residency program's health center practice sites. An example uncertainty case focused on management of a challenging patient who frequently called the clinic and sought care in the emergency department for inappropriate reasons. In the PI group conversation, the team speculated that one contributing factor to the patient's behavior could be inadequate relationships with key care providers in the clinic. To test this, a "micro team" (a designated medical assistant, nurse, integrated care manager, and resident physician) was created for this patient as consistent contacts. At each phone call, the patient would be connected exclusively with at least one of the micro team members. For each of the more frequently scheduled visits with the patient, several micro team members interacted with the patient either sequentially or together. This approach allowed the individual disciplines to give coordinated inputs. The patient was very satisfied with "her team." In providing consistent messages to the patient while sharing the responsibilities of care, the team members felt supported. The patient's phone calls and ED visits diminished substantially, and the team and patient decided to decrease visit frequency.

A qualitative research project is underway to understand how meeting as a PI group adds value to the clinical teams. Team members' observations have yielded these representative comments:

- "(PI) has given me a new appreciation for my fellow team members and my role."
- "Taking time to reflect on what I am doing has made me more aware of how I can work better (with the team)."
- "I think more about what could be behind a patient's behavior."
- "Knowing that others have some of the same challenges as I do have helped me a lot."

University of Virginia

While PI at UVAFMR is well established, it is also still in evolution. The residency program has demonstrated commitment by providing bimonthly meeting time and funding for food. Facilitating residents' timely arrival at meetings is challenging, but attendance overall is good. The PI group as a safe and secure place is built on the foundation established by a long-standing, first-year resident support group.

In the coming year, the program will experiment with other PI methods (e.g., a second-year resident asking a third-year resident to serve as a consultant for an uncertainty case in the PI group; see Box 10.1).

Contra Costa

At CCFPR, expanding the PI model to include third-year residents as well as second-year residents is under consideration and seen as a way to promote an emphasis on uncertainty engagement into postresidency practice. While trainees could potentially benefit from starting PI in their first year, the second-year resident group's prior clinical experience appears essential for enriching the experience. Experimenting with the "rapid reflections" and "clinic session review" discussion formats are also planned (see Box 10.1).

The Educational Inquiry (EI) format is used with the clinician faculty who work with the residents in the clinic settings. The three annual faculty retreats include discussion of the challenges in teaching relationships with residents. Similar to PI with patients, this approach encourages support and wisdom from teaching colleagues. It helps identify why "this resident" is particularly challenging and incorporates literature for offering intervention strategies.

Recommendations for Practice Inquiry Implementation in Residency Programs

Creating an Atmosphere of Trust

Similar to the requirements for a positive clinician-patient relationship, group members' trust in one another is critical for group effectiveness. This necessitates special efforts when resident groups have trainees from different years who do not know each other well or when faculty with various backgrounds and program tenure are together in one group. Clear, explicit expectations around confidentiality should be provided at a new group's first meeting.

Introducing Practice Inquiry in a Residency Program

Observing PI group sessions is invaluable for anyone interested in introducing PI at their residency program. Providing a very brief description of PI attributes followed by involving the clinicians in an actual group is an effective introductory approach. Formats such as the "appreciation case format" can offer a positive initial experience (see Box 10.3).

Box 10.1 NH Dartmouth Family Medicine Residency at Concord Hospital (NHDFMR)

I. Small Group Discussion Formats[1]

Rapid Reflections Format

- "Take-home" patients (Patients thought about after workday)

  - Facilitator lists residents' short descriptions: "22-year-old who is pregnant and homeless – how can I help her?"
  - Group reviews list for commonalties across patients
  - Uncertainty themes emerge (setting limits)
  - Reflection identifies challenging populations (refugees, children with special needs) and reasons residents "take patients home"

- Specific clinic sessions (brief reviews of all patients seen in a half-day clinic to identify issues in workflow, communications with interdisciplinary team members, handling documentation needs)
- "Surprises" (patients that behave differently than expected)
  Example: A patient on a chronic pain treatment regimen transferring care from another practice asked about alternative treatments for a muscle strain other than the option of more medication. The resident entered the exam room ready to set limits around medications but instead explored the use of heat, physical therapy, etc. The visit evolved in a completely different direction than the resident imagined.

Consultation Format ("I Am Your Consultant")
Third-year residents learn to rely on each other as a practice group and have opportunities to "think out loud":

- One resident becomes consultant to presenter
- Computer and projector used
- Presenting resident gives patient summary and/or reviews patient's computerized record and identifies uncertainty type (e.g., diagnosis, treatment, relationship)
- Resident "consultant" uses computer, explains literature search strategy, and facilitates conversation to support presenter in addressing questions
  Examples: (1) Consultant resident selects unique literature search strategy new to presenting resident; (2) Consultant resident demonstrates use of new risk calculators in patient visit when discussing lifestyle modification.

---

[1]At least one session per format required; residents' choice of formats for remaining sessions.

(continued)

Box 10.1 (continued)

Individual Uncertainty Case Format

- Focuses on individual patients (previously identified through other discussion formats) or patient recently seen
- Presenter accesses electronic medical record to review needed parts of record (e.g., medication list)
- Use of five-part "Inputs to Judgment Table" to structure conversation (see Chapter 9). The table highlights inputs to clinical judgment to include clinical experience of other participants, patient's context, clinician's context, patient/clinician/team relationship, and "evidence"

  Example: A resident discusses the care of a 17-year-old female, pregnant for the second time. The resident was curious about why his interactions with her were not going well. Not knowing the source of his discomfort presented a challenge. The group and presenter used the Table for considering the patient's and the resident's unique contexts. The resident talked about his personal difficulties accepting the reality of teenage girls being sexually active. The risk of pregnancy and their lack of maturity led him to believe they should practice abstinence until later in life. As the conversation evolved, the resident became aware of how his beliefs and biases could lead him to unintentionally "lecture" teens about sexual activity and contraception. This approach could make establishing rapport with teens difficult. The facilitator asked the presenting resident and other group members to identify different approaches that would honor the resident's beliefs and promote better interactions with teens around sexual activity. At subsequent meetings, the resident reported that his awareness of these attitudes helped modify his style with teens. He worked more collaboratively with his clinical team members and requested feedback about subsequent patient interactions.

Generic Features Across Formats

- Designed to promote individual/collaborative reflection
- Treatment plans confirmed with faculty physicians after PI sessions
- Use of traditional residency resources (e.g., customizing elective time, consulting literature, and specialists) when knowledge gap identified
- Patient follow-up provided at subsequent sessions; consultant teaching points shared

(continued)

Box 10.1 (continued)

II. Group Composition

- First PI group: 2007
- Third-year residents – rationale:

    - Two years' experience building relationships with peers
    - More clinical exposure
    - More patients in panel
    - Higher confidence level, awareness of vulnerabilities
    - Value consultation and exposure to reflective skills

III. Facilitation

- Faculty member with nursing/behavioral health background as sole facilitator
- Residents' preference for nonphysician faculty; value of peers as consultants modeling postresidency practice

IV. Meetings[2]

- Monthly 1-hour meetings; session occurs during seminar afternoon (released from patient care duties)
- Attendance: 7–8 (8 maximum)
- Conference room setting; refreshments periodically
- Confidentiality terms regularly reinforced

V. Evaluation
Focus group
Questions:

- What are the major things you have learned from Practice Inquiry?
- What did you learn during this curriculum relevant for your future practice?

Representative Comments (36 Residents)
Reframing Perspective

"I was able to reframe my way of thinking about complex patients."
"Learned to ask the questions in a different way."
"Not just looking at what I do but how what I do affects everyone."
"Self-awareness helps me move forward in a new way."

---

[2] Residents also attend monthly Balint groups with peers in their class.

(continued)

Box 10.1 (continued)

Practicality of PI

"Being able to have 'real life' experiences in dealing with multidisci-
plinary issues with patients is helpful."
"(PI offers) an opportunity to look at the system more closely."
"Reflection on my patterns and how they compare to what others are
doing is helpful."

Collegiality

"It's a very nice forum to bring an interesting or frustrating case to your
peers and say what would you do"
"It points out how important it is to be in a group of trusted colleagues."
"Relying on each other in the PI meetings has helped me think through
complex situations."
"I look forward to PI because I get great ideas from my group."

Future Learning/Practice

"That's something I would love to continue in future practice."
"Good model for the future – I hope my new practice is interested in making this happen."
Reflection tool: (Completed at end of third year; identifies practice challenges, e.g., certain types of patient communications, time management)

End-of-the Year Resident PI Session
Representative Comments about PI: (Shared During Session)

- "Collaboration matters"
- "I need to ask for help and that is OK"
- "Others feel the same as I do"
- "I have something to offer others from my experience or
  perspective"
- "Challenges can be exciting and thought-provoking instead of
  discouraging"
- "Self-awareness helps me move forward in a new way"
- "I don't have to have all the answers"
- "There is a structure for pausing to look at things in a new way"
- "It opens up so many more choices which reduces my feelings of
  powerlessness and/or incompetence"
- "My schedule has not allowed me to attend as many sessions as I
  had hoped"
- "We don't always have enough time to explore more than one
  dilemma in a session"
- "If we could make the sessions longer, even just a few times a year,
  that would be helpful"

Box 10.2 University of Virginia (UVAFMR)

I. Small Group Discussion Formats

Individual Case Format

- Used most commonly
- Prompt: "Think of a patient who you have 'taken home'" (e.g., someone you think about after workday)

Case Example

A third-year resident describes a 29-year-old female patient presenting with poorly controlled asthma and pain who is applying for disability coverage. The resident expresses frustration with the patient who seems more interested in gaining disability designation than in taking steps he thinks would help her feel and function better and could prevent the need for disability. He explains how he has tried to convince the patient to take these steps without success. Other residents express frustration with similar patients. The facilitator notes this distress and asks: "What is the hardest part of caring for patients like this?" One resident shares that it can be difficult to keep from blurting out to the patient that he or she is not disabled and to "just get out!" A second resident explains that he became a doctor to help people get better and how demoralizing it is to work with patients when it is unclear if they want to get better. A third resident notes that the hardest part is feeling manipulated by patients who want something different than what they say they want. Group discussion leads to the observation that perhaps physicians are not sufficiently straightforward regarding what they are thinking so as to avoid offending patients and how this may not be helping patients or physicians. Discussion ensues about how to be appropriately honest and how to word difficult messages. It is suggested that the presenting resident share his real concern with the patient rather than continuing to persuade her to comply with treatment (e.g., "I'm worried that applying for disability isn't going to actually be good for you...") The resident agrees and will provide follow-up at the next session.

Positive Surprise Format

- Prompt: "Recall a recent patient interaction that surprised you in a good way" (e.g., tricky interaction went well, patient's outcome better than expected)
- Residents use index cards to write descriptive phrases per patient:

  - Parent expressed appreciation when resident explained reasoning for not prescribing antibiotics to child

(continued)

Box 10.2 (continued)

> – Family asked specifically for resident rather than waiting for physician supervisor
> – Teenage mother followed up on her child's care with unexpected diligence
> – Thanked by family member of very sick patient in intensive care unit

- Residents read cards aloud
- Group makes observations
- Value: opportunity for positive feedback

Case Example

Colleagues observe that the resident (who talked about her "surprise" regarding a diligent teen mom) speaks respectfully and personally to teen patients and inferred that her communication style encouraged the teen mom to collaborate fully with the resident.

"Pooling Questions" Format

- Designed to increase residents' general comfort revealing uncertainty and sharing knowledge/resources with peers
- Process:

  – Residents write clinical question on cards
  – Cards collected, shuffled, and passed around
  – Each resident reads one card
  – Value: answers *and* information sources shared

Example Questions

– What to do about hyperglycemia not responsive to treatment? (Patient's nausea, headache, and malaise persist.)
– What is the next step in working up a patient with low back pain and an x-ray consistent with spondyloarthropathy?
– A patient describes symptoms of anxiety and depression and is prescribed two medications. She claims that one of them makes her symptoms "ten times" worse. Why would that be?

II. Group Composition

- First PI group: 2008
- Second-and third-year residents only – rationale:

  – Residents requested PI as augmentation of existing "Intern Lunch"(support group)

(continued)

Box 10.2 (continued)

- – Resident-perceived value: increased reliance on peer support as a step toward independent practice

III. Facilitation

- Original approach – two faculty (one physician, one behavioral scientist)
- Since July 2009 – two behavioral scientist faculty members
- Resident preference for nonphysician faculty:

  - – Allows for heightened responsibility for clinical issues
  - – Avoids MD faculty bailout
  - – Increased comfort in sharing (e.g., disagreements with faculty; personal shortcomings)

IV. Meetings

- Every other week at noon, 1 hour, department-funded lunch
- Format: (1) informal conversation, (2) facilitator introduces format
- Attendance: 8–10 residents, 1 fellow (Maximum potential – 18 residents, 2 fellows)
- Text-paging reminders on meeting days
- Confidentiality terms reinforced regularly

V. Evaluation

- 2011 Written Survey N = 13 residents
- Statement: "Practice Inquiry sessions were of great help to me"
  69%: Strongly agree or agree;   23%: Neutral;   8%: Disagreed

Representative Responses to Question: "How Is PI Helpful?" (29 Comments Grouped into Categories)

Emotional Connection and Support

"These sessions relieve tension – helps to realize we aren't the only ones dealing with these kinds of issues."
"Excellent time to share gripes and challenges."
"These are one of the most important and special parts of our department…Every resident needs this forum just to even TALK about problems, much less troubleshoot."
"One of the factors that makes our program unique."
"They are tremendously helpful to de-stress, connect with your colleagues."
"Keep the food!"

(continued)

Box 10.2 (continued)

Learning from Colleagues

"I look forward to these sessions to learn from my colleagues."

"Helpful to…find solutions in a group dynamic."

"These sessions give [us] a chance to learn from each other in a safe environment."

Engaging with Challenge

"Good supportive opportunity to discuss tough patients, helps to guide [us] more regarding patient communication."

"They help us overcome or understand how to deal with difficult patient encounters or situations."

"It gives us a chance to *all* share some of our challenging patients and situations."

"The sessions help us know how to handle situations in the future."

Constructive Criticism

"The location is inconvenient."

"Sometimes redundant with same residents discussing same issues over and over."

"Maybe have some unstructured PI sessions that take us back to intern lunch-style meetings."

"Better when we help solve problems…instead of just talking about the incident."

"Did not feel comfortable discussing issues dealing with physician supervisors when there was a physician supervisor there."

"Hard to get to the sessions on time."

Facilitation

Behavioral health professionals as well as physicians make good PI facilitators provided they are seasoned clinician educators with small group teaching experience. Either type of educator can facilitate a group or co-facilitate as a team. Resident preference for physician, behavioral health professional, or both should be a consideration in making facilitation decisions. Very importantly, PI group facilitators who are well liked by residents are valuable assets to the residency program. (See On-line Resource #4 and #6 for PI group facilitation methods and small group discussion formats, respectively).

Box 10.3 Contra Costa Family Medicine Residency (CCFMR)

I. Small Group Discussion Formats

Individual Uncertainty Case Format

- Facilitator requests follow-up on last session's case
- Facilitator asks, "Does anyone have a case?"

Case Examples

A second-year resident presented a patient with severe obesity and arthritis who walked with great difficulty. After reviewing what he had done to investigate her medical issues and offer weight loss and exercise options, he had run out of ideas. Other residents expressed their frustration with caring for similar patients. Several residents offered ideas both within the system and in the community to help the patient lose weight and exercise. Residents struggled over why some patients seemed to exercise and diet but could not lose weight. One resident responded that patients were always lying about their dietary intake. Another resident referred to studies in the literature about patients who simply cannot lose weight despite tight diet control and exercise. Through this process, the presenting resident realized this patient is one of several who wanted and expected him to "fix everything." He shared his own expectations that he should fix problems for his patients. That dynamic made those clinic encounters very stressful. The group identified ideas to move the responsibility back to the patient, using patient logs, motivational interviewing techniques, and assessing the possible contribution of depression.

A resident presented a patient with mental health issues, chronic pain issues, and significant opioid narcotic and benzodiazepine use. The patient is a high emergency care utilizer and sees many different doctors for controlled medication prescriptions. Through the group process, the resident delineated more appropriate boundaries for the patient, developed strategies for getting the patient the necessary mental health care, and made a formal care plan for subsequent visits.

Appreciation Case Format (Used Routinely in the first PI Session of the Year)

Residents:

- Identify 2–3 clinic patients with whom they now have positive doctor-patient relationships after much special effort
- Write one-line patient descriptions
- Residents share case challenges and relationship change stories

(continued)

Box 10.3 (continued)

- Facilitator helps residents summarize key drivers of relationship change
- Themes identified: importance of feeling appreciated, importance of acknowledging hard work, acknowledgement of special connections with certain patients, and value of letting oneself be vulnerable
- Value: morale booster and a reminder of gratifications gained from working with challenging populations

Case Example

A resident presented an obstetrics patient with frequent ER visits and hospital admissions for recurrent headaches. By seeing the patient frequently and checking in by telephone, she developed a strong rapport with the patient, learned about her history of abuse, understood the patient's strengths in surviving past violence, and redirected the patient toward more healthy behaviors. Despite the need for ongoing narcotics (which did not feel like a perfect result), the resident experienced herself as a partner in the patient's growth

Panel Reflection Format

- Facilitator asks residents to list patients recalled from recent clinic sessions with brief descriptor phrases
- Residents group patients into categories they create (e.g., age groups, likeability)
- Group discusses categorization schema (e.g., similarities, differences, overlaps)
- Participants explore categorization usefulness for panel management.
- Value: identification of patients who "stand out" (e.g., chronic pain, favorites, medication-seeking)

II. Group Composition

- First PI group: 2009
- Second-year residents only – rationale:

    ° Sufficient clinical experience to not be overwhelmed by uncertainty
    ° Open to new ways of approaching challenges

- Average attendance: 11–12 (14 maximum)

III. Facilitation

- One family medicine physician faculty, one to two behavioral scientist faculty

(continued)

Box 10.3 (continued)

IV. Meetings[3]

- Location: resident lounge, refreshments sometimes
- 1.5 hours monthly for nine consecutive months; scheduled after resident support group, reinforces PI as different kind of support
- Text-paging reminders on meeting days
- Confidentiality terms reinforced regularly

V. Evaluation

2009–2011 Representative Comments on Feedback Form
N = 24
Questions: "What Do You Value About Practice Inquiry?" (Representative Comments)

- *Expanding Ideas About Patient Care*

  "Getting different perspectives, different management styles."
  "Ability to help colleagues."
  "It's very interesting hearing how other people managed their patients and different resources people know about and how there are different approaches – helps step back from situations."

- *Improved Well-Being and Confidence in Practice*

  "Good to sympathize with peers"
  "Gave me confidence I was doing ok managing my patients"
  "Saw group change to become more confident"
  "Improved and relieved I was not screwing up"

- *Improved Interaction with Patients*

  "There are some patients to whom I now listen to without thinking about how to treat them or meeting certain goals."
  "Helped me prepare better for a home visit I did by myself."

- *Constructive Criticism*

  "Having a case to prepare prior to scheduled day would be useful and probably better for learning."

---

[3]Residents also attend monthly support group made up of residents in all three training years.

Role of Organization Support

Availability of organization resources to support PI is critical. These should be devoted to creating a positive, relaxed environment that fosters exploration and the ability to discover and push one's limits. Providing dedicated time for consistent learner participation with a planned meeting schedule (at least monthly) contributes to the group's ability to engage and develop trust.

Conclusion

From training through advanced practice, uncertainty is inherent in medicine. Practice Inquiry presents a versatile and effective approach to help participants actively identify, manage, and live with uncertainty. In creating the time and space for the explicit engagement of uncertainty, a void in primary care training is filled. There are challenges to introducing new and different ways of learning. Resident acceptance could increase as faculty, teams, and other groups in the organization are observed using uncertainty engagement methods. Learning uncertainty engagement during residency training, a most significant educational and socialization period, can go far to sustain these skills throughout a career in medicine.

References

An, P. G., Rabatin, J. S., Manwell, L. B., et al. (2009). Burden of difficult encounters in primary care: Data from the minimizing error, maximizing outcomes study. *Archives of Internal Medicine, 169*(4), 410–414.

Atkinson, P. (1984). Training for certainty. *Social Science & Medicine, 19*, 949–956.

Bovier, P., & Perneger, T. (2007). Stress from uncertainty from graduation to retirement – A population-based study of swiss physicians. *Journal of General Internal Medicine, 22,* 632–638.

Dornfest, F., & Ransom, D. (2012). American Balint Society website.

Evans, L., & Trotter, D. R. (2009). Epistemology and uncertainty in primary care: An exploratory study. *Family Medicine, 41*(5), 319–326.

Fox, R. C. (1957). Training for uncertainty. In R. K. Merton, G. G. Reader, & P. Kendall (Eds.), *The student-physician: Introductory studies in the sociology of medical education*. Cambridge: Harvard University.

Fraser, S., & Greenhalgh, T. (2001). Coping with complexity: Educating for capability. *British Medical Journal, 323*, 799–803.

Geller, G., Faden, R. R., & Levine, D. M. (1990). Tolerance for ambiguity among medical students: Implications for their selection, training and practice. *Social Science & Medicine, 31*, 619–624.

Ghosh, A. K. (2004). Dealing with medical uncertainty: A physician's perspective. *Minnesota Medicine, 87*(10), 48–51.

Griffiths, F., Green, E., & Tsouroufli, M. (2005). The nature of medical evidence and its inherent uncertainty for the clinical consultation: Qualitative study. *British Medical Journal, 330*, 511.

Hewson, M. G., Kindy, P. J., Van Kirk, J., et al. (1996). Strategies for managing uncertainty and complexity. *Journal of General Internal Medicine, 11*, 481–485.

Kelly, A. V. (2004). *The curriculum: Theory and practice* (Vol. 5, pp. 5–6). Thousand Oaks: Sage.

LaBarre, P. (2011). Developing mindful leaders. Harvard Business Review. http://blogs.hbr.org/cs/2011/12/developing_mindful_leaders.html.

Launer, J. (2007). Moving on from Balint: Embracing clinical supervision. *British Journal of General Practice, 57*(536), 182–183. March.

Light, D., Jr. (1979). Uncertainty and control in professional training. *Journal of Health & Social Behavior, 20*, 310–322.

Pink, D. H. (2009). Drive: The surprising truth about what motivates us. In LaBarre, P. (Ed.), *Developing mindful leaders*. New York: Harvard Business Review. Retrieved Jan 26, 2012, from http://blogs.hbr.org/cs/2011/12/developing_mindful_leaders.html, 11 Dec 2011.

Richmond, M. E. (1922). *What is social case work? An introductory description*. New York: Russell Sage.

Rizzo, J. A. (1993). Physician uncertainty and the art of persuasion. *Social Science & Medicine, 37*, 1451–1459.

Schor, R., Pilpel, D., & Benbassat, J. (2000). Tolerance of uncertainty of medical students and practicing physicians. *Medical Care, 38*, 272–280.

Sommers, L., Morgan, L., Johnson, L., et al. (2007). Practice inquiry: Clinical uncertainty as a focus for small-group learning and practice improvement. *Journal of General Internal Medicine, 22*, 246–252.

Wayne, S., Delimore, D., Serna, L., et al. (2011). The association between intolerance of ambiguity and decline in medical students' attitudes toward the underserved. *Academic Medicine: Journal of the Association of American Medical Colleges, 86*(7), 877–882.

Weick, A., Rapp, C., Sullivan, W. P., et al. (1989). A strengths perspective for social work practice. *Social Work, 34*, 350–354.

Chapter 11
"We're All in the Same Boat:" Potentials and Tensions When Learning Through Sharing Uncertainty in Peer Supervision Groups

Charlotte Tulinius

In Denmark, GPs have participated in peer supervision groups for more than 30 years. Nowadays it is taken for granted that a newly qualified GP will join a supervision group within a few years of settling into a GP surgery. A recent study (Nielsen and Söderström 2012) has shown that approximately a third of all GPs participate in supervision groups, two thirds have been active in a supervision group at some stage in their professional life, and in 2003 95% of all GPs were organized in a peer group for supervision or professional development. The groups have different names, but have very often started as a "*Tolvmandsgruppe*," later developing into a supervision group or a continuing professional development (CPD) group (Nielsen and Tulinius 2009).

Tolvmandsgruppe directly translated means "12-man group." The concept has been used for at least 200 years in Denmark in many professions from cycle racing to editorial boards, describing the sharing of knowledge and decisions in a group of people. For Danish general practice this means groups of up to 12 GPs formed within a geographical area, the groups functioning as local professional peer support groups. Practicing within the same area, members can discuss their challenges within the local context and conditions of practice. Although some groups do not use a specific supervision model, I use the term "peer supervision group" throughout the chapter to simplify the description. (See Fig. 11.1 for an overview of GP education in Denmark, and Figs. 11.2 and 11.3 for an overview of the GP's role in Danish primary care.)

These groups are so much a part of the discourse of GP education that being part of and learning how to work in a peer supervision group has been mandatory in medical specialist training for general practice since 2007. As part of its medical educational

C. Tulinius, MD, PhD, MHPE, MRCGP (✉)
Associate Professor of Postgraduate Education, The Research Unit and Department of General Practice and Department of Public Health, Faculty of Health Sciences, University of Copenhagen, Denmark

St. Edmund's College, Cambridge University, UK
e-mail: rxs667@sund.ku.dk

L.S. Sommers and J. Launer (eds.), *Clinical Uncertainty in Primary Care: The Challenge of Collaborative Engagement*, DOI 10.1007/978-1-4614-6812-7_11,
© Springer Science+Business Media New York 2013

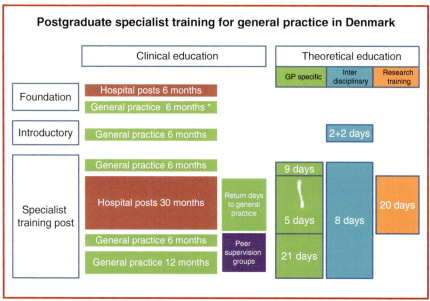

Fig. 11.1 Overview of GP education in Denmark. Medical School in Denmark lasts 72 months. All medical graduates go through foundation training of 12 months, 6 months in a hospital post and 6 months in a general practice post (or two posts within two different hospital specialties). After foundation training the young doctor has the possibility of applying for an introductory post in up to two different specialties, making it possible to ensure the right choice of medical specialty. These posts are of 12 months duration in all specialties except general practice where an introductory post is normally only 6 months. However, if a young doctor has not been employed in general practice during foundation training, he or she qualifies for an introductory post in general practice of 12 months. The trainee has to prove mastery of eight basic competencies gained during the introductory post to qualify for application to a specialty training post. Specialty training posts are directed by a national competency-based curriculum, and consist of a clinical education and a theoretical education as illustrated in the figure

reforms in 2002 the Danish National Board of Health chose the "seven roles of the doctor" from the Canadian CanMEDS-2000 project as the educational framework for the construction of new curricula for all medical specialties in Denmark (Royal College of Physicians and Surgeons of Canada 1996). When constructing the new national GP curriculum, participation in a peer supervision group was suggested as a possible learning strategy for GP trainees to develop their roles as scholars, communicators, and professionals. A group of GPs already functioning as supervisors in GP peer groups from all parts of Denmark developed a description of core values and a training program for supervisor faculty development for these new trainee peer groups.

Before the educational reforms, an important factor in the breakthrough of peer supervision groups was a regulatory initiative to educate GPs in counseling to manage the increasing number of patients with mental illness (Nielsen and Tulinius 2009). The supervision initiative might have been triggered by other professional issues, but a change in the management of mental health just happened to be the incident that in general made many GPs aware of their need for peer support to sustain their professional development. The groups were also approved very early on in their development as a legitimate form of CPD, releasing (symbolic) funding for GPs.

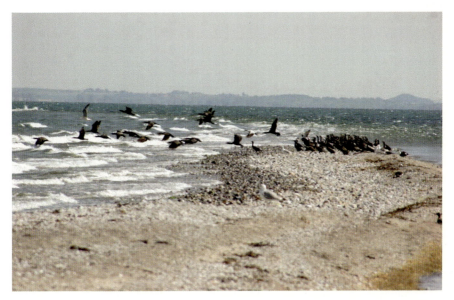

From one of the many islands of Denmark: Sejrø. (Photo Arthur Hibble)

No matter where you are in Denmark, it takes no more than half an hour in a car to reach the sea. In Danish history living with, from, and on the sea has played a very prominent role in Danish everyday lives. Although industrial production and agriculture took over dominance of the national economy a long time ago, sailing and being close to the sea are still important parts of the culture in sports, the preferred summer holiday location, and in the language. To allow the reader to get a little more of the cultural flavor, I have employed some of the maritime metaphors used in Denmark to describe experiences with Danish GP supervision.

The chapter is divided into four parts.

In Part 1, *"The Journey of a Peer Supervision Group,"* there are examples of how a Danish GP supervision session might be run. I describe some common features of the different methods used in Danish GP peer group supervision sessions.

In the second part, *"The Waters to Navigate,"* I enumerate the cultural conditions and perceptions of GP professionalism that support the development and maintenance of supervision groups in Denmark. An essential feature seems to be the double focus on teamwork between the group members and the supervisor, and on the role of the supervisor, issues that are also explored in this chapter.

Part 3, *"Is It Worth the Journey?"* explores the published effects of supervision sessions, including some of the research results from a study following three groups over a period of 2 years.

Numbers

• **GPs in the country**	Approx. 3.500
Patients per GP	Approx. 1.500

Admission

• **Daytime**	8 am to 4 pm
• **Out of hours' services**	Coordinated and delivered mainly by GPs.
Payment	No fees for patients in daytime or out of hours, apart from a few services related to documentation of health (e.g. driver's license) or travel related services (e.g. vaccinations).
Listing	Theoretically patients can choose GP freely within 10 –15 kilometers of their home, but with limitations when there is a lack of GPs in the area.
Reimbursement	Capitation and fee for services delivered

Closest partners in care

• **Other GPs**	In the same surgery or within the same geographical area
• **Other medical specialists**	Mainly from the medical specialties of gynecology, pediatrics, psychiatry, ENT, ophthalmology, and neurology, and practicing in the local community, as part of the secondary care, but outside hospitals. No fees paid by patients if referred by a GP.
• **Nurses**	Either as part of the surgery staff, or as part of the community team as visiting nurses
• **Midwives**	As part of the community teams. Visiting all families with a newborn at least once, and on a needs basis
• **Medical laboratory assistant**	As part of the surgery staff, or as part of the community service
• **Dieticians**	As part of the surgery staff, or as part of the community service

Fig. 11.2 GPs and their role in Danish primary care

The fourth and final part of the chapter, *"Voyages of Discovery, or Just Staying in the Same Professional Duck Pond?"* will draw on examples from the earlier parts of the chapter and on my experience of being part of several peer supervision groups as a member, a researcher, and as an educator. Here I discuss potential tensions and challenges when peer supervision groups are set up to support learning through the sharing of uncertainty in "the Danish way".

The Journey of a Peer Supervision Group

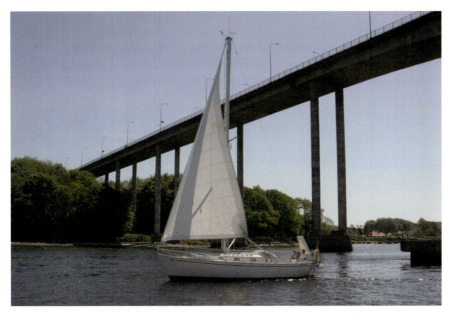

Many Danes have sailing as a hobby. From Svendborg Sund (South Funen), Denmark. (Photo Arthur Hibble)

The Focus and Method May Vary

At least two methods are commonly used among Danish GPs, the Balint method (Balint 2000; Kjeldmand 2006) and reflecting teams (Andersen 1996), but there are several other approaches used around the country (Nielsen and Söderström 2012). Some groups are mainly focused on clinical updates, others are focused on professionalism in more general terms, and some are mainly social.

No matter what the approach, one thing seems to be the same: implicitly or explicitly sharing uncertainty among GPs regarding the management of their daily work, challenges in working with patients, regulatory bodies, implementation of new treatments, guidelines or new educational reforms, changes in local services for their patients, and so on. In groups that are mainly focused on professional development, group sessions can provide room for a systematic approach to the work, based on a challenge or question that has created uncertainty in one of the group members. In groups that are mostly focused around social networking, group sessions will provide a room for the individual GP to vent ideas or challenges in a less systematic way, but on a needs basis.

In Denmark the GP is at the heart of primary care. The figure is from the Danish GP Curriculum, describing the GP's role as a leader, collaborator, and administrator. This illustration is one of 15 conceptual maps constituting the Core Curriculum of the Danish GP Curriculum summarising the educational interpretation of the seven roles of a doctor in a general practice perspective. The entire Curriculum can be found at http://www.dsam.dk/flx/uddannelse/videreuddannelsen/maalbeskrivelser/maalbeskrivelse_for_start_efter_1_jan_2004/

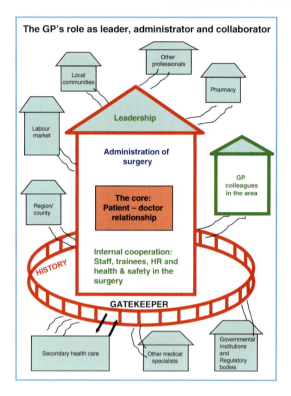

General practice resembles other parts of the health care system in many ways, but it also has a number of distinctive features. The red house illustrates one of these differences:

The general practitioner's role as leader, administrator and manager also comprises his or her role as self-employed in his or her own firm. The firm is a small unit with nonselective admittance for patients. The fence encircling the house illustrates that the practitioner also acts as gatekeeper vis-à-vis the rest of the health care sector; it is important to keep those patients within the house for whom general practice offers the best monitoring and treatment and to refer those who need treatment elsewhere to the right locations within the health care sector. The presence of the surrounding houses illustrates that the gatekeeper function involves extensive collaboration with numerous other health care organisations and institutions outside the health care sector.

However, being self employed also requires internal organisation of the firm in the form of leadership, practice management, and administration. The management function is captured by the green color and it spans from internal collaboration within the practice to collaborative relations with the colleagues who represent a rich source of help in solving problems.

Fig. 11.3 General practice in Denmark

The methods, learning objectives, and aims of peer supervision groups are the focus of continuous discussion. The use of a wide spectrum of methods, and different perceptions of what peer group supervision is among GPs, became apparent when the Danish College of GPs advertised for possible facilitators/supervisors for the trainee supervision groups. GPs came forward who were part of (or trained to facilitate) groups using the Balint method, the reflecting team model, the Bendix method, and a model called "TERM." The Balint method is described in detail in Chapter 4 of this book; the reflecting team model is a "fishbowl" type of model described in Fig. 11.4 (see also Chapter 7).

The Bendix method and the TERM models have been used to train GPs in the management of difficult encounters with patients, with a specific focus on communication skills and strategies. The Bendix model is based on audio recordings of the GP and patient, and at these supervision sessions the GPs train in active listening, often with the tape recording as the point of departure (Bendix 1991). The TERM model (The Extended Reattribution and Management Model) is used as a training program for doctors managing so-called "functional disorders" in general practice (Fink et al. 2002). On the business cards of course organizers and trainers across the country you can see an even wider spectrum of supervision activity described as "psychotherapeutic supervision," "cognitive therapy," or "mindfulness."

The implementation of mandatory supervision still leaves much to be desired. In fact this learning strategy has only been fully implemented in half the country; evaluation of the initiative where it has been implemented is very sparse. The important issue, however, is that the Danish College of GPs now acknowledges supervision as paramount in the training of GPs in order to learn how to manage their CPD, defined as "professional development, personal development, development of self care, and taking part in supervision."

The Common Core of Supervision Sessions

For groups I have been part of, have observed, or set up, a common element is that the sessions are experience-based, allowing the individual GP to present, explore, and discuss a selected problem in depth as a case, and with a supervisor as part of the set-up. The supervisor is sometimes labeled "the facilitator" or "the interviewer," and in the descriptions of the sessions, I have chosen to use the term "supervisor" or "facilitator" for the person who leads and has the main responsibility for the process of the session. The presenting GP works with the problem as a "case" throughout the session, supported by the rest of the group. Through exploring questions, the supervisor supports the case presenter in refining the description of the problem. The rest of the group members listen to the case presentation, reflect and make associations with what they hear, and offer their reflections in parts of the session. The case presenter is then offered the possibility of reflecting and perhaps integrating the

This requires a supervision group of 7-10 peers with practical experience of the topic that the supervision is focussing on (e.g. practical experiences in clinical practice). The set-up allows protected time for these practitioners to reflect and learn from the experiences by sharing them in the group. A reassuring, comfortable, undisturbed room is essential. Establishing the trust in a 'safe to share' space is paramount to achieve learning in the 'zone of proximal development.'

What are the roles?

All participants have a role in every session. The roles shift with every session. The roles are:

- A case presenter
- An interviewer
- A reflecting team

How does the session run?

Some groups start with an ultra-short 'round'. This allows everyone who would like to present a case to come forward, and for the group to choose one or two of these to address within the session. Someone is assigned the role of interviewer, and everyone else becomes a member of the reflecting team. The point of departure is a critical incident presented as a case; a positive or negative event which has made an impression on the case presenter. All participants will have reflected before the session in order to identify a possible case. Participants are encouraged before the session to write down keywords or dilemmas perceived in relation to this case.

The interviewer and case presenter sit in a 'fish-bowl' with the reflecting team observing them. Together the case presenter and the interviewer explore the incident, unfolding what the case is about. The interviewer will ask supportive questions to help the case presenter clarify the elements of the case. The reflecting team will not be allowed to comment or interrupt the interview. Instead they will listen until the interviewer decides that their input is necessary to clarify the case further.

When the interviewer pauses to invite their comments, the reflecting team does not address the two directly. Instead they discuss among themselves the thoughts generated during the interview they have just heard: how did the interview affect the members of the reflecting team; what associations did they have; how did they feel when they listened to the interview? The reflecting team will NOT give advice to the interviewer or the case presenter, only communicate with each other their associations, reflections, feelings provoked by the interview. Meanwhile the interviewer and case presenter listen to the discussion and get ideas for how to take forward the interview. There is a structured time line for the session, but the interviewer can extend or shorten the elements of the session based in the needs in the individual case.

What is a suitable 'critical incident' to bring?

This is a case or a situation which surprised you in a positive or negative way; a situation different from the routine situations you normally encounter; something that made you think or even change perception of your work. Starting a session with such an event makes it possible to uncover your own and your colleagues' practical knowledge and non-verbalised strategies in order to strengthen the strategies and strengthen the awareness of possible ways forward. The critical incident should be related to the focus of the group

Fig. 11.4 Working with a reflecting team

(eg clinical practice). The case discussion will give you the opportunity to discuss situations and experiences that are difficult for you with competent colleagues and peers. Working in groups like these over several years, each of you will however experience critical incidents in your personal lives too, and if such an event is flagged up in the round, the group should offer to run a session with this as the focus. We are in this boat together, and if one of the team is bereaved, in a family conflict or otherwise personally in crisis, the function of this crew member is not optimal. We have to take good care of each other to keep the boat floating. It is important though to remember that the reflecting team sessions are NOT therapeutic set-ups. The interviewer is not expected to go into in-depth psycho-analytic interpretations of the case presenter's story, but instead to stimulate and encourage the case presenter's reflection. The aim is for the case presenter to be able to clarify their thoughts and to make absolutely explicit 'what this is a case about'. During a session it is very common that the problem is redefined several times indicating that the case presenter is developing a deeper understanding of why this particular situation was a critical incident, and how to approach the problems related to the incident.

Time table of a session
The structure of the reflecting team is always the same, but the time allocated for a reflecting team session varies. From my experience you will need at least an hour for each critical incident to be discussed in a way that feels calm and safe for the case presenter. Typically this will mean the following time schedule (for convenience I refer to the case presented as male and interviewer as female):

- The case presenter tells as much as he can about the critical incident (10-15 minutes)
- The interviewer asks questions to stimulate reflections to get the case presenter to clarify 'What is this a case about' (5-10 minutes)
- When the interviewer feels the need for input from the reflecting team, she asks for permission from the case presenter to open the fish bowl to include the reflecting group. (5-10 minutes)
- The interviewer closes the discussion and continues the interview, using ideas or themes that have arisen from the reflecting group's discussion in the pursue to widen their understanding of what this is a case about and ways forward (5-10 minutes)
  The interviewer invites in the reflecting group again for reflections as described above (5 minutes)
- The interviewer and case presenter end the dialogue. The case presenter describes what he has learned about the critical incident, and how he is going to take the work with the challenge forward. (5 minutes)
- The process of the session is evaluated by the interviewer describing her perception of how the session went: were there any challenges for her in the interview, in what way was the reflecting group's discussions helpful, and what has she learned from the session. The reflecting group is invited to join in with comments of the process, but no more remarks or reflections on the content are allowed (5 minutes)
- Everybody gets up, and changes position and chairs. Physical activity is necessary to underline that the session is over.

(Adapted from Kjær and Tulinius, 2004; appendix 6)

> **Important**
> **Feeling safe in the reflecting team session is paramount to the success of these sessions as a learning strategy.**
> **It is therefore extremely important to remind the group members after each session that everything they have heard and discussed in the session, cannot be discussed outside the four walls of the room. You can tell others about your own insights in relation to your own new understanding, but you can never mention names or the original case content to others.**

Fig. 11.4 (continued)

group's reflections and associations in order to come closer to an understanding of what the case is about, as well as possible ways forward. Based on the grass roots, bottom-up ethos of development and often self- directed learning, peer group supervision demands a lot from both members and facilitators.

Cases brought to peer groups are typically about clinical challenges or the difficulties of interaction, collaboration, and teamwork between GPs and other colleagues, other professions, and patients. A typical case in a peer supervision group working with *clinical challenges* could be described as the "heart sink" patient, the patient who makes your heart sink by just seeing him on the list of the day's encounters (O'Dowd 1988). It could be the patient who challenges your professionalism implicitly or explicitly: the patient encounter that makes you realize that your clinical knowledge or skills have become a bit rusty. Or it could be the patient with a need that puts you in a professional or perhaps ethical dilemma. If the patient is a child, how do you protect and support the patient at the same time as supporting a complex family situation that is part of the patient's problem?

Cases focusing on *cooperation difficulties* might be experiences with another colleague inside or outside the GP surgery, with team members within or outside the medical profession, or they could be of a professional–political character, for example, "How do you handle a surgery when your secretary is on long-term sick leave?" or "How do you handle a hospital doctor refusing to receive a patient you refer to her?" Cases may also be of a more *organizational or philosophical character*, for example, "who takes care of the pastoral needs of my patients if I don't?" or, "Am I a healer?"—a "suburban shaman" as Cecil Helman (2006) described it—rather than a medical "techno-rational professional," to use Schön's (1987) term. Some groups will also discuss issues that are less clinical and more within the role of the academic. Critical appraisal techniques, management models, or ethical and medico-legal cases would be typical for these discussions.

In some peer supervision groups, GPs pay a supervisor to facilitate their group. It is possible to apply for financial support to establish a new peer supervision group, but the funding will only pay parts of the costs. These supervisors are very often psychologists, psychiatrists, or GPs with supervisor training of some kind. Many groups, however, work with one of the GPs in the group as the facilitator on a rota system. This arrangement works well for several of the models, such as the reflecting team model.

Different Kinds of Expertise Are Involved

Many groups will have chosen the model they use to run the group, but these models do not themselves direct the focus of the discussions. Learning in groups of peers is dependent on different kinds of expertise in the group. As a part of the national GP curriculum the Danish College of GPs needed to write an educational program for the supervision element of GP training. Not surprisingly, this was not easy. The solution therefore was to ensure the faculty development of GP supervisors, giving them a shared understanding not of a specific model to be used, but a set of general values, and the competences for working in teams to be achieved through the program. These reflected the experiences of GP peer group supervision in all their diversity.

Seen from an educational perspective, Danish peer supervision groups are designed to allow learning to happen not because a professional expert is "telling" the learners, but because nonprofessional experts are sharing their experiences in order to gain a common understanding of a phenomenon. The learners are clinical experts, and experts on their working conditions, situations, and experiences gained from their work, but educationally they are seldom experts. The empowerment of clinicians through the peer group work consists not necessarily of widening their clinical content knowledge (although it might), but definitely widening their understanding of how to learn and develop as professionals, managing their clinical knowledge in their specific work settings. Fish and Coles (1998) have very elegantly described how to give professionalism back to professionals, a principle that very nicely captures the values of Danish peer group supervision.

Theoretically, nonprofessional expertise can also be understood through the lenses of social anthropology. The ethnographer, J. P. Spradley (1979). defined the "good informant" as a person who is a living part of the phenomenon you are studying, one who is able and willing to describe the phenomenon in nontheoretical terms, and who has the time to work with the researcher. The anthropologist learns from sharing knowledge and interpreting the shared knowledge together with the informant, negotiating an understanding that is neither the researcher's original understanding nor the informant's, but an understanding they have developed together, and is understood by both.

This phenomenological point of departure provides a good theoretical basis for understanding learning in peer supervision groups as the process of sharing experiences, adjusting professional/clinical behavior into alignment with the peer-acknowledged consensus. All doctors are experts on the clinical settings and situations they have experienced and bring to the group, and they are all good communicators, willing to give time, and most often communicating these in an (educationally) nontheoretical way. For supervision sessions, GPs bring their understanding to the group, share their understanding, and are open to negotiate their understanding by listening to peers.

The Waters to Navigate: Peer Supervision as a Culturally Embedded Professional Activity

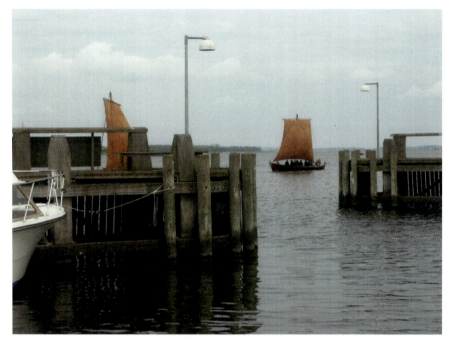

The Danish Viking ship Museum in Roskilde offers the chance of going out in a boat like the ones used by the Vikings. (Photo Arthur Hibble)

This part of the chapter is about the key contexts, cultural conditions, and perceptions of GP professionalism that support the development and maintenance of Danish GP peer supervision groups.

There are probably several reasons for the popularity of peer supervision groups among Danish GPs. From the literature I cannot claim to know exactly why they are popular, but in this part of the chapter I describe possible professional and cultural factors contributing to the development of peer supervision as an activity that is taken for granted as part of professional life among GPs:

- The development of Danish general practice as cooperatives
- The inspiration from abroad and the cultural perception of GP professionalism
- The cultural concept of sameness
- Reflection and reflexivity
- Uncertainty as a general condition of work (and life)
- Striving to keep the human being at the center, including for the professionals themselves

The Development of Danish General Practice as Cooperatives

Denmark is a very small country, where good ideas can spread fast. Societies, unions, and cooperatives where ideas can be discussed have thrived for more than a century. In some parts of the country it will still be taken for granted that you are a member of at least one society, and if you are a homeowner, you are very often part of and expected to be active in the homeowner's association covering your small local area. The foundation of the family doctor arrangement was *sygekasserne* ("disease societies"), based on the cooperative ethos, and established in the second half of the nineteenth century. Here people with a low to average income could be insured to have parts or all of their medical expenses paid by the disease society when seeing the disease society doctor with whom they were signed up (Vedsted et al. 2005).

In many parts of the Danish society there is a high acceptance of solving problems in small groups with similar interests, values, ideas, or perhaps similar challenges, translating into GPs working in group surgeries, and the *tolvmandsgrupper* described above.

Inspiration from Abroad and the Cultural Perceptions of GP Professionalism

Danish GPs have searched for inspiration from UK general practice for more than two generations, even before general practice was given medical specialty status in 1993. Since the mid-1960s individuals or groups of GPs have come to the United Kingdom to visit GP surgeries in the search for inspiration on professionalism, and work by Colin Coles, John Launer, the Tavistock Clinic, and Balint are always coming up when you discuss supervision in Danish general practice.

If a group of GPs decides to start a new supervision group they are entitled to approximately 2,750 Euros (US $3,600) per year to cover their expenses for supervision sessions. Of this they can use a maximum of 25 Euros (US $32.50) per person per day for refreshments, making it possible for groups to have a sandwich when they meet and meet at least 10–12 times a year. Thus being part of a supervision group, meeting regularly with the same group of peers is today acknowledged among Danish GPs, and perceived as a CPD method authentic for general practice and efficient for self-directed professional development (Tulinius and Hølge-Hazelton 2010).

The Cultural Concept of "Sameness"

The acceptance of professional development through sharing experiences in a peer group may also be supported by what anthropologists would call Scandinavian "sameness" (Haastrup 1990; Hervik 1994). Sameness in the Scandinavian contexts describes how people take the notion of being equal for granted. The concept of Scandinavian sameness demonstrates a strong linkage between equality and alikeness—homogeneity—among Scandinavian people. Sameness has been used to explain the strong development of feminism in Scandinavian countries as well as the development of legal regulations of work, for example, the Nordic worker–carer model which has given support to equal access of affordable day care for all children, maternity leave for fathers, and equal opportunities for both genders in the labor market (Boyle 2011). Although there is a fluid border between sameness and otherness in anthropological terms, it has also been suggested as one of the drivers for the political tendencies of nationalism, and as a way of understanding these (Hervik 1999).

When working with GP trainers I have met the influence of Scandinavian sameness in GP trainers' discomfort in assessing trainees. When a trainee works in the GP surgery he or she is welcomed as a peer, an equal professional, and the concept of sameness seems to contradict the judging of your peer in the assessor role. In this way "sameness" might also support the flat hierarchy of a peer supervision group, making every experience equally worthy of discussion among GPs. No perception, no attitude, or no case could ever be described as less necessary to discuss in the peer group if of concern to any of the members of the group.

Reflection and Reflexivity

The use of reflection in relation to work-related experience is connected with an understanding of the consultation as patient-centered. In Danish general practice, a common understanding of the consultation includes the concept of inner dialogues and *reflexivity*. Reflexivity I define as "a self-conscious account of the production of knowledge as it is being produced" (Baarts et al. 2000). It means being aware of your own contribution to the way you and the other person construct meaning as you talk. Supervision groups using the Balint method or the reflecting team model allow GPs to bring the inner dialogues and understanding gained from their reflexivity during their day-to-day work so they can continue the reflective process, extending their dialogues from inner ones to explicit case discussion. For some GPs and GP trainees this will mean preparing for the supervision session, using a reflective log book in an e-portfolio, or reviewing the little yellow stickers on their desks. These will help to remind them of the issues they want to discuss with their peers, so they can extend their inner dialogues in the surgery into the external forum of peer supervision (Hoelge-Hazelton and Tulinius 2012).

Reflexivity is also paramount for the supervisor facilitating the session. The supervisor has to support the case presenter in getting a more detailed case description and hence understanding of what the case is about. If the case is understood in the same way and brings out the same feelings in the supervisor as in the case presenter, the supervisor may not sufficiently challenge the presenter's perspective. It will be equally problematic if the topic of the case is morally or emotionally unsettling for the supervisor. No matter what kind of experience or attitudes she has in relation to the case, the supervisor will inevitably contribute to the way the case does or does not unfold. If her contribution to the understanding of the case is not made conscious, or is not taken into account by the supervisor herself during the session, her perceptions, attitudes, and behaviors in the situation can actually block the case presenter from unfolding the case the way that is needed in order for the presenter to develop professionally.

Used as a tool in anthropological research, reflexivity is described as "the conscious use of self as a resource for making sense of others" (Hervik 1994, p. 68). In the setting of a supervision group I would extend this to "…and for the supervisor to understand the process of supervision and her contribution to the development of the process as the session is taking place." The aim of an anthropological study is to gain understanding of other lives and to produce new knowledge shedding light on everyone's life. In peer group supervision, the aim of the supervisor is to use her own awareness of herself, and of her interaction with the people in the group, to help everyone become wiser, with the help of each other's insights, about situations and dilemmas similar to the ones presented.

Here is an example of reflexivity in action in a peer group. As a supervisor in a group of doctors I was interviewing Sharon, who presented the case of a 12-year-old girl who had come on her own to her surgery. She described the situation in highly morally colored terms: "What mother would allow her 12-year-old daughter to see the GP on her own?" Sharon asked, thus judging the girl's mother as irresponsible, and unfit as a parent. The harsher she spoke of the girl's mother, the more irritated I became. Or perhaps even angry. At least, I was uncertain about the truth of the statements Sharon was making. "My own mother would have sent me alone to the GP when I was 12," I thought, "not because she was a bad mum, but because she would have been working during GP opening hours! And yet, would I myself have sent my daughter alone to the GP? Would it not be dependent on how worried I was myself?"

As Sharon was unfolding the case I knew that I would find it hard to support her opinion and her pursuit of establishing that the mother was unfit, especially if no more information was available on *why* the girl had come alone. I asked myself: "How can I make sure that the next question allows Sharon to develop in her own pace, with her own perspective?" In the next second, Sharon looked at me with a glimpse of uncertainty. "I am sitting here listening to your case," I said, "and wondering if you know why the mother was not with her? Did the mother actually know that the girl had gone to see you?" I felt the tension in my question, and although this was an attempt to open Sharon's perception towards a broader explanation, I was also pushing her towards at least thoughts of a possible justification for the girl being in her surgery on her own. My experiences and feelings had made me less open and forthcoming in my role as the supervisor, and I had had to decide whether I would communicate this to Sharon at this stage or later. Whether helpfully or not, I was now putting my own fingerprint on the process of her journey to discover what this case was about.

When the reflecting group was invited to reflect, several of them gave stories of how they themselves had had to send their teenage children off to an appointment on their own. Would they have contributed in this way, if I had not pushed in that direction? At the end of the process I finally had the chance as interviewer to talk about the challenges I had faced in the conversation. This gave me the opportunity to describe my uncertainty about my response as the supervisor, and how I knew this had had an impact on the situation.

Uncertainty as a General Condition of Work (and Life)

Danish general practice was originally set up as it was in most western European countries, getting doctors out from the capitals and into the rural communities, close to where the patients lived and worked. Until 1993 general practice was not a medical specialty in Denmark. The perception among a lot of Danish doctors was exactly like Lord Moran's description of English doctors "falling off the ladder" when leaving a hospital career to go into general practice (Royal Commission on Doctors' and Dentists' Remuneration 1960). Some doctors came from broken dreams of surgical or physician careers, others had grown up as countryside doctors' children, knowing what their father's or mother's lives offered. A common condition for all of them was that "the path was made as they walked." This description was used by the Norwegian professor of general practice Kirsti Malterud when she gave a lecture describing her career of becoming a researcher, doing research relevant for general practice work (Malterud 1988). In my opinion it is a very good description of all professional development in general practice.

To get a picture of the culture of general practice it is also helpful to listen to a group of doctors visiting but not yet fully embedded in GP culture. Studies have explored the perceptions of young doctors having their first encounter with general practice during their foundation training years, or later as GP trainees/registrars. In a focus group study of learning in general practice, a GP trainee described the constant need for professional development in general practice:

> What I had heard at the hospital departments before I started was that general practice was some sort of "low-level-a-little-of-a-lot-of-specialties," but I very quickly realized that general practice is everything that is not described in the textbooks we read at medical school. I really admire the GPs now, they just have to learn all the time. (Kjær and Tulinius 2004)

Another feature of general practice that fits with the use of peer group supervision might also be the existing learning environment in general practice, and the ethos of learning embedded in the work there. Again the fresh eyes of a young foundation doctor described this perfectly:

> [In general practice] I think you learn a lot about how you work as a doctor, as an individual doctor. You detect your limitations because there is room for it. … [T]he older GPs tell you that they sometimes are uncertain and how they have experienced being afraid in professional situations. At the hospital departments the doctors don't talk about this. You are more alone at the hospital. You are running around with the "beeper" afraid of making mistakes …. (Kjær and Tulinius 2004)

Uncertainty was and is still a given condition when working in general practice. This has been beautifully described theoretically as "finding your way through the swampy lowlands of general practice" (Schön 1987). Philosophically it would be difficult to argue against the anticipation of uncertainty as a given condition of life in general practice. The postmodern human being is described as being constantly searching for certainty in an uncertain life, minimizing the uncertainty whenever possible. It is my perception that GPs are so close to people's everyday life, that the conditions of everyday life in general constitute an important contribution to their medical professionalism. The uncertainty of the patients' lives is shared with and by the GP.

When asking GP trainees what they learn from patients during their training, the essence was an insight into how people in general manage the uncertainties of life, and understand and maneuver in a framework of lay knowledge to handle the challenges of illness (Tulinius, unpublished data). Sharing uncertainty in peer groups makes it possible to integrate uncertainty as a natural part of the professional development of this specific professional group, and it makes it possible for GPs to sustain professionalism despite carrying their own as well as their patients' uncertainty in life.

In their book about producing knowledge in health and welfare through reflective practice, Taylor and White (2000, p. 200) describe how practicing reflectively may be seen to produce uncertainty, whereas working with the certainties of evidence-based research and applying them to practice can seem to be much easier. Their point is, however, that reflective practice switches the *application* of the technical knowledge to *managing* it in the encounters with the individual patient. In this way reflective practice as seen in Danish peer group supervision can support practitioners in establishing how to manage knowledge. There may be a cultural expectation for doctors these days to be professional robots in the way they perform: over the last few decades they have come under continuous public scrutiny. However, doctors are in some ways protected by their professional robe, and holding on to uncertainty could be a consequence of culturally embedded expectations for them as one of the classical professions.

Striving to Keep the Human Being at the Center, Including for Professionals Themselves

Part of modern GP professionalism is to practice evidence-based medicine, to apply the newest guidelines, working within a fixed health care budget that contributes to the needs of the health care service. This is in accordance with expectations from regulators and patients, and within a society that is changing every minute. CPD activities support updates of knowledge and clinical skills, but dealing with the pressure of keeping abreast is itself often not seen as part of CPD in Denmark. The normal human responses to these demands, pressures, and continuous developments are not addressed in CPD activities.

In fact, a normal human response to these demands is very often described as pathological in relation to professionalism: How often have you heard feedback on a professional issue start with "Now there is no reason to personalize it!" How often have you heard someone talking about an "emotional response" as opposed to "being professional"? In our culture showing anger, sorrow, or any other emotion as a reaction to a professional problem is seen as *un*professional. You are supposed to continue smiling and behaving in a way that does not distinguish you from any of your peers in terms of personality, and act as if you were stripped of emotions. However, a doctor, a human being without emotions striving to practice empathically, is an oxymoron, creating paradoxes in the understanding and management of what it means to practice professionally.

Doctors are heavily socialized from the start of medical school and throughout their careers. Being a doctor is so closely linked to identity that distinguishing between you as the doctor and you as the person is very often just not possible. If not supported, the doctor will not be able to manage the pressure and burnout and compassion fatigue have been described as consequences (Figley 2002). In peer group supervision you can take off your coat of professional armor, and allow yourself to be human with a mixed professional and personal identity, integrating the feelings of a normal human being.

Is It Worth the Journey?

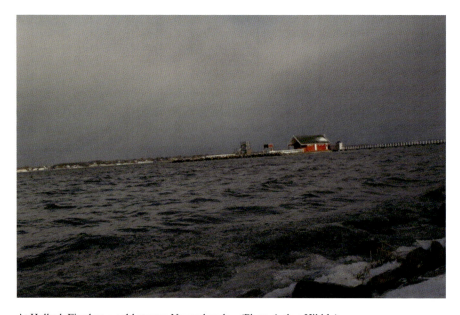

At Holbæk Fjord on a cold stormy November day. (Photo Arthur Hibble)

In Peer Group Supervision You Can Work with a Broad Range of Professional Challenges

Not much has been published on the effect of supervision within Danish GP peer groups. In this part of the chapter I explore some of the reported effects of GP peer group supervision. Although the study described below relates to a specific project that took place in three supervision groups, its findings may be relevant to Danish peer groups generally.

Over a 2-year period we studied three peer supervision groups of GPs. Their supervision had a topic as its focus: children in need. The aim of the project was to prevent the neglect of children by early and competent action and to strengthen the professional identity of the participating GPs in children's cases. The specific learning objectives were to strengthen the GPs' competencies in:

- Identification (of a child case)
- Referral (of a child to relevant local initiatives or parts of the social and health care system)
- Intervention (relevantly in a child case)

The groups met for peer supervision 8–10 times a year. They were observed and interviewed and also contributed to the evaluation of the study by written evaluation forms. The analyses of all their cases showed four general themes in relation to the challenges raised by the cases (Tulinius and Hølge-Hazelton 2010).

The general themes were challenges involving:

- Definition and maintenance of personal and professional boundaries. Examples of questions asked in this category were:

  "How can the GP express or point out to the parents that the behavior of their child when present in the surgery shows that the parents are not setting boundaries for the child?"
  "How can the GP approach the discovery of parents' medicalization of a child?"
  "What can a GP do if parents 'experiment' with alternative treatments for their child, rather than following the more conventional treatments prescribed?"

- Feelings of doubt, powerlessness, or uncertainty related to the GPs' own professionalism. Examples of questions asked in this category were:

  "Within the time and legal limitations of general practice, creating risks of misjudgments, how can the GP put herself forward as a resource person?"
  "How do you approach a young person in crisis when there is a history of self-mutilation?"
  "How do you as a GP support a child who functions as an interpreter for a seriously ill mother?"

- Directing attention to problems that the child or his or her family had not brought up themselves. Examples of questions asked in this category were:

  "How do you as a GP talk about obesity in a family not aware of the issue, without coming across as moralizing or condemning?"
  "How do you as a GP ensure the safety of children of drug-abusing parents?"

- Collaboration with other professionals working with children and families. Examples of questions asked in this category were:

  "How does the GP deal with frustration when parents are sent by other professionals to ask for referrals from the GP?"

"What does the GP do when there is no action taken on a referral to the social authorities concerning a child's safety?"

We do not know whether these themes would replicate across other topics and in supervision groups without a topic focus. However, a key ingredient of all the themes is uncertainty about the full range of GP professionalism: from uncertainty regarding specific clinical situations and the relationship with the patient, to those regarding personal and wider professional issues.

Using a mixed method evaluation design it was possible to categorize the 70 cases presented and discussed in the study. They primarily described problems concerning the parental roles, such as behavioral problems, and problems related to events such as death, divorce, war, and torture. It was characteristic that almost half of all the presented cases were brought up in the supervision because of the doctor's anticipation of a potential problem or worry for the child/family, and not because the parents themselves presented the topic as a problem to the GP.

Many of the cases could be described as a form of indirect consultation for children, occurring when the GPs became aware of a patient's problematic family circumstances. Several cases even described potential problems for an unborn child. The analysis and detailed cases can be found in Hølge-Hazelton and Tulinius (2010), but below are a few examples:

- "Since her divorce the mother of two teenagers has started drinking a little. The father does not want contact with his children. The GP can see the whole family feels terrible and the GP is frustrated because there is nowhere suitable to refer them."
- "Mother with preschool child. The problem is access to the father, whom the mother describes as a psychopath. The mother wants to go 'undercover' with the child and consults the GP."
- "Toddler spoils things in the GP's office while the parents are completely passive. The GP is irritated at the child but does not want to expose the parents."
- "A concerned neighbor of an alcoholic divorced mother of two children calls the GP. The GP knows the mother but not the children."
- "Young pregnant women with a violent boyfriend: the doctor is concerned about the woman's capability for motherhood."

Although all participants in this study described tremendous professional development gained from the peer supervision sessions, the groups had an uneven result when studied at an individual GP level. There are many possible explanations for this. One explanation could be the GPs' different experiences both in terms of clinical experiences, and experiences in the use of supervision as a CPD method. GPs with long clinical experience and prior experience of peer group supervision were more likely to develop to a higher level of professionalism and in accordance with the curriculum for the intervention, than GPs with short clinical experience and/or no prior experience with supervision

One of the more inexperienced GPs seemed to have set his expectations too high or perhaps wished for more complicated learning to happen. Referring to himself as being a novice GP, he also expressed the need to develop his own experiences rather than what he described as "transferring knowledge" from the more experienced GPs (Hølge-Hazelton and Tulinius 2012). This particular GP did not experience the supervision group as a group of peers. This might reflect that age, clinical experience, perhaps gender, and perhaps other parameters are important to consider when a new group of peers is started. It is, however, to me, also a sign of a dysfunctional peer supervision group, possibly influenced by the skills, attitudes, and professionalism of the supervisor.

Supervisors from Within or Outside the Profession Might Make a Difference to the Outcome

No matter whether the facilitator has another educational background, or is a GP himself, the task is to allow for the case presenter to get to a better understanding of the presented case: "What is this case about?" The facilitation skills comprise the same kind of openness to the structure and content of the session as an ethnographer's acceptance of the phenomenon as it is presented to her. The ethnographer will have to follow wherever the phenomenon takes her, and explore the aspects of the phenomenon presented to her, and go with the description evolving in the collaboration between the case presenter, the supervisor, and the rest of the group. During the phase of exploration of "what is this case about?" listening and analysis skills are paramount to allow the GP to unfold the case. The learning potential is not just in understanding how to manage the specific case, but to understand the different aspects of professionalism that the case illustrates, see possible transferable aspects, and to unveil possible learning needs for the case presenter as well as the rest of the group members.

In the evaluation study of the three groups of GPs referred to above, two groups had a GP as their supervisor, and the third group had a psychologist (Hølge-Hazelton and Tulinius 2010). It is not possible to generalize from this study to all peer supervision groups in Denmark. It is, however, interesting that comparing the psychologist supervisor-led group with the GP supervisor-led groups, the learning processes and outcomes were very different: in the group with the psychologist supervisor the GP members of the group established a common understanding of holes in their collective knowledge, the learning potentials of the group, the learning needs, and how and where to go to improve their professionalism.

The groups facilitated by the GP, on the other hand, developed a strong sense of praxis and professionalism among their peers in the group (see Chapter 3) and felt supported by the development of "a collective we," but they never reached the point of defining gaps in their knowledge or new learning objectives. In the group where the facilitator was a psychologist, the protective "collective we" did not set in as a solution to the same extent. This is not to say that psychologists are better facilitators than GPs who have gone through supervision training, but to raise awareness that the focus of professional development is different within different disciplines, and to underline that unless the supervision method is supported with clearly described processes and outcomes, the perception of what is professional development will influence the group dynamics and learning processes in the peer supervision groups.

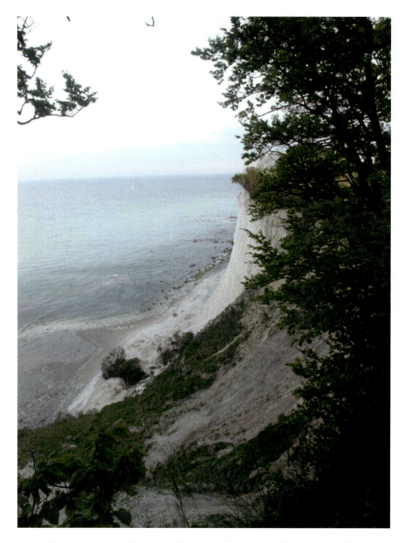

Every year a few centimeters of Denmark disappears into the sea (Photo Arthur Hibble)

Preventing Burnout

Dr. G: '... Do I want to be part of a research study on life style advice in general practice!!!?? And it "only" takes three hours! Are you aware what it is like being a GP in a single
handed surgery?! (Speaking very fast). I see a new patient every ten minutes, my secretary
left two months ago and I haven't found a replacement yet. I have no breaks, I work from
eight in the morning till ten at night, I am behind schedule for sending in my claims, my tax
accounts have to be sent in by next week, my husband is asleep when I come home at night
and when I leave in the morning. I just can't take it anymore ... (starts crying).'

Dr. G was one of almost 200 randomly picked Danish GPs we talked with over the phone to recruit 40 GPs for five focus groups on lifestyle advice in general practice (Tulinius and Dencker 2001). The project was unrelated to supervision groups but its findings have implications for them.

Most of the GPs just explained that they were too busy to participate in more activities, but four others reacted like Dr G, yelling or crying on the phone with me or my colleague, a total stranger on the other end of the line. We asked for 3 hours of their lives to describe their needs and opportunities for CPD within the context of GPs giving lifestyle advice. To me it was terrifying and a very clear sign of just how much psychological pressure these professionals experienced. Did they have anyone with whom to discuss this? Who were supporting them? How close were they to breakdown or even burnout?

Evaluation reports have shown that Danish doctors who are part of a supervision group experience better communicative skills, that they develop personally and professionally; that they have better job satisfaction, and that they find supervision to have a preventive effect on a feeling of burnout (Firth-Cozens 2001; Soler et al. 2008). When examining GPs from other countries, preliminary results of studies point in the same direction as this finding: when Balint-group–trained they have better job satisfaction, higher awareness of their own feelings, better psychological skills, and more tolerance with patients with uncertain diagnoses. However, looking at other professions such as private practicing psychologists the picture is not so clear, and among these professionals it has not been possible to confirm supervision as a significant predictive factor for burnout and compassion fatigue (Clarke 2007).

Voyages of Discovery, or Just Staying in the Same Professional Duck Pond?

This final part of the chapter draws mainly on my experiences of being part of several peer supervision groups as a member, a researcher, and as an educator. Here I discuss potential challenges when peer supervision groups are set up to support learning through the sharing of uncertainty in "the Danish way".

The Construction of the Professional "Collective We" for Better and for Worse!

"We are all in the same boat" was a Danish revue song from 1944 describing solidarity during hard times (and an only slightly concealed resistance message). It was performed during the Occupation, has been carried forward colloquially for generations, and is used today with the same meaning. It builds nicely onto the idea of Scandinavian sameness: no one is more than me, hence no one is going to tell me how to run my surgery. On the other hand, if I have a problem, other GPs will have the same problem, and we will have to solve the problem for the profession. Using the peer group as a safe place to disclose your challenges and problems, it becomes possible to find solutions that all agree on, and the professional "collective we" is born.

The "collective we" can be used as a claim for professionalism in certain groups, thus giving clout to a statement. For example, in Denmark I very often hear GPs say "in general practice we . . .," as the start of a description of work practice, attitude, perceptions, educational practice, and the like. In Danish grammar this "we" is not describing specific persons, but rather the professional we, the cooperative concept of any GP. This concept has both advantages and disadvantages when used in a peer group learning setting.

Where uncertainty rules or at least colors every action, the need for certainty and approval rises. Postmodernist life has been described as an attempt to minimize the size, impact, and number of risks that we all unavoidably meet in life (Fox 1999). Establishing a common "we" in the group of equals then supports the development of the identity of the profession. This is how *we* do it in our profession, in *our* part of the profession, in *our* part of the country, in *our* peer group of the profession. Acknowledging solutions to cope with uncertainty offers a kind of counterweight certainty against chaos. So does agreement on what is good medical practice, as seen in the examples from peer groups.

In the study mentioned above, evaluating learning in Danish supervision groups (Hølge-Hazelton and Tulinius 2010) it was also clearly shown that the construction of a "collective we" can also have the opposite effect: limiting the development of professionals. Medicine is one of the classic professions, characterized by a monopoly on knowledge, a codified language, autonomy, authorization, self-regulation, and adherence to an ethical code of practice, giving a certain status in the society (Cruess 2006). Classical professions such as medicine can, however, also be perceived as under threat, stimulating the profession's need to maintain its privileges, and this can possibly draw members of the profession in two directions: the establishment of new platforms; development of the original base of knowledge, language, and status; or a tightening of the original regulations and classifications, making sure that the profession is not diluted by any factors, by other professions or nonprofessions (Figley 2002).

In this connection, Saltiel (2010, p. 141) writes about reflective practice in the health care sector as follows: ". . . [L]anguage constitutes rather than reflects reality. Reflective accounts are as artfully constructed, as storied, as any other usage of language. They give access to how professionals construct their identities (and those of service users) and their practices but they are not, by themselves, enough." There is no doubt that this sets high demands on the methods and structure of supervision groups to maintain the potential for professional development.

In the same study, the development and outcome of supervision was also examined (Tulinius and Hølge-Hazelton 2010). The aim was for GPs to use peer

In one of the groups in the study (Tulinius and Hølge-Hazelton 2010) the supervisor was a GP, who frequently used the strategy of supporting the GPs' feeling of doing well within the frames of the existing health care system to support their development of the GPs' professional identities. In one of the sessions a GP described frustration that a family had not come to her when there were problems in the family, and the fear that she had overlooked something in earlier encounters.

Supervisor: "But we are normally not challenging, we expect people to come to us, and then we act!"

The group then discussed the emotional side and the moralities involved in professional action.

Supervisor: "You have to be realistic, not idealistic.... It is a condition for our work; we need constantly to make decisions. A lot of things you are not allowed, not expected to do, but the everyday in a GP surgery looks different!"

By contrast, in another group the supervisor was a psychologist with an overall strategy to challenge the presented perception of practice in order to develop the GPs' professional identities. In one of the sessions a GP was worried about how to support a family where he could see a situation potentially developing into abuse of a child.

GP: "I feel like saying something about it to the mother, but where are the limits for my intervention? I mean, I could ask her, if I should talk with their dad?"

The reflecting team then discussed what GPs in general could and could not say.

Supervisor: "Are you ready to proceed? Tell me, how would you define the child abuse in this case?"

The following debate moved the whole group's definition of what it means when you talk about safeguarding children, widening their understanding of the concept.

Fig. 11.5 Two kinds of supervisor

group supervision as part of their CPD in order to develop their professional identity, with the specific focus of supporting children with special needs. Several of the GPs in the groups felt challenged when working within this field. Actual knowledge was sparse in all the groups, and the experiences of dealing with these cases were at best patchy. The scarcity of professional knowledge within the topic and the focus on the "collective we," the "us" as normal human beings in the room, meant that the GPs drew on their own family values and experiences. Moral perceptions very often took over the session, and almost no new knowledge was allowed into the forum, let alone requested as a possible learning need for the group.

In Fig. 11.5 you can see an example of the difference between the construction of a "collective we" consolidating professional identity but limiting development (Group 1), versus challenging the identity and opening the possibility for development of the "collective we" (Group 2). In the (probably unconscious) attempt to keep professional control of the GPs' knowledge base, praxis, and cooperation with partners in supporting children with special needs, the "collective we" became protective of the current profession in some of the groups rather than challenging the professionalism of this area. The psychologist supervisor more often challenged the knowledge within the group than the GP supervisors. In this way the psychologist-led group members were sent out into more open waters than the GP supervisor-led group.

We do not know how common a lack of challenge is in GP peer supervision groups in Denmark. In the groups where the challenge of professionalism is not happening, change is probably going to be difficult because peer group supervision in Denmark is perceived as an integrated part of the professional life and characteristics of being a good GP. A way forward for supervisors who use the "collective we" as professional protection, would be to allow themselves to include competencies from the field of medical education to a higher degree. In this way they would be able to use educational principles such as the zone of proximal development (Vygotsky 1978) and an understanding of education towards professionalism as dynamic and evolving as described by Stenhouse (1967) and Jarvis (2002, 2006) to support the group's professional development beyond the current praxis of general practice. The boat would not have to stay in the protected lakes and bays of the fiords; it would be able to go out to open sea with all the security installations needed to make for safe travel.

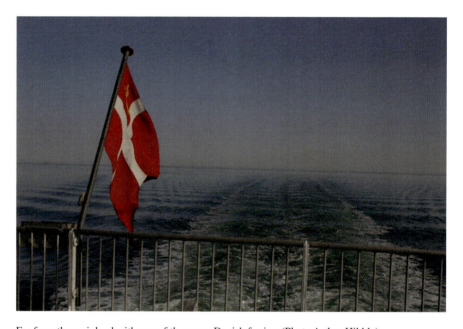

Far from the mainland with one of the many Danish ferries. (Photo Arthur Hibble)

Conclusion

The development of professionalism through Danish peer group supervision depends on the banks surrounding the water. The potentials of peer group supervision as established in Denmark are not difficult to spot: supporting self-directed learning in how to improve professionalism among individual doctors who have to make the path as they go about their daily work, navigating in different kinds of uncertainty within a broad range of challenges. The grass roots bottom-up design allows "giving professionalism back to the professionals" (Fish and Coles 1998), developing authentic questions and authentic answers to support GPs in their every-day clinical work.

But (because there is a "but") unless there is an explicit educational strategy decided by the group and the supervisor in order to counteract it, this way of working is also likely to stimulate the construction of a "collective we" that can be more pro-tective of current praxis than stimulating the development of future practice. The boat can certainly be controlled by all the rowers, but there is a difference as to whether the boat is led out into the open sea, looking for solutions and inspiration from a wider world, understanding what is not already understood by the individual crew members; or if the boat stays in the same duck pond, the crew carefully monitoring and describing the calm surroundings and unchanged depth of water, to reassure themselves that the crew is still able to maneuver in this particular pond, while their capacity to get out into the open sea is unrecognized, unchallenged, and untrained.

Doctors need to be responsive to changes in society, patient expectations, current evidence of best practice and the needs of the health service. I have no doubt that peer group supervision—supported by a supervisor and conducted in accordance with educational principles—can provide one of the best training methods for the professional survival of doctors.

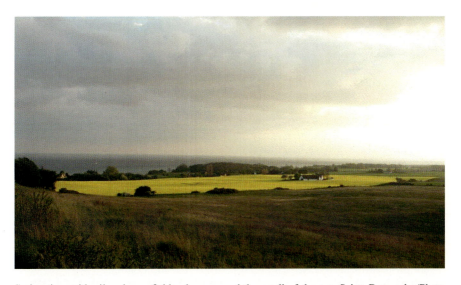

Spring time with oilseed rape fields, showers, and the smell of the sea. Sejrø, Denmark. (Photo Arthur Hibble)

References

Andersen, T. (1996). The reflecting team: Dialogue and meta-dialogue in clinical work. *Family Process, 26*, 415–428.

Baarts, C., Tulinius, C., & Reventlow, S. (2000). Reflexivity – A strategy for a patient-centred approach in general practice. *Family Practice, 17*, 430–434.

Balint, M. (2000). *The doctor, his patient and the illness*. London: Churchill Livingstone.

Bendix, T. (1957). *Din nervøse patient. [Your nervous patient]*. Copenhagen: Lægeforeningens forlag.

Boyle, K. (2011). *Taking sameness for granted through the Nordic worker-carer model. Thinking Gender Papers*. Los Angeles: UCLA Center for the Study of Women.

Clarke, M. M. (2007). *Private practice psychologists' use of peer supervision groups and experiences of compassion fatigue, burnout and compassion satisfaction*. Dissertation. Chicago: Loyola University.

Cruess, S. R. (2006). Professionalism and medicine's social contract with society. *Clinical Orthopaedics and Related Research, 449*, 170–176.

Figley, R. C. (2002). Compassion fatigue: Psychotherapists' chronic lack of self care. *Psychotherapy in Practice, 58*, 1433–1441.

Fink, P., Rosendal, M., & Toft, T. (2002). Assessment and treatment of functional disorders in general practice: The extended reattribution and management model–an advanced educational program for nonpsychiatric doctors. *Psychosomatics, 43*, 93–131.

Firth-Cozens, J. (2001). Interventions to improve physicians' well-being and patient care. *Social Science & Medicine, 52*, 215–222.

Fish, D., & Coles, C. (1998). *Developing professional judgement in health care*. Oxford: Butterworth Heinemann.

Fox, N. (1999). Postmodern reflections on 'risk', 'hazards' and 'life choices'. In D. Lupton (Ed.), *Risk and sociocultural theory: New directions and perspectives* (pp. 12–33). Cambridge: Cambridge University Press.

Hastrup, K. (1990). The ethnographic present: A reinvention. *Cultural Anthropology, 5*, 45–61.

Helman, C. (2006). *The suburban shaman, tales from medicine's front line*. London: Hammersmith Press.

Hervik, P. (1994). Shared reasoning in the field: Reflexivity beyond the author. In K. Hastrup & P. Hervik (Eds.), *Social experience and anthropological knowledge* (pp. 60–75). London: Routledge.

Hervik, P. (1999). *Den Generende Forskellighed – danske svar på den stigende multikulturalisme. [The annoying otherness: The Danish response to an increasing multi-cultural society]*. Copenhagen: Hans Reitzels Forlag.

Hølge-Hazelton, B., & Tulinius, C. (2010). Beyond the specific child. What is a 'child case' in general practice? *The British Journal of General Practice, 60*, 9–13.

Hølge-Hazelton B., & Tulinius C. (2012) Individual development of professionalism. A multiple case study of GPs in group supervision. *International Journal of Family medicine* 2012, 13. Article ID 792018, doi:10.1155/2012/792018, can be accessed freely at http://www.hindawi.com/journals/ijfm/2012/792018/. last 17th March 2013.

Jarvis, P. (2002). Practice-based and problem-based learning. In P. Jarvis (Ed.), *The theory of practice of teaching* (pp. 123–131). London: Kogan Page.

Jarvis, P. (2006). *Towards a comprehensive theory of human learning: Lifelong learning and the learning society* (Vol. 1). London: Routledge.

Kjær, N. K., & Tulinius, C. (2004). Learning in general practice in Denmark: Trainees' and trainers' perspectives. Masters thesis. Maastricht: MHPE, Maastricht University.

Kjeldmand, D. (2006). The doctor, the task and the group: Balint groups as a means of developing new understanding in the physician-patient relationship. Ph.D. thesis. Uppsala: Uppsala University.

Malterud, K. (1988). Veien blir til mens du går [The path is made as you walk it]. In G. Almind, D. Bruusgaard, N. Bentzen, B. Hovelius (Eds.), *Forskning i nordisk allmennmedisin [Research in Nordic general practice]* (pp.169–176). Oslo: Universitetsforlaget.

Nielsen, H. G., & Söderström, M. (2012). Group supervision in general practice as part of continuing professional development. *Danish Medical Journal, 59*(2):A4350.

Nielsen, H. G., & Tulinius, C. (2009). Preventing burn-out among GPs – Is there a possible route? *Education for Primary Care, 20*, 353–359.

O'Dowd, T. (1988). Five years of heartsink patients in general practice. *British Medical Journal, 297*, 528.

Report of the Royal Commission on Doctors' and Dentists' Remuneration. (1960). Evidence of Lord Moran of Manton. *The Journal of the College of General Practitioners, 3*, 133–134.

Royal College of Physicians and Surgeons of Canada. (1996) Skills for the new millennium: Report of the societal needs working group – CanMEDS 2000 project. *Annals Royal College of Physicians and Surgeons of Canada, 29*, 206–216.

Saltiel, D. (2010). Judgement, narrative and discourse, a critique of reflective practice. In H. Bradbury, N. Frost, S. Kilminster, & M. Zukas (Eds.), *Beyond reflective practice: New approaches to professional lifelong learning*. London: Routledge.

Schön, D. (1987). *Educating the reflective practitioner*. San Francisco: Jossey-Bass.

Soler, J. K., Yaman, H., Esteva, M., et al. (2008). Burnout in European family doctors: The EGPRN Study. *Family Practice, 25*, 245–265.

Spradley, J. (1979). *The ethnographic interview*. New York: Holt, Rinehart and Winston.

Stenhouse, L. (1967). *Culture and education*. London: Nelson.

Taylor, C., & White, S. (2000). *Practising reflexivity in health and welfare: Making knowledge*. Buckingham: Open University Press.

Tulinius, C., & Dencker, A. (2001) Patienterne ville jo tro, at jeg var monoman, hvis jeg tog rygning op hver eneste gang.. [The patients would think I was suffering from monomania if I talked about smoking in every encounter…] A study of GPs' attitudes, work and expectations for the work as life style advisers. Copenhagen: Department of General Practice, University of Copenhagen.

Tulinius, C., & Hølge-Hazelton, B. (2010). Continuing professional development for general practitioners: Supporting the development of professionalism. *Medical Education, 44*, 412–422.

Vedsted, P., Olesen, F., Hollnagel, H., et al. (2005). *Almen lægepraksis I Danmark [General practice in Denmark]*. Copenhagen: Maanedsskrift for almen praksis.

Vygotsky, L. S. (1978). *Mind in society: Development of higher psychological processes*. Cambridge, MA: Harvard University Press.

Chapter 12
Case-Based Learning in Swedish Primary Health Care: Strengths and Challenges

Gösta Eliasson

Introduction

This chapter describes how managing uncertainty is addressed through case-based training in small groups for family physicians. Many family physicians in Sweden now belong to these. They are called FQ groups, where "F" stands for the Swedish word for continuing professional development (CPD) and "Q" for quality development. An FQ group is a group of five to ten family physicians, including the leader, who meet regularly to exchange experiences and to develop knowledge. They offer structured problem-based, self-directed learning, facilitating life-long learning helping doctors to maintain and develop ideas, skills, and attitudes. They achieve this by the use of case reports and narratives from patient encounters, which are analyzed and discussed in the group.

In Sweden, the initiative to start FQ groups came from the profession itself. Since 1992, the Swedish Association for General Practice (SFAM), the Swedish counterpart to AAFP in the United States and RCGP in the United Kingdom, has developed a nationwide educational program involving local FQ groups. The aims of these FQ groups are to:

- Inspire individual learning
- Enable the exchange of knowledge and experience between family physicians
- Identify learning needs and organize further learning from those needs
- Promote professional identity and support
- Contribute to quality development

Electronic supplementary material: The online version of this chapter (doi:10.1007/978-1-4614-6812-7_12) contains supplementary material, which is available to authorized users.

G. Eliasson (✉)
Swedish Association for General Practice, Björkhagsringen 13, Falkenberg SE-311 72, Sweden
e-mail: gosta.eliasson@telia.com

Members often come from different centers. Meetings are meant to occur regularly, at least once a month, with a duration of 1–3 hours. FQ groups are democratic and members decide together about structures and processes such as group size, the appointment of a group leader, rules for discussions, and the choice of topics.

The concept of small group learning is not new. Problematic "heart-sink" patients have for a long time provided doctors with a reason for joining Balint groups. However, in Sweden, Balint groups have never been used on a large scale, probably due to their time-consuming sessions and the need for skilled supervisors and because the focus is on psychologically complex patients: these are undoubtedly important but constitute just one facet of daily work in family practice. Patients discussed in Balint groups are ones with whom the clinicians may have trouble communicating or who cause them strong emotional reactions. By contrast, patients discussed in FQ groups are more likely to be those who raise straightforward clinical dilemmas such as "What is causing my patient's symptoms?" "Why isn't my patient getting better?" or "How would you handle my patient?"

In Sweden, being able to join a group where you can present patients with any kind of dilemma has provided the answer to a growing demand for collegial dialogue in which family physicians can help each other to cope – not only with problematic patients but also with common tasks and problems coming up in their everyday practice. In addition, group discussion is a facet of quality and organizational development.

In the first section of this chapter, we meet David, a group leader, telling us about his experiences as an FQ group leader. He will describe his group, how their discussions proceed, what kind of cases members bring, and what a group leader has to do. The section finishes with his own ideas on how groups handle uncertainty and how they acknowledge "not knowing."

The second section is an overview of features characteristic of the Swedish program for learning in FQ groups, as launched by the Swedish Association of General Practice (SFAM) in the 1990s and still in use. The section includes details of the reasons for launching the program, with an outline of the learning structures, the methods used, and aspects of group leader maintenance as well as management and ownership of the program – together with the author's personal opinions on how groups deal with uncertainty.

The third section is an outline of the precautions necessary to make groups survive and flourish in the future. It highlights the strengths of group learning as well as threats and challenges. The sections end with an account of measures to secure the national program.

For readers unfamiliar with Swedish primary care, Box 12.1 offers a brief glimpse, and Box 12.2 gives details of SFAM and the origins of FQ groups.

Report from an FQ Group Leader

I'm a family doctor and have been a leader of an FQ group for about two years, although I joined the group five years ago. Up until then I had only read about FQ groups and didn't know much about them. When I was at a conference for family

> **Box 12.1** A Glimpse of Swedish Primary Care
>
> Almost all Swedish public health care, including hospital and primary care, is financed by taxes. Twenty-one separate county councils charge the population and distribute money to health care.
>
> A Swedish primary care unit is a health center, where at least two but sometimes up to eight or more family physicians work together. There are also a number of nurses, district nurses, and secretaries employed. Besides these people there might also be occupational therapists, counselors, and psychological expertise as well as orthopedic and other specialists connected, depending on need.
>
> Primary care units are accredited and contracted by county councils which are local authorities regulating payment, services, care quality, etc. In 2012, a visit to a family doctor cost the patient about 13 €.
>
> According to a new law on freedom of choice, people are encouraged to choose a primary care unit and/or a named doctor in a system, in which all inhabitants are listed on a record kept by the health care center and by the county council. Reimbursements to the center are given by the county council, according to the number and ages of individuals on the list and in some areas also by the number of visits they do.
>
> Most of Swedish family physicians' encounters are with acute nonemergencies or with chronically ill patients. In addition, many family physicians offer basic child and maternal health, school health, rehabilitation, and care for the elderly at home and in nursing homes. Cooperation with district nurses plays an important role. In rural areas, there might be emergency patients and the possibility of caring for patients in hospital-like wards. Almost all Swedish primary care units are well equipped for minor surgery, proctoscopy, eye and ear microscopy, spirometry, ECG, etc.

physicians, I met some colleagues who told me about learning in small groups and that they were able to get feedback from colleagues on their own cases. On my way home I sat thinking about my development as a doctor, and I found that the main sources of my own learning were courses, conferences, and medical journals. At that time I didn't see my frequent occasional and short consultations with colleagues as learning opportunities. But I would have been delighted if, now and then, I had had an opportunity to dig a little deeper into a problematic case and have my colleagues' opinions about it.

With this in mind I made a proposition to some colleagues to start an FQ group to find out if it could help us learn in a better way. We asked our primary health care (PHC) manager if we could do that, and after some negotiation, we ended up with an agreement saying that half of the time should be taken from work time and the other half from private time. Then we had our first meeting, agreeing about practical rules for the group. We persuaded an older colleague to take the group leader position and from that day onwards we have been meeting every month.

Box 12.2 The Swedish Association of General Practice (SFAM)

As in many other countries, Swedish primary care has its roots in hospital care. Until about 1970, family doctors were specialists educated in hospitals who had left the hospital to work in the community. At that time most doctors were happy if they could get sporadic lectures from medical authorities and experts on science, drugs, and treatments.

In 1978, an investigation of family doctor's education concluded:

> ...the family physician gets a lot of new experiences every day. This might lead to the formulation of new ideas and hypotheses about correlations, but these hypotheses are very seldom tested and discussed. If this were done. doctors would have a better chance to develop their unique field of knowledge. This could be a starting point for a better definition of family medicine.

The mission of The Swedish Association of General Practice (SFAM) is to support the development of education, quality, and research in primary care. Today, SFAM has about 2,300 members, organized in local associations. Financing come from member fees, in 2011 it was about 170 € a year.

In 1993 SFAM applied for financial support from the Swedish government for an extensive CPD project directed to family physicians including structures for local, regional, and national educational activities. Recommended methods and content included FQ groups using an Irish model for small group learning (Boland 1992). Group leader courses were introduced on a large scale.

Two years ago I was asked to take over as group leader because the existing leader was going to retire. I didn't find that problematic at all, because I already knew what would be expected from me: a person with responsibility for booking a conference room, bringing refreshments, and – the most tricky task – keeping our group discussions on track.

Our meetings have always been on Tuesdays. They go on for 2 hours and nowadays we are lucky enough to be able to meet in work time. We are eight colleagues including me, and all work as family physicians. Three of us are female, two come from the same health center, and the other doctors come from different centers. As we meet at my place, some people have to drive by car for about 20 minutes.

As primary care teams include many different professions it could be argued that these too should be in the group. There are two arguments against this. First, I believe that tasks, problem presentations, and beliefs differ between professions. Secondly, there is a risk that openness would suffer if other professionals were involved. This would be a disadvantage, at least in discussions about mistakes and shortcomings and in revealing "not knowing." In some regions, nurses and social workers do use similar methods and have formed groups of their own. The common opinion among people here is that accepting other professions in this kind of group would have no advantages.

This is how we spend our session time:

We make a point of starting the group meeting on time. The first 5 minutes will be spent on "socializing," gossiping, and informal talk. If we didn't do that, we might have to talk about these things during the session, which would be rather annoying.

More often than not, people recall interesting cases from earlier meetings and want to hear what happened to the patient. Members in our group are strongly encouraged to bring information back to the group about cases discussed earlier. We spend about 15 minutes presenting short case reports, getting brief comments in return. Also, every colleague will present "the second patient I had yesterday," and how this case was handled.

For example:

1st doctor: My second patient yesterday was a 16 year old boy who had had a little traffic accident on his way to school. He got entangled with another bicycle and fell to the ground. Abrasions of both palms but nothing more. He needed some comforting. After he had gone, I asked myself: why did he have to see a doctor? A nurse would have been good enough, or what do you think?

2nd doctor: My second patient came without booking to renew her sick-leave certificate which had expired two days earlier. I refused to see her as an emergency and told her to ask the reception for a scheduled encounter. Wow, she got soo angry…!

3rd doctor: My second patient was a teenager with a sore throat. It was obviously tonsillitis. Strep-A-test was positive and I gave her penicillin. I knew her from before, she is a very quiet and shy person. I wonder if she heard what I said about the tablets….

As these examples show, we often present and highlight trivial cases like a patient asking for sick leave or how to treat a sore throat. The value of presenting such cases is that we are encouraged to question our routines, revealing to colleagues how we handle common problems. This will often start a discussion on how to handle routine cases in the most effective way and with a minimum of resources.

During the next 45 minutes, there are opportunities for those of us who wish to present a more complex case, in which we may have got stuck. Our case discussions are very different from each other. They may range from a presentation of a successfully treated patient to a very complex case, in which difficult decisions about priority, investigations, and treatment must be done. Now and then, one of us wants to get an opinion on how to give a seriously ill patient bad news. The motive for us bringing such cases into the group is not to get an unequivocal answer but to try out some possible alternatives and sometimes to get support for acting in a certain way. Feedback and support from other group members often relieve a lot of anxiety due to difficult decisions.

This is an example of a complex case:

The patient is 81 years old. She has taken tablets for diabetes type 2 for 15 years, now and then she has somewhat high blood glucose. She's also got mild hypertension and some kind of mysterious recurring arthritis making her unable to walk during relapses. Last year she had a stroke and now she is partly immobilized due to weakness of left arm and leg. I have also noticed some signs of dementia. Now her daughter is insisting that I should try to convince her mother that her diabetes will be treated better if she moves to a nursing home. I think so too, but this old lady is obstinate and I can't do this against her will, can I? I also wonder how important it is to keep her sugar low. And what is "low" in this case? I can't understand what's in her aching joints. Rheumatoid tests are all negative. I'm doubtful whether I should prescribe diclofenac, I think it might increase her blood pressure.

Normally, we have time to discuss two or three complex cases during a session. After we have been talking for a while, I often notice that the agenda we agreed on from the beginning drifts away and the focus gets lost. In such circumstances, I have to get people back on track, telling them we have two options: keep talking about the new upcoming topic or return to the original one.

Everybody in a group should be able to talk. The more individual members contribute and engage in discussions, the more likely it is that group members will thrive. The atmosphere in the group is crucial; we want it to be permissive, nonjudgmental, and supportive. Giving criticism is easy, for instance, telling a colleague "…you ought not to have done that…." However, the person who makes these critical comments does not have all the information about what has been done and said in the consultation room. Instead we should try to be helpful and supportive, saying, for example: "What made you do that?" "Tell us more!" "How did you feel when…?"

Often, but not always, a group member will document important reflections, decisions, and recommendations that have come up during a session. All notes are archived for later follow-up. Here is an example of such a note:

Case presentation by Johanna 2008/04/09

Background: 62 year old man, not married, former captain of a ferryboat, diabetes, treated with diet and tablets. On sick-leave for a year due to low back pain.

Doctor's problem: HbA1c 9, B-Glucose 16, patient not compliant to recommended diet, neglecting prescribed treatment.

Reflections in the group: Well-recognized problem. Consensus that no quick fix exists. Ethically correct to accept unwillingness to follow recommendations? What feelings does he evoke in doctor? Is patient fully informed about consequences? Referral to hospital for dose adjustment? See another doctor? Will he benefit more from frequent contacts with a nurse? Insulin might help him realize the seriousness of his disease.

Recommendations and decisions: Johanna asks a diabetes nurse to see patient within a few days keeping frequent contacts with him for at least three months. Then Johanna will give us feedback.

During the last 5 minutes, we evaluate the meeting, talking about lessons learned, and we plan for coming meetings. Some members may have some homework to do, which they are asked to present next time. Among all the homework tasks we have given ourselves, I recall one in particular. It was to search the internet for papers on how mortality rates are affected by treating moderate hypertension with angiotensin II blockers in patients over 80 with diabetes. That was because one of us had been visited by an elderly patient who asked what the odds would be if he stopped taking the prescribed tablets. Of course we were unable to find an unambiguous answer in this particular case, but at least we learned to search for and handle scientific results and how to bring best evidence into our practice.

Another homework task included making telephone contact with three specialists in geriatrics, asking them for advice on when to refer patients with osteoporosis to bone densitometry and to see to what extent their advices were congruent. As we had expected, advices varied to such a great extent that we decided to adhere to existing national guidelines.

A third homework task included finding out the incidence, diagnostics, treatment, and prognosis for cold urticaria; this was triggered by a patient suffering from recurring hives. If the results of such homework are presented during the next meeting, I think facts are easier to remember than information acheived from traditional sources.

Sometimes we spend an hour or so discussing a clinical entity or a general problem, for instance, the drug treatment of diabetic patients with concomitant hypertension and renal failure. I often notice a surprisingly high level of know-how coming up during case discussions in our group, but sometimes we find ourselves to be short of the knowledge we need to solve a problem. In such cases, we get missing information by temporarily asking a hospital specialist to attend our group. Our guest will be asked to answer our unresolved questions. This approach has the advantage of bringing hospital doctors and family physicians closer to each other and promoting the exchange of knowledge, shared care, and better logistics between primary care and hospital. Here is an example of this:

"How to treat patients with a red eye" was a recurrent agenda in our group for years. Knowing when to refer a patient to an eye-specialist was a problem for all of us. Therefore, a few years ago an ophthalmologist was invited to one of our meetings. First we asked her what sort of signs should be taken seriously and referred to hospital as emergencies. She gave us a short list of such cases and showed a couple of pictures of red eyes, illustrating examples of emergencies. Then we discussed how to treat less serious conditions like bacterial conjunctivitis and allergy in primary care. Finally, we agreed on what information referrals to an eye-clinic should contain. The ophthalmologist asked us for tips on how to get in contact with us in case a patient needed follow up in primary care. I think all of us learned something during that meeting.

Some discussions of clinical entities have been thoroughly documented and processed further, to be used as "home-made" guidelines. An example of this is our local guideline about acute otitis media. In that document there are useful recommendations about how to diagnose otitis; how long to wait before starting antibiotics, the recommended dose, and preferred antibiotics; how to examine small children; when to follow up; and when to refer to a specialist. Merging our own experience with a knowledge of local conditions and with established sources of information (in this case national guidelines and the opinions of a local ENT specialist), we were able to write up a practically useful guideline.

Real cases are seldom hard to find. But when our FQ group was new and we wanted to discuss how lower back pain should be treated, people had some difficulties in presenting cases coming from their own practice. Some had difficulties recalling a "typical" patient; others felt uneasy in presenting a complex and elusive case in a concise way in front of other colleagues. Therefore, before the next meeting, all members were asked to download a "study letter" on low back pain from SFAM's webpage (see below for an account of study letters). In that study letter we found a couple of case histories of patients suffering from lower back pain, which felt familiar to all of us. We went through a few cases and discussed treatment alternatives. We read the brief summary of what evidence there was for different treatment options, and finally we landed on a treatment alternative. After some time, a colleague recalled a patient with pain he had met in his surgery. He vividly described the uncertainty he had felt during that encounter. He was in great doubt whether he should order an investigation for malignancy or if he could wait and see.

During that lower back pain session, we learned things from each other about how we cope with uncertainty. For instance, we found it a relief to hear other group members talk about moments of hesitation and doubt. The problem, as I see it, is that we always try to "play the game" and hide our uncertainty. We also concluded that uncertainty and doubtfulness, though stressful, make us creative, because we then think about a problem for a longer time before making a decision. Acknowledging uncertainty, regarding it as a natural part of care, makes us feel more secure and satisfied.

People's willingness to talk during our meetings varies considerably. I often have to stop a colleague who takes over the talking, but I also have to encourage quiet members to talk. Two group members may engage so deeply in a subject that they forget about other people, talking exclusively to each other instead of addressing the whole group. It can be tricky to stop such "sideshows" without being impolite. Most of the time we talk about patients in the third person, that is, "…she told me I was a bad doctor and that she wasn't given what she needed." If case presentations contain such emotional stuff, I often suggest the case should be presented as a role-play. This means that the owner of the case either plays the role of the patient, mimicking his or her behavior, or plays the doctor role while a group member plays the patient. Even if a colleague gets into role-play for a short while, he or she tend to revert to the storytelling mode. Nevertheless, role-play training has reduced the sense of threat, and I think we will use it more in the future.

Now and then I notice that there are private topics coming up. Hidden conflicts are not unusual and may come into sight through small, sticky comments and nonverbal signs. If they occur just once or twice, I don't comment it but if they tend to recur I will confront group members with the problem. Up till now, this strategy has been successful. The chemistry between group members must be taken into account and I have found that handling group dynamics is not as easy as it appears. A permissive group climate can be undermined in overt or subtle ways. A new colleague can make other group members behave differently or evoke conflicts due to different kinds of political and personal views. For instance, a member who pleads for a religious or feminist approach can be a challenge to others and can at worst make the group dysfunctional.

Our group is performing quite well, and I think we have found an important platform for learning and a way for professional development that fits all of us. In a functioning group, members will like each other and will tolerate and appreciate divergent opinions. The possibility of group members choosing each other increases the chances of group thriving. Personally, I wouldn't think of joining a group in which people are chosen by anyone outside the group.

Defining clear rules for group work seems to be a prerequisite for group achievements. For instance, in our group we have put an effort into deciding what will happen if a member persists in arriving late to meetings, how disagreements about topics for discussion will be handled, and how the group leader should be elected. It is also important that members agree on confidentiality about things said and done in an FQ group.

When our group was new, we were rather afraid to talk about patients we thought we had handled inadequately. But after some time, we were ready to lower our guard and talk freely about our shortcomings and problematic patients. In most physicians' minds, uncertainty about having made the right decision and insecurity about the ability to treat patients is a gnawing reality. Today we do not hesitate to tell each other what silly things we have done, just because we trust each other and feel confident.

In my experience, listening to case presentations will reveal uncertainty in almost all case reports. People in our group are still anxious to show that they are knowledgeable and capable of making correct decisions. In time, we will be able to talk more about "not knowing" in front of colleagues as well as with patients without losing respect or self-esteem. We learn a lot more from analyzing mistakes than from announcing success. Yet, discussing critical incidents and shortcomings has proven to be rather easy compared to acknowledging uncertainty, doubt, and "not knowing."

An Overview of FQ Groups

The following section focuses on doctors' expectations and beliefs and on the relationship between continuing professional development, learning, and the use of FQ groups. As there is no robust evidence on these topics, most statements rest on the author's own observations and on personal messages from colleagues who lead FQ groups. Background details relating to vocational training and CPD for Swedish family physicians, the number of FQ groups, and their funding appear in Boxes 12.3, 12.4, and 12.5.

Stages to Pass for a Group to Be Productive

An FQ group is not just a number of doctors talking about their patients; the goal must be set higher because a group has the potential to be a continuously developing, unpredictable endeavor for achieving professional development. Research on group psychology shows that there are four distinct phases in the development of a group over time: forming, storming, norming, and performing (Elwyn et al. 2001).

In the first stage, *forming*, the group will decide about logistical matters including where and when to meet and who should be responsible for room bookings and that, for example, during the first 10 minutes, time should be devoted to socialization.

In the next phase, *storming*, FQ group members will get to know each other more and they start to express opinions on, for example, how much work they are ready to invest

Box 12.3 How Are Swedish Family Physicians Educated?

Physicians who work in Swedish primary care units are almost exclusively specialists in family medicine, even if other specialists are allowed to work and cooperate with family physicians in primary care settings.

To become a Swedish family physician, qualified graduate physicians have to go through a 5-year training period, employed by a health care unit. More than half of the training is devoted to practicing in primary care under supervision. Time is also spent in hospitals, on joining a number of obligatory courses and on writing up a small scientific paper. There is no obligation to go through an examination to become or to remain a specialist, but SFAM offers an optional examination process.

As a rule, county councils and health care units share the costs of trainees.

on group work and what kind of items they should discuss. Visible conflicting interests may now emerge in the group, some of which are discussed and neutralized.

In the next, *norming,* phase, most group members adapt to agreed goals of achievements, for example, how many different topics they should cover during a year, to what extent they should discuss these, and how they should present results. Members now begin to accommodate to each other's peculiarities, eager to find accepted norms for working together smoothly, finding it rather pleasant to be together in a group. They may have created explicit or, more often, implicit rules for interaction and social behavior – for instance, how private, intimate, or provocative a person can be.

Eventually the group will arrive at the *performing* phase, in which all group members work effectively together towards an agreed goal. Having learned how to handle and neutralize conflicts the group is now capable and productive.

When an FQ group has reached the performing stage, group members take on two different key roles. First, they contribute to the objectives of the group by task achievement, that is, being productive in developing knowledge and finding new solutions to problems. Secondly, they contribute to the cohesion of group processes and to group maintenance, that is, they will support each other in making the group a pleasant, enjoyable, and social endeavor. Both roles are essential in order to make an FQ group perform well.

Discussion Content and How Learning Happens

Topics for discussion in an FQ group are up to the individual group to decide on, but the group process itself is invariably characterized by interactive problem-based and self-directed learning. Case discussions are by far the most common activity in an FQ group, and cases retrieved from real life or from study letters (see Boxes 12.6 and 12.7) are a natural starting point in the development of knowledge. Cases may

---

Box 12.4 How Many FQ Groups Are There in Sweden?

In a national survey in 1998, the number of FQ groups was 220, which suggests that about 1,500 physicians were active FQ group members. Less than half of the group leaders had undergone training courses. Case discussions were by far the most popular agenda.

A national survey in 2010 indicated that there are now about 110 active FQ groups left. This means approximately 770 family physicians joining an FQ group. The reason for the falling number might be recent radical changes in organization of primary care in Sweden. The old system, in which county councils were suppliers and managers of primary care centers, has been abandoned and is replaced by a customer choice, competitive system leading to emergence of many new private driven units. On top of this, there is a substantial lack of Swedish family physicians.

An investigation in Stockholm County 1997 showed that the average meeting frequency for FQ groups was 1–2 times a month and attendance rate 70%. Eighty percent of participants judged the educational value of groups to be greater or equal to "activities sponsored by drug industry." Compared to the existing big range of traditional CME, the benefits of FQ groups were rated rather low, covering only up to a fourth of their learning needs. In the County of Halland, a similar survey identified 78 out of a total of 112 family physicians as FQ group participants (Eliasson and Mattsson 1999).

National surveys of physicians' education activities show a constant decrease in time used for CPD. Moreover, Swedish physicians' engagement in education has been more on supervision and vocational trainees, that is, on doctors who undergo training to become specialists. On the other hand, there is now a clear trend towards greater interest in education among Swedish physicians, backed up by professional associations and physicians' trade unions. This interest might be triggered by an ongoing discussion about patient security. If this increasing interest in education continues, it may lead to calls for interactive and problem-based approaches in education like FQ groups.

---

present as complex and problematic as well as uncomplicated and trivial. They often trigger discussions around common clinical problems like diabetes care and the treatment of hypertension, but at times they give rise to debates about the benefit of using guidelines, about the importance of shared care between family doctors and hospitals, etc.

In addition, critical incident analyses, personal shortcomings, and failures have a place in discussions. But the group will also scrutinize trivial problems, which represent a great proportion of family physicians' encounters. There are preconditions for having fruitful discussions about the effectiveness of treatment routines and whether doctors could handle these patients in alternative ways. This type of

---

Box 12.5 Who Owns the Program and Who Pays?

Family physicians have been owners of the Swedish FQ group project, which has given it a high degree of credibility. Financial support has come from the Swedish government. Future maintenance and development of new pedagogic methods may require financial resources from other stakeholders. While not letting go of the leading position for the profession, it would be wise to incorporate health authorities, client organizers of health care, patient organizations, employers, and managers.

Use of groups for learning is not restricted to family medicine. Other specialists and professions face the same kind of diffuse problems even if contexts differ. They all have a professional body of knowledge, and practical, experience-based knowledge is as important as scientifically grounded knowledge. Furthermore, accountability and the skill to tolerate uncertainty is a common denominator. Therefore, it is not surprising that nurses and social workers have adopted the pedagogy of learning in FQ groups.

---

discussion could also be regarded as quality development, as it contributes to new ideas about how to improve patient care.

Once group members are confident and know each other well, they will be eager to present their own cases. In an insecure group, members tend to be shy and cautious, focusing on facts and neutral issues. In new FQ groups, insecure members often experience such difficulties, and they are often reluctant to bring cases from their own practice. A remedy to this can be the use of study letters in order to initiate and facilitate a discussion.

In FQ group discussions, individual knowledge can be made "collective." All knowledge and experience that people bring to a group discussion will be picked up by the other group members. Eventually, group members are able to share a common pool of collective knowledge. However, sometimes the pooled knowledge of the group members is insufficient to deal with a problem, and there is a demand for more information. In this case they can invite an expert, often a hospital specialist, and ask him or her to answer unresolved questions.

The initiative for this kind of "seminar" and the process for it must come from group members themselves. One-way and teacher-led knowledge transfer should be avoided. As has been pointed out, there are additional benefits for the visiting person as well. Hospital specialists learn how to cooperate and apply shared care. They also get a better understanding of how family doctors think and deal with medical problems in primary care.

Box 12.6 What Is a Study Letter?

SFAM has published a number of study letters, which are documents, usually not bigger than ten pages, containing material for group discussions on a topic that should be relevant to most family physicians. The reason is that many FQ groups ask for brief summaries of treatment options and typical cases, which can be used to start a discussion. Besides a number of case reports, they often contain a brief summary of updated scientific evidence and a short introduction to a clinical entity. A study letter has no guideline status, and it does not constitute a comprehensive source of facts on the subject.

Patients' concerns in study letters are presented as ambiguous, which means they can be handled in alternative ways. The final part of a study letter is usually a summary of alternative ways to handle the cases, and sometimes the actual course of the disease is revealed to the reader. Study letters are free of charge, publicly available, and downloadable from SFAM's website.

Some study letters refer to recommendations from the Swedish Council on Health Technology Assessment (SBU), an independent public authority for critical evaluation of methods to prevent, diagnose, and treat health problems. SBU compiles available evidence and some reports are particularly important to primary care. Cooperation between SBU, SFAM, and family physicians has made it possible to supply family physicians with study letters built on SBU reports.

In the future, study-letters will probably be replaced by interactive e-learning.

Organization and Facilitation

The success of an FQ group depends on how well group members work together. This, in turn, is dependent on the group leader's ability to handle group psychology. The designation "group leader," which is commonly used in Sweden, may be misleading. The leader of the group is not a formal chief, responsible for the achievements and well-being of the group. Instead, he or she should act as a facilitator, helping the group to stick to its initial decisions about rules, agenda, and topics. On the other hand, while encouraging shared responsibility, the group leader is still responsible for "keeping the group on track" and for practical things like room booking, refreshments, and notes on attendance. During meetings, the group leader has to ensure that all members have a chance to talk, balancing the discussion and keeping talkative persons from dominating. To be a supportive leader and at the same time a full member of the group, sharing the need for new knowledge and listening to case presentations requires multitasking competence. To be able to handle this, the group leader should attend a group leaders' course.

Box 12.7 Topics of Study Letters in Early 2012. (See On-line Resource #8 for Insomnia in adults and elderly)

Asthma and COPD
Calculating cardiovascular risk
Dementia
Drugs and elderly
Dyspepsia and reflux
Epidemiology
Handling of critical incidents
Home health care
How to manage our FQ group
Lower back and neck pain
Muscle and tendon pain
Preventive health
Prioritizing patients in PHC
Prismatic consultation analysis
Registering diagnoses
Rheumatoid arthritis
Risky drinking
Sleep disturbances
The sit-in consultation
Thrombosis
Treating children with tympanostomy tubes
Treatment of prolonged pain
Urinary incontinence

Because all FQ groups make up their own agenda, we do not know how they spend their time. A good guess is that most groups devote more than half of the available time to case discussions and comparatively less time to discuss general medical topics, research, and evidence based medicine (EBM). The group process is not the same in all groups or in all sessions of a group. Discussions may be structured or fragmented, neutral, or emotive. They may follow a previously agreed agenda or constantly jump from one subject to another. No group process can be said to be right or wrong, as long as it maintains performance. It is important that members of the groups feel that the group is making progress and that they find discussions important and relevant. Some meetings end up in huge ethical and philosophic debates which can be quite stimulating.

Addressing Uncertainty

Even a trivial complaint can evoke uncertainty if the doctor smells that "there is a rat here." Differential diagnoses may turn up. The patient may have looked disappointed, leaving the doctor confused. Such case presentations are common in FQ groups.

Do FQ groups address uncertainty? The answer is yes – and no. In some FQ groups, uncertainty is never recognized or explicitly discussed while other groups are more or less aware of its existence. Arguably, case presentations in an FQ group regularly show elements of uncertainty; otherwise cases would never be interesting enough to bring to the group. Thus, an FQ group has the potential to highlight, analyze, and dissect the concept of uncertainty. The group environment may even be a prerequisite for uncovering issues of uncertainty. Knowing that uncertainty exists as a part of medicine is an important aspect of medical education as well as in CPD.

The culture of medicine, medical training, and expectations from care organizers may be responsible for the common belief that uncertainty and the use of intuition lead to dangerous and unnecessary care, suboptimal outcomes, and iatrogenesis. At the same time, uncertainty can also be regarded as a motor in decision-making processes and may have saved many lives. Family physicians often make statements like "I felt insecure, so I sent her to X-ray." Thus, recognizing uncertainty often turns out to be of great help, telling us that it may play an important role in family medicine.

A good physician is expected to provide unambiguous information and not to show signs of hesitation in decisions. Today, medical students are given no opportunities to discuss uncertainty and doubt. If they do, they find themselves ignorant and inexperienced, making them stressed and annoyed. No wonder that uncertainty is considered a negative and unwanted manifestation of care! Yet if they recognize uncertainty, students may be more prone to search for information and collegial dialogue in their pursuit of the best solutions to complex clinical problems.

When a group is new, members will usually not recognize uncertainty. When group members get to know each other, they show confidence and a willingness to discuss things they usually keep to themselves. The big challenge to group members, including the group leader, is to try to put words to feelings and to acknowledge uncertainty. According to many group leaders, the longer a group exists, the more situations will occur where uncertainty is acknowledged.

A willingness to talk about doubts, one's own mistakes and uncertainty may increase with the number of years spent as a family physician. Also, many group leaders have noticed that family physicians close to retirement use wait-and-see strategies more than younger doctors. Wait-and-see can be a powerful instrument in two ways: first, if a patient is seen on a follow-up visit, there is potential for learning from observation of the course of a disease. Secondly, when a wait-and-see approach is used, there are opportunities to train to handle and tolerate uncertainty.

Uncertainty can also be a link between guidelines and clinical uncertainty. Uncertainty about how to handle a patient during an FQ group discussion (and in real life), means a stimulus to search for relevant scientific evidence. In this situation, guidelines can be of help, as one of many sources of knowledge.

As every FQ group is different, the extent to which uncertainty is tolerated, recognized, or expressed in each one varies. Training people to recognize uncertainty and making this a tool in CPD are not very common issues today, but may be in the future. In any case, research in this field is needed.

Strengths of FQ Groups and Challenges Ahead

Time for Reflection

Donald Schön once postulated that professionals, while they work, unconsciously reflect on what to do next in the problem-solving process, which he named reflection-in-action (Schön 1995). During a reiterating process, new ideas are scrutinized, tested, and evaluated in order to find an acceptable solution. A similar process called reflection-on-action can occur afterwards. These processes facilitate experience-based learning, which leads to the development of new, practice-based knowledge. However, a booked-up surgery and a full waiting room seldom allow for reflection or discussing a problem with a colleague. In most situations colleagues do their best to help and give advice, but this is often done without a reflective discourse. In contrast, FQ groups offer a protected place for discussion, built on reflection-on-action.

Self-Directed Learning

A clear strength of FQ groups is that they use self-directed, problem-based learning that fulfills most criteria of modern adult pedagogy. Learning in an FQ group means "reflection-on-action". It means learning in close relationship to the tasks and problems emerging in daily practice, and is different from being taught things by passive listening or reading textbooks. FQ group members soon discover that knowledge is to be found not only in libraries, textbooks, and guidelines but also in the minds of experienced and reflective colleagues.

Blind Spots

Another strength is that FQ group work will uncover unknown ignorance and increase motivation to learn. No doctor can avoid "blind spots," that is, unconscious gaps in medical knowledge. If, during a case discussion, my colleagues seem to master something that I haven't even heard of, I will become aware of my ignorance and try hard to find ways to fill the gap. Many group members testify that case discussions help them to be aware of learning needs, which in turn leads to planning of educational activities.

FQ Groups and Benefits of Guidelines

Guidelines and recommendations based on scientific evidence tend to flood health care. Many physicians say that they welcome recommendations. But when trying to apply recommendations to an individual patient, they often get stuck. Guidelines may be of help if the problem is formulated as a well-defined question, but individual patients in family practice do not always allow for this. Frustrated by the lack of time and inability to find the relevant search question, doctors tend to downgrade the value of EBM.

If doctors find guidelines to be of limited value, they try to marginalize their impact on care. But when a case is discussed in an FQ group, guidelines can be used as one of many sources of knowledge contributing to the process of reflection, finally leading to a well-informed decision. The doctor's intuition, the patient's preferences, and social or psychological facts may contribute to the final decision. If guidelines are used in this way in FQ groups, they may be appreciated as a support for decisions.

Some of SFAM's study letters (see Boxes 12.6 and 12.7) provide cases representing a clinical entity which is also elaborated in a national guideline. Guidelines sometimes tend to complicate things, as doctors have to take into consideration not only clinical evidence and treatment advice but also individual variations, patient preferences, and ambiguous symptoms. Study letters, providing cases that address topics in guidelines, will probably stimulate reflective discussions about how to use guidelines in daily practice.

Defining the Core Values of Family Medicine

Defining the core values of family medicine as well as explaining its practical implications in health care has been an endeavor for family physicians for many years. Explaining the contents of family medicine to lay people will be more difficult than defining the work of a hospital specialist. In defining the core values and limits of family medicine, FQ groups are important as platforms for keeping the debate about family medicine theory flowing. Hence, an effect of FQ group work and case-based training might be a deeper understanding of what Iona Heath denotes "the mystery of general practice," by exploring, explicating, and developing the art of family medicine (Heath 1995).

Challenges to Overcome in Organization, Culture, and Climate

If a doctor has to negotiate with the chief and with colleagues every time before joining an FQ group session, motivation will soon vanish. This can be avoided if all involved, including managers, try to create a permissive educational culture, closely related to quality development. Participation in collegial groups will then be regarded as much a duty as seeing patients.

Political and personal standpoints may obstruct group work and be a strain to group cohesion, but in a permissive climate, these may equally be beneficial and enable group members to exchange views and opinions, leading to creative discussions.

A shortage of physicians in primary care and the recruitment of locums can be a challenge not only to good care but also to FQ groups. Doctors working only for a short time are seldom fully accepted as team members, and locum doctors will have to focus on the production of care rather than on CPD. In a center with many locums, reflection, motivation to learn, and opportunities to join FQ groups will be absent.

Shortness of time is what many physicians rate as the most important obstacle to embarking on CPD. Family physicians are loyal and will prioritize availability for their patients before leaving for education. Finding protected time to join an FQ group will often be a challenge, both to managers and physicians. In a prosperous educational culture, all team members are open about their own professional development and regard it as a collective task. Staff, including those colleagues who haven't yet joined a group, should therefore be informed by group members about what groups do and why it is important to meet regularly.

Recruiting and Training Group Leaders

Presumptive group leaders often hesitate to assume leading roles, fearing that this would require extensive clinical expertise – but group leaders are not supposed to be more knowledgeable and clinically experienced than other FQ group members. However, specific group leader training is essential for the survival of groups, and regular courses on national and local level have been essential for the Swedish program to develop.

During an FQ group leader course, participants learn about group psychology, pedagogic methods, facilitating, interactive problem-based learning, and how to tackle dysfunctional groups. Group leaders need encouragement, both from group colleagues and from employers. There should be financial compensation for time spent and for the responsibility of keeping the group together.

FQ groups may drift away from their original educational agenda and finally end up in social chatting. Dysfunctional leadership is a serious threat if members feel they spend time on discussion without learning. Also, if groups meet too seldom, continuity is lost and the result may be poor motivation, feelings of alienation, and group dissolution. This can be prevented by an exchange of experiences and material during separate meetings for group leaders.

Overcoming Physician Resistance

Doctor's beliefs can impede the development of FQ groups. Some doctors argue that joining an FQ group is a waste of time, believing that any knowledge that really matters will be found in guidelines, academic institutions, and textbooks. Early influences in medical education undertaken in hospitals might have contributed to this. In a biomedical context ruled by EBM and guidelines, many doctors believe that practicing medicine is equivalent to applying acquired knowledge to patients.

Accordingly, many doctors meet their learning needs in a passive way, where lectures provided by experts and views of authorities represent the main sources of knowledge. Experiences acquired in everyday work are belittled and perceived as unpredictable and unreliable. Marketing of FQ groups by the use of social networks and multifaceted measures including outreach visits, lobbying, and invitations to "Try-a-group" seminars can be a way out of this.

Introducing a new concept of learning to physicians who are not aware of their learning needs can be a challenge. If an organization wants to implement a new behavior (for instance, changing prescription habits), it often uses one-way communication and written material. Information coming from anonymous organizations will have a low impact on a physician's routines (Fraser and Plsek 2003). If, on the other hand, people are informed face-to-face or by the use of social networks and if recipients are given time to reflect and discuss pros and cons, they will be more prone to adopt new ideas (Lomas 1991).

Evidence of Impact

Politicians and officials may be right in asking for proof that time and money spent on a certain pedagogic method is worthwhile. To this end, there is some evidence supporting the benefit of education in general and education using interactive methods in particular.

A Cochrane review concludes that "interactive workshops" can result in moderately large changes in professional practice and that didactic formats (lectures, instructions, etc.) alone are unlikely to change practice (O'Brien et al. 2001). There is also evidence that educational meetings (courses, conferences, workshops, seminars, etc.) alone or in combination with other interventions can improve both practice and health care outcomes (Forsetlund et al. 2009). There is a consensus among educationalists that interactive educational workshops can change practice, while listening to lectures is likely to have no effect at all. In a long-term study, case-based education in primary care using small groups to implement evidence-based treatment with lipid-lowering drugs was found to reduce 10-year mortality significantly in patients suffering from CHD (Kiessling et al. 2011). The findings of Kiessling et al. suggest that case-based training possesses a potential to save lives (Davis 2011).

Searching for evidence of efficacy or best practice should be a rule when it comes to patient care. Therefore, one could argue that evidence for the efficiency of FQ groups is needed before implementation. Possible methods for measuring the effects on physicians might include objective structured clinical examinations (OSCEs), self-evaluation schemes, and assessments by colleagues and staff members. Other variables might include a combination of data on referral rates, patient satisfaction questionnaires, patient enablement instruments, and scoring of patient-centeredness in consultations (Howie et al. 1999; Kinnersley et al. 1999). Measuring the impact on quality of care from FQ group work has many sources of error and will need multifaceted and qualitative methods.

FQ group discussions, case-based training, and problem-based activities do not in any way rule out listening to lectures, attending conferences, and reading textbooks. However, the pedagogy of FQ groups can release creativity, energy, and curiosity that will stimulate learning with the use of other methods.

It is important not to forget that an FQ group is a social endeavor and as such it will satisfy many people's need for socializing and communication. FQ group members often mention the beneficial effect group work has on their satisfaction, self-esteem, well-being, and sense of coherence (Antonovsky 1987). Social aspects are important to groups as they act as key factors for the maintenance and performance of groups (Elwyn et al. 2001).

Conclusion

For a long time, education of family physicians has rested upon didactic methods mediating knowledge developed in academic institutions and hospital environments. To develop skills in solving the common problems of daily primary care, small collegial discussion groups based on case discussions (FQ groups) have been used in Sweden. Experiences are positive and a nationwide structure for the maintenance of small groups has been built up. In contrast to didactic methods, case-based learning may facilitate the acknowledgement of uncertainty and of "not knowing." Due to these qualities and high credibility, FQ groups have potential to be the hub around which other parts of family physicians' CPD rotate.

References

Antonovsky, A. (1987). *Unraveling the mystery of health – How people manage stress and stay well*. San Francisco: Jossey-Bass.

Boland, M. (1992). *Continuing medical education for general practitioners: A review of the CME tutor scheme after 10 years*. Dublin: The Irish College of General Practitioners.

Davis, D. (2011). Can CME, save lives? Results of a Swedish, evidence-based continuing education intervention. *Annals of Family Medicine, 9*, 198–200.

Eliasson, G., & Mattsson, B. (1999). From teaching to learning. Experiences of small CME group work in general practice in Sweden. *Scandinavian Journal of Primary Health Care, 17*, 196–200.

Elwyn, G., Greenhalgh, T., & Macfarlane, F. (2001). *Groups: A guide to small group work in healthcare, management, education and research*. Oxford: Radcliffe Medical Press.

Forsetlund, L., Bjørndal, A., Rashidian, A., Jamtvedt, G., et al. (2009). Continuing education meetings and workshops: Effects on professional practice and health care outcomes. *Cochrane Database of Systematic Reviews*, (2). Art. No.: CD003030. doi: 10.1002/14651858. CD003030.pub2.

Fraser, S. W., & Plsek, P. (2003). Evidence into practice: External spread or personal adoption? *Education for Primary Care, 14*, 129–138.

Heath, I. (1995). *The mystery of general practice*. London: Nuffield Provincial Hospitals Trust for John Fry Trust Fellowship.

Howie, J., et al. (1999). Quality at general practice consultations: Cross sectional survey. *British Medical Journal, 319*, 738–743.

Lomas, J. (1991). Words without action? The production, dissemination, and impact of consensus recommendations. *Annual Review of Public Health, 12*, 41–65.

Kiessling, A., Leewitt, M., & Henriksson, P. (2011). Case-based training of evidence-based clinical practice in primary care and decreased mortality in patients with coronary heart disease. *Annals of Family Medicine, 9*, 211–218.

Kinnersley, P., Scott, N., Peters, T. J., et al. (1999). The patient-centredness of consultations and outcome in primary care. *The British Journal of General Practice, 49*, 711–716.

O'Brien, M. A., Freemantle, N., Oxman, A. D., et al. (2001). Continuing education meetings and workshops: Effects on professional practice and health care outcomes. *Cochrane Database of Systematic Reviews*, (1) Art. No.: CD003030. doi::10.1002/14651858.CD003030.

Schön, D. A. (1995). *The reflective practitioner*. New York: Basic Books.

Chapter 13
Afterword

John Launer

The explicit subject of this book is helping clinicians to engage with uncertainty through collegial dialogue. The implicit subject is how to improve patient care by doing so. Quite appropriately, Trish Greenhalgh opened Chapter 2 with narratives about patients. I want to begin this "Afterword" with a story too.

A young woman came to my clinic some time ago complaining of a rash that looked like scabies. I gave her a prescription for a suitable lotion and printed off some guidance about how to apply it. Within a few minutes we were talking about all sorts of other things: dissatisfaction with her job as a teacher, a love affair that had gone wrong, and a general lack of direction in her life. I told her that I hesitated to make the suggestion because I didn't want to make her feel she was going over the edge, but I wondered if she had considered seeing a counsellor. 'It's funny you should say that', she answered, and she went on to explain that a friend had already put her in touch with one. As the consultation ended, she paid me a nice compliment. 'You do read between the lines', she said. I wondered how to respond and then said by way of explanation: 'I've known your parents for twenty years'. She had no difficulty in understanding what I meant. 'I guess that's right', she replied. According to my computer, the encounter lasted about 10 minutes.

This encounter, like so many in primary care, was entirely unlike anything the patient or I might have predicted in advance. To an outsider, it might have looked rambling, more like a social exchange than a scientific one. Yet almost any primary care physician might recognise it as having many of the elements that are most characteristic of our work, including trust on both sides. Perhaps the most notable characteristic was the fact that this single short consultation might have taken so many different directions. Just as Greenhalgh describes in her own encounters,

J. Launer (✉)
Tavistock Clinic, 120 Belsize Lane, London NW3 5BA, United Kingdom
e-mail: john.launer@londondeanery.ac.uk

L.S. Sommers and J. Launer (eds.), *Clinical Uncertainty in Primary Care: The Challenge of Collaborative Engagement*, DOI 10.1007/978-1-4614-6812-7_13,
© Springer Science+Business Media New York 2013

I don't think I was conscious of uncertainty as this encounter took place. The word 'uncertainty' never even crossed my mind. Yet in retrospect, the whole conversation – on my part and probably on the patient's too – had so many aspects of uncertainty that it is scarcely possible to enumerate them. It would be no exaggeration to say it was *suffused* with uncertainty.

In the few minutes the encounter lasted, I had to consider (consciously or subliminally) whether the obvious diagnosis was the right one. Perhaps I recalled occasions when I had confused scabies with a staphylococcal skin infection, or even shingles. As I printed out the prescription, I may have considered for an instant whether the latest guidelines still recommended that particular lotion – and I made an instantaneous decision to assume my knowledge was up-to-date. In doing this, I was also making a crucial professional judgement, of the kind that Colin Coles identifies in Chapter 3: to use the short amount of time to focus on a wider discussion of the young woman's life and personal contexts.

As the next part of the conversation proceeded, the choices I faced and the decisions I made were moral ones. I have no active memory of doing so, and yet I no doubt wondered whether to ask about a possible connection between her skin condition and her love life. Was she perhaps concerned she had caught the infestation from her unfaithful lover? She didn't mention this, and I chose not to inquire. Sensitive to the unspoken elements in such encounters, raised by Henry Jablonski and his co-authors in Chapter 4, I needed to manage my own feelings in relation to her. She was someone I had known as an infant but was now displaying the vulnerability of an attractive young woman, recently disappointed in romance.

When I broached the possibility of counselling, I needed to do a different kind of emotional calculus in my mind. Was I perhaps imposing my own prejudice in favour of 'talking treatments', or even acting out my ambivalence about whether I wanted to be spending that day as a family doctor, or in my other professional role – as a family therapist? And heaven knows what elements in my mind – or in hers – converged in order for us to construct, jointly, such a poignant and human ending to our meeting. As the consultation wove in and out between the biological and biographical, the personal and the professional, both she and I were making continual and instantaneous choices and taking risks in doing so.

Managing Uncertainty

Greenhalgh's new taxonomy of uncertainty in her chapter and Coles's typology of professional judgement are tremendously helpful, especially in the context of research and training. Yet here I want to argue that these schemas, essential as maps, are not the territory itself. In the 'swampy lowlands' identified by Donald Schön and cited by so many of the authors here, uncertainty doesn't come occasionally, singly, or in isolated categories (Schön 1987). To change the metaphor, it is the ocean in which we swim in primary care for most of our working lives. Contrary to the algorithmic assumptions that often dominate medicine nowadays, the most significant dilemmas in our encounters with patients may not be the ones that occur every 10 or 15 minutes and take the form of 'Lotion A or Potion B'. They are the moment-to-moment ones and they are of a far more subtle nature.

The dilemmas addressed in textbooks and journals are about diagnosis and treatment. In real life, the far commoner ones are these: do I speak or do I remain silent? If I speak, do I ask a question or give advice? If I ask, should I phrase my question warmly and risk seeming overfamiliar, or in a detached manner that may equally offend? It is from such split-second dilemmas and the choices we make about them that the overall truth emerges. Such truth may indeed partake of some of the evidential truths of scientific medicine: at any given time there will be a lotion that overcomes resistance in *Sarcoptes scabiei* and many outdated remedies that do not. Some of the approaches described in these pages, like Practice-Based Small Group Learning and Practice Inquiry, (Chapters 6 and 9) rightly emphasise the importance of respecting this.

But there is another kind of truth also – one that is fragile, dialogical, and emergent. This truth exists not in some objective, eternal domain but in the actual words and feelings that pass between doctors and patients as they meet each other. Most patients will probably be aware of how these different kinds of truth intermingle. Doctors may vary in their ability to do so. At least some of them will constantly monitor this through their scrutiny of self, the conversational choices they make, and the possible effects they anticipate: a disciplined process that Charlotte Tulinius accurately terms 'reflexivity' (Chapter 11).

When Lucia Sommers and I set out to collaborate on this book, we shared a conviction that uncertainty lay at the centre of the medical enterprise and everything it involved. It wasn't just that kind of uncertainty so well addressed in textbooks. It was the complex and constantly shifting mixture of the technical and the existential that Lucia Sommers describes in the opening paragraphs of her Introduction to this book and that characterised my encounter with the young woman described above. However, the shared conviction we had as editors went beyond that. As the Introduction states, we believed as educators that the work needed to address uncertainty of this nature wasn't something that any physician could – or should – ever do alone for virtually all of the time, without recourse to reflective collegial help for at least the more complex and challenging cases.

From my own experience as a family physician, I knew that I couldn't possibly have engaged with encounters of this kind unless there were colleagues in the consulting rooms on either side of mine, to whom I could turn (during the consultation if necessary) if I had doubts about diagnosis or treatment that I couldn't resolve through looking at the Internet or in reference books. I also knew that I could turn to them for reassurance or advice afterwards, for example, if I emerged from the encounter feeling I had said something awkward or mistimed. If truth is something that evolves in the space between doctor and patient, it does so equally in the concentric space that surrounds this: the dialogue between doctor and doctor (Gabbay and LeMay 2010).

For over 20 years I worked alongside four other family physicians at a health centre within a deprived area of north London, in a location called Forest Road. Jokingly, we used to refer to it as the 'University of Forest Road'. But we also knew we weren't joking. We learned vastly more from interchanges with each other (and with the nurses and other co-workers) than any of us had ever learned at a 'real' university, or in any formal continuing professional development (CPD) we received as established practitioners.

As editors, Lucia Sommers and I both knew from our educational experience that many doctors in primary care were not so privileged. The conversations they had with their colleagues about their clinical work were brief, sporadic, and banal – or quite simply non-existent. In consequence, the quality of conversation they were able to have with their patients, or indeed with themselves, appeared to be significantly impoverished. We believed that in such cases (and even where doctors were adequately supported within their medical teams) it was essential to have some regular forum, preferably in the workplace and preferably with a skilled and trained facilitator, where the more challenging uncertainties of professional encounters could be aired and addressed.

These convictions – the centrality of uncertainty in primary care, the inseparable link between collegial dialogue and quality of care, and the essential place for facilitated case-based discussion among peers – were not ones for which we had evidence. They were based on a view of the world of medicine as constituted not by disembodied facts but through real-life interactions. This in turn was supported by our personal experience of running such groups in primary care practices and elsewhere and our observation of the significant difference this has made to the culture of medical practice where we have done so.

Once we set out on the project itself, we learned many things. Some of these, as the Introduction describes in detail, we learned as we tried to map out the scale and nature worldwide of the kinds of activity we were interested in: primary care physicians getting together, with or without a facilitator, to spend extended time in dialogue about specific cases causing them uncertainty. As we made contact with colleagues in primary care in different countries who shared our passion – some already known to us, others not – we learned even more. And as we exchanged dozens (and sometimes a hundred or so) of emails with each of the authors appearing in these pages, our learning continued to advance. It still does so.

One of the things we learned is that sustained and regular case-based dialogue of the kind we wanted to promote remains *the activity of only a small minority of primary care clinicians*. While we cannot assess the richness or otherwise of the conversations that individual physicians or groups of physicians have with each other informally about their patients as I did with my colleagues at Forest Road, we know for a certainty that most do not have the time, the motivation, the funding or perhaps even the wish to set aside formal periods to discuss clinical cases, and the challenges and complexities inherent in them. One focus for future research might therefore be to try and discover how much learning, and how much professional development, actually takes place in the informal exchanges that doctors so often described to us – and how much the quality of patient care is related to the quality of those exchanges.

Another thing we learned is that clinicians may spend quite a great deal of their time in discussions of one sort or another about individual patients – perhaps in meetings or over the phone with colleagues – but these conversations are by and large *technical and solution-focussed rather than reflective*. The kinds of extended case-based conversations that take place regularly – and are sometimes mandated – within parallel professions such as psychologists and counsellors, falling under the general heading of reflective peer supervision, are a rarity in primary health care. Yet they do take place in some places, most notably in Scandinavia. As Gösta Eliasson and Charlotte Tulinius describe, along with colleagues from the Balint movement, we are just beginning to discover what happens to doctors' learning when this happens. We need to know more. In particular, we need sustained and scholarly research into whether it makes a difference to patient care and, if so, what kinds of difference.

Perhaps the biggest surprise for us as we carried out our explorations was that *there are abundant theoretical models for conceptualising how to manage uncertainty in the consultation but few opportunities for doctors to discuss how they apply these models in practice*. Indeed, one of the paradoxes of education in medicine is that undergraduates and trainees may have countless opportunities to present cases at length and discuss how they have used their theoretical learning to deal with these, whereas established physicians may never do so again once they have left medical school. It seems likely that regular, case-based collaborative engagement of the kind described in this book is an effective way of allowing clinicians to learn from each other how best to put such models into practice – especially where the approach to case discussion and consultation are congruent with each other, as with Narrative-Based Supervision. Here too, we do not know for certain that this is the case, and we need to find out.

Models of Collaborative Engagement in Primary Care

There is now a *wide range of approaches* for helping physicians in primary care to hold extended case-based discussion in groups in order to address their uncertainties and improve patient care. These extend from those with a primary emphasis on *technical decision-making* to those with an emphasis on emotional attunement and understanding *what is happening between doctor and patient in the encounter*. However, all of them allow for both forms of learning to take place.

The approaches with a more technical focus may use printed sample cases (as in the case of the 'study letters' from the Swedish Family Medicine Association or the 'educational modules' used in Problem-Based Small Group Learning). Yet even in these instances, there appears to be a great deal of flexibility so that the more mature or confident groups may use these less than newer ones that are finding their way. What is noticeable is the extent to which even the approaches with roots in psychoanalysis or psychotherapy, such as Balint groups and narrative-based supervision, can nowadays offer the space to seek and find technical solutions to the problems that group members bring.

All these approaches are applied in the great majority of instances *outside the workplace of the practitioners themselves*. Whatever theoretical advantages there might be for these discussions to take place within health centres or the other primary care premises where doctors work, they choose to do so elsewhere. One can only speculate on the mixture of factors making this almost universally the case. Possibly physicians feel more comfortable exposing their uncertainties to local colleagues who are not their daily co-workers – although clearly there are instances when two or more doctors from the same workplace belong to the same peer group too. In some instances, only a minority of doctors from any particular locality will wish to spend time in such a group. Conversely, some of these doctors may come from workplaces that have achieved 'in-practice' learning in other ways, but they come to peer groups because they want something separate as well. Possibly there are logistical factors: someone is always needed to 'mind the shop' while a group meets. Whatever the actual factors involved, it would be fascinating to try and establish the reasons for this phenomenon and what doctors perceive the advantages of an external venue to be.

The nature of *facilitation* varies from one approach to another. Some of them – including especially Balint groups and Narrative-Based Supervision – assign considerable importance to the selection and training of facilitators. Others choose 'home-grown' facilitators from among themselves – with or without sending them off for additional training in their leadership role, however this is construed. An issue of particular interest is whether facilitators should be doctors (as appears to be the case with PBSGL) or from outside, including professionals with a background in the social sciences, psychology, or psychotherapy. Without pressing the case for their superiority, Charlotte Tulinius in Chapter 11 puts forward a persuasive argument for considering the advantages that arise from having a facilitator who can take an ethnographic view of the way that a group of doctors may choose to see or describe the professional realities around them. As some Balint groups have found, the combination of having a medical and non-medical facilitator working alongside each other can also be highly effective.

Some of the most interesting descriptions in this book relate to *national systems of peer group learning* for established physicians in primary care – either using a single unified model or encouraging a plurality of models. Some have spread so widely as to have become effectively universal, as in Denmark, or they have been made obligatory, as in Sweden. In Scotland and Canada, PBSGL appears to have gained so much momentum as to be well on its way to becoming part of a 'de facto' national system of this kind. Those of us who share enthusiasm for this type of work may look with envy on such systems, but here too it is worth noting Tulinius's alert: universality brings its own risks – including complacency, collusion between group members, and the risk of CPD degenerating into 'convivial pizza dinners'.

For me, especially as I examined the final drafts of chapters for editing, one fact stood out from all the others: *the close connection between the scale and nature of peer group activity, and the social context*. It cannot have escaped the attention of many readers that both the countries represented in the book where peer group supervision has been most successfully established are Nordic social democracies, with strong traditions of public welfare provision – and an apparent willingness among citizens to pay taxes commensurate with this.

By contrast, in the most powerful and wealthiest nation described in these pages, the United States, the sole model that appears to have emerged – Practice Inquiry – is a relative newcomer and is striving for even a small part of the recognition that similar approaches to peer group learning have achieved elsewhere. Without labouring the point, it is hard not to surmise a systemic relationship between mutual support among physicians, collectivism among citizens, and the better health outcomes seen in northern Europe than in the US. For those of us who live in countries that are moving rapidly – some might say uncontrollably – from a European tradition of 'welfarism' to a more American, market-based model of health care, this apparent equation is a cause of great concern.

Research into Collaborative Engagement

The challenges of research into complex educational interventions are well known (Kirkpatrick and Kirkpatrick 2006). Inviting participants to indicate points on a Likert scale or to tick 'smiley faces' to show their satisfaction with a learning event is easy and almost invariably gratifying – but lacks serious scientific value. Showing that participants will use their learning to change their clinical practice, improve the quality of their patients' lives, and even prolong them is formidably difficult. This is not universally understood. As Coles points out in Chapter 3: 'Even those who regulate professionals may not fully appreciate the complexities of what professional practice actually entails and how becoming a professional practitioner can best be achieved educationally or within what time-scale'. The same holds true for the agencies that support and offer grants for research. If they are willing to fund any research at all into educational interventions for established practitioners (a very big 'if'), they may still have naïve and unrealistic expectations about what can be achieved and how quickly.

In spite of these obstacles, the *proponents of virtually every model in this book have been able to cite sound educational research* associated with their approaches, at a number of different levels. To mention just some of the examples that appear in these pages, Balint groups can bring about significant changes in doctors' attitudes and their performance in psychological approaches to treatment (Chapter 4); doctors who acquire a narrative approach can become more deeply involved with the patient and exhibit a greater engagement (Chapter 8); PBSGL learning modules can lead to significant and sustained improvements in prescribing (Chapter 6); case-based education in small groups in Sweden significantly reduced 10-year mortality from CHD (Chapter 12).

In keeping with the collegial stance that infuses this book, many chapter authors suggest that *future research should centre on shared good practice* rather than the (possibly small) ideological and technical differences in their educational approaches. As Greenhalgh points out in Chapter 2, 'the commonalities between the approaches described in this book are more noteworthy than their differences'. Similarly, Kjeldmand's review of Balint research includes this proposal: 'Perhaps, if small group enthusiasts of different persuasions could set aside their concern with theoretical differences and concentrate on what they have in common, more meaningful research might follow' (Chapter 5). This seems an excellent starting point for considering how to move a research agenda forward.

As most of our authors emphasise, *much future research will need to be qualitative*: we need to know more, both within models and across them, about the kinds of clinicians who do and do not attend, the day-to-day problems that most commonly evoke uncertainty, how groups (and their facilitators) go about exposing this to analysis and discussion, what group participants find most helpful, and how they alter their practice as a result. There is already 'cross-fertilisation' of ideas and skills across different models (e.g., the adoption of 'reflecting team' methods within Balint, NBS, and other approaches and a willingness among 'affect-based' groups to engage with clinical evidence, and vice versa). A deeper knowledge of what actually happens in different forms of collaborative engagement and what constitutes good educational practice could hasten that process – while at the same time allowing adaptation for local and national contexts. Intellectual honesty also demands that we take note of the ways that collaborative engagement can foster negative effects, like the collusion Tulinius describes when people take refuge in the collective identity of 'we doctors' (Chapter 11). Sound qualitative research can help us learn both what we do well and what we do merely through habit and need to correct.

In addition, *we need to grasp the nettle of quantitative research*. Long-term practitioner groups are subject to many influences that can potentially disguise or distort numerical results, but these can be taken into account. While strictly randomised double-blind controlled trials might not be possible – because doctors know if they are attending groups and cannot prevent patients from discovering this too – there are other valid methodologies for showing how educational input for clinicians can lead to an impact on patient health and well-being (Norman and Eva 2010). These include case control studies comparing matched cohorts of patients from practitioners who are either trained or untrained in a particular method. There is no reason for educators to fear outcome measurements at the level of practitioner activity (e.g., the number of difficult psychological cases a doctor is able to carry, or the capacity to change prescribing habits) or measurable effects on patients (an improvement on depression scales or a reduction in CHD events).

One of the most crucial areas we need to examine, using both qualitative and quantitative methods, is *the wider systemic relationship between the case discussion group and the practice or locality setting* in which it takes place. So far, research into collaborative engagement has largely been unconnected with research into such questions as how improved relationships in a practice can lead to a better quality of care (Lanham et al. 2009) or how to build a learning organisation within the primary care clinic or 'patient-centred medical home' (Nutting et al. 2009). There is a persuasive case for including 'in-practice' learning of the kind described by Coles

(Chapter 3) or the '*Inquiry Practice*' envisioned by Lucia Sommers (Chapter 9) within programmes of organisational development and quality improvement that are emerging in many places in primary care. We need to discover more about the contribution that collaborative engagement of this kind can make to such programmes. It would be good to see enough evidence to justify putting collaborative engagement at the very heart of practice development.

The phrase 'more research is needed' is often a mere mantra, designed to evoke further extravagant funding for some infinitesimal advance in pharmacology. In the context of collaborative engagement, I believe it has a far more valid meaning. The budgets needed for high-quality educational research are minimal by comparison with pharmaceutical trials. The potential gains in terms of long-term, systemic change in clinical practice and outcome may be huge.

Conclusion

Health is indivisible. Although none of the authors in this book say so directly (since they have other immediate preoccupations), all hint at different aspects of the medical enterprise that are split apart and need to be reunited. Looking after patients is inseparable from looking after ourselves as professionals. Doing so means that we take mutual responsibility for each other: for our successes, our errors, and above all our learning from both of these. And so it goes on. Different writers in this book allude to the inseparability of mind from body, of physical illness from mental distress, and of primary from secondary care. In grappling with the unified field of human experience and human suffering, we also cannot separate the clinical service we provide from the training and collaborative engagement among colleagues that supports this service.

Peer group supervision among doctors, whether it is in the workplace or not and whether it is facilitated or not, is a systematic attempt to join together some of the fragmented parts of the medical enterprise. It does so by enacting one of the most central activities of human life: telling stories, listening to them, questioning them, joining in the storytelling, and collectively generating new stories. Scientific knowledge plays a part in this, and so do expertise and the giving of advice. Evidence certainly does, but so do the many contexts to which the evidence must be applied – personal contexts, social ones, and moral ones.

What weaves all of this together is the search for meaning and the articulation of that search through dialogue. It is our belief and a belief that has been strengthened by editing and producing this book that peer group, case-based supervision offers the potential for enriching the professional lives of doctors and hence of bringing about a qualitative change in the care of patients. We look forward to a time when the models of continuing learning described in this book, or the successors to these models, become just as established as the training we undertake to become primary care clinicians in the first place.

References

Gabbay, J., & LeMay, A. (2010). *Practice-based evidence for healthcare: Clinical mindlines*. London: Routledge.

Kirkpatrick, D. L., & Kirkpatrick, J. D. (2006). *Evaluating training programs* (3rd ed.). San Francisco: Berett-Koehler.

Lanham, H., McDaniel, R., Crabtree, B., et al. (2009). How improving practice relationships among clinicians and nonclinicians can improve quality in primary care. *Joint Commission Journal on Quality and Patient Safety, 35*, 457–466.

Norman, G., & Eva, F. (2010). Quantitative research methods in medical education. Chapter 21. In T. Swanwick (Ed.), *Understanding medical education: Evidence, theory and practice* (pp. 301–322). London: Wiley-Blackwell.

Nutting, P., Miller, M., Crabtree, B., et al. (2009). Initial lessons from the first national demonstration project on practice transformation to a patient-centered medical home. *Annals of Family Medicine, 7*, 254–260.

Schön, D. (1987). *Educating the reflective practitioner*. San Francisco: Jossey-Bass.

Index

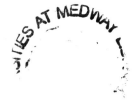

Printed by Printforce, the Netherlands